# Clinical Pharmacology

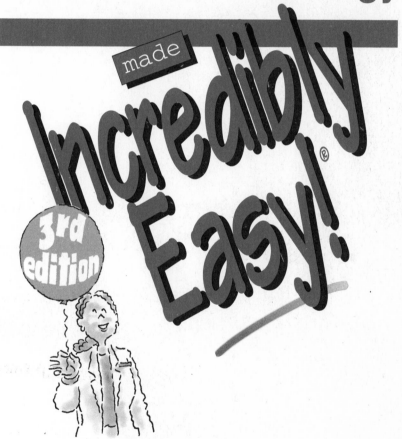

# Clinical Pharmacology

made

## Incredibly Easy!®

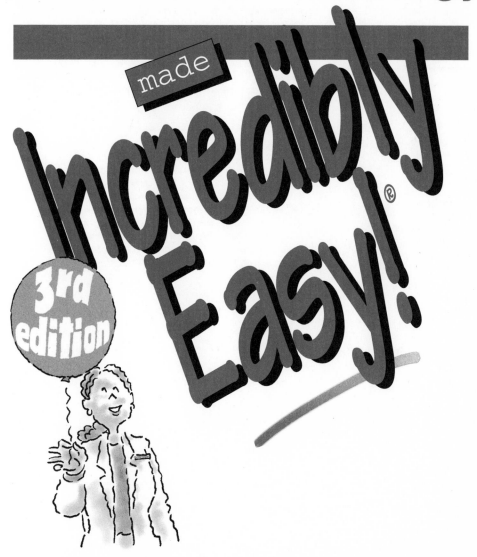

**3rd edition**

Wolters Kluwer Health | Lippincott Williams & Wilkins

Philadelphia • Baltimore • New York • London
Buenos Aires • Hong Kong • Sydney • Tokyo

## Staff

**Executive Publisher**
Judith A. Schilling McCann, RN, MSN

**Editorial Director**
David Moreau

**Clinical Director**
Joan M. Robinson, RN, MSN

**Art Director**
Mary Ludwicki

**Clinical Project Manager**
Jennifer Meyering, RN, BSN, MS, CCRN

**Editors**
Margaret Eckman, Diane Labus

**Copy Editors**
Kimberly Bilotta (supervisor), Jane Bradford,
Shana Harrington, Lisa Stockslager,
Dorothy P. Terry, Pamela Wingrod

**Designer**
Georg W. Purvis IV

**Illustrator**
Bot Roda

**Digital Composition Services**
Diane Paluba (manager), Joy Rossi Biletz,
Donna S. Morris

**Associate Manufacturing Manager**
Beth J. Welsh

**Editorial Assistants**
Karen J. Kirk, Jeri O'Shea, Linda K. Ruhf

**Indexer**
Barbara Hodgson

**Library of Congress Cataloging-in-Publication Data**
Clinical pharmacology made incredibly easy!. — 3rd ed.
    p. ; cm.
    Includes bibliographical references and index.
    1. Clinical pharmacology — Outlines, syllabi, etc.
    I. Lippincott Williams & Wilkins.
    [DNLM: 1. Pharmacology, Clinical — methods — Handbooks. 2. Drug Therapy — Handbooks. 3. Pharmaceutical Preparations — Handbooks. QV 39 C6417 2008]
    RM301.28.C556 2008
615'.1—dc22
ISBN-13: 978-0-7817-8938-7 (alk. paper)
ISBN-10: 0-7817-8938-9 (alk. paper)    2008009967

# Contents

Contributors and consultants      *vii*

Not another boring foreword      *ix*

| | | |
|---|---|---|
| 1 | Fundamentals of clinical pharmacology | 1 |
| 2 | Autonomic nervous system drugs | 21 |
| 3 | Neurologic and neuromuscular drugs | 49 |
| 4 | Pain medications | 93 |
| 5 | Cardiovascular drugs | 119 |
| 6 | Hematologic drugs | 155 |
| 7 | Respiratory drugs | 175 |
| 8 | Gastrointestinal drugs | 195 |
| 9 | Genitourinary drugs | 223 |
| 10 | Anti-infective drugs | 237 |
| 11 | Anti-inflammatory, anti-allergy, and immunosuppressant drugs | 293 |
| 12 | Psychotropic drugs | 311 |
| 13 | Endocrine drugs | 339 |
| 14 | Drugs for fluid and electrolyte balance | 359 |
| 15 | Antineoplastic drugs | 371 |

Other major drugs      414

Vaccines and treatment for biological weapons exposure      421

Treatment and antidotes for chemical weapons exposure      422

Herbal drugs      423

Selected references      *426*

Index      *427*

Internet drug updates      *eDruginfo.com*

# Contributors and consultants

**Tricia M. Berry,** PharmD, BCPS
Associate Professor of Pharmacy Practice
St. Louis College of Pharmacy

**Victor Cohen,** BS, PharmD, BCPS
Assistant Professor of Pharmacy Practice
Arnold & Marie Schwartz College of Pharmacy & Health
  Sciences
Clinical Pharmacy Manager & Residency Program Director
Maimonides Medical Center
Brooklyn, N.Y.

**Jason C. Cooper,** PharmD
Clinical Specialist, MUSC Drug Information Center
Medical University of South Carolina
Charleston

**Michele A. Danish,** PharmD, RPH
Pharmacy Clinical Manager
St. Joseph Health Services
North Providence, R.I.

**Glen E. Farr,** PharmD
Professor of Clinical Pharmacy & Associate Dean
University of Tennessee College of Pharmacy
Knoxville

**Tatyana Gurvich,** PharmD
Clinical Pharmacologist
Glendale (Calif.) Adventist Family Practice Residency Program

**Catherine A. Heyneman,** PharmD, MS, ANP
Associate Professor of Pharmacy Practice
Idaho State University College of Pharmacy
Pocatello

**Samantha P. Jellinek,** PharmD, BCPS
Clinical Pharmacy Manager for Medication Reconciliation &
  Safety
Clinical Coordinator, Pharmacy Practice Residency Program
Maimonides Medical Center
Brooklyn, N.Y.

**Christine K. O'Neil,** PharmD, BCPS, CGP, FCCP
Professor of Pharmacy Practice
Duquesne University
Mylan School of Pharmacy
Pittsburgh

**Jean Scholtz,** PharmD, BCPS, FASHP
Associate Professor
Department of Pharmacy Practice and Pharmacy Administration
University of the Sciences in Philadelphia

**Anthony P. Sorrentino,** PharmD
Assistant Professor of Clinical Pharmacy
Philadelphia College of Pharmacy
University of the Sciences in Philadelphia

**Suzzanne Tairu,** PharmD
Clinical Specialist
The Medical Affairs Company/Consultant for Pfizer
Kennesaw, Calif.

**Karen Jo Tietze,** BS, PharmD
Professor of Clinical Pharmacy
Philadelphia College of Pharmacy
University of the Sciences in Philadelphia

# Not another boring foreword

If you're like me, you're too busy caring for your patients to wade through a foreword that uses pretentious terms and umpteen dull paragraphs to get to the point. So let's cut right to the chase! Here's why this book is so terrific:

 It will teach you all the important things you need to know about clinical pharmacology. (And it will leave out all the fluff that wastes your time.)

 It will help you remember what you've learned.

 It will make you smile as it enhances your knowledge and skills.

Don't believe me? Try these recurring logos on for size:

 *Now I get it!* illustrates normal physiology and the physiology of drug actions.

*Warning!* alerts you to potentially dangerous adverse reactions.

*Yea or nay?* sorts through current issues related to drug risks and benefits.

*Safe and sound* explains how to administer medications safely.

 *Memory jogger* reinforces learning through easy-to-remember mnemonics.

See? I told you! And that's not all. Look for me and my friends in the margins throughout this book. We'll be there to explain key concepts, provide important care reminders, and offer reassurance. Oh, and if you don't mind, we'll be spicing up the pages with a bit of humor along the way, to teach and entertain in a way that no other resource can.

I hope you find this book helpful. Best of luck throughout your career!

*Joy*

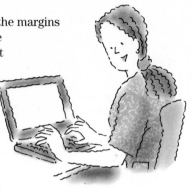

# 1

# Fundamentals of clinical pharmacology

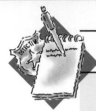

## Just the facts

In this chapter, you'll learn:

♦ pharmacology basics
♦ routes by which drugs are administered
♦ key concepts of pharmacokinetics
♦ key concepts of pharmacodynamics
♦ key concepts of pharmacotherapeutics
♦ key types of drug interactions and adverse reactions.

## Pharmacology basics

This chapter focuses on the fundamental principles of pharmacology. It discusses basic information, such as how drugs are named and how they're created. It also discusses the different routes by which drugs can be administered.

### Kinetics, dynamics, therapeutics

This chapter also discusses what happens when a drug enters the body. This involves three main areas:

   pharmacokinetics (the absorption, distribution, metabolism, and excretion of a drug)

   pharmacodynamics (the biochemical and physical effects of drugs and the mechanisms of drug actions)

   pharmacotherapeutics (the use of drugs to prevent and treat diseases).

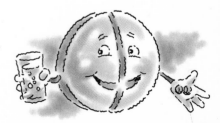

Read on to find out what happens when a drug enters the body.

In addition, the chapter provides an introduction to drug interactions and adverse drug reactions.

## What's in a name?

Drugs have a specific kind of nomenclature—that is, a drug can go by three different names:

- The *chemical name* is a scientific name that precisely describes its atomic and molecular structure.
- The *generic*, or nonproprietary, name is an abbreviation of the chemical name.
- The *trade name* (also known as the *brand name* or *proprietary name*) is selected by the drug company selling the product. Trade names are protected by copyright. The symbol ® after the trade name indicates that the name is registered by and restricted to the drug manufacturer.

To avoid confusion, it's best to use a drug's generic name because any one drug can have a number of trade names.

In 1962, the federal government mandated the use of official names so that only one official name would represent each drug. The official names are listed in the *United States Pharmacopeia* and *National Formulary*.

## Family ties

Drugs that share similar characteristics are grouped together as a *pharmacologic class* (or family). Beta-adrenergic blockers are an example of a pharmacologic class.

The *therapeutic class* groups drugs by therapeutic use. Antihypertensives are an example of a therapeutic class.

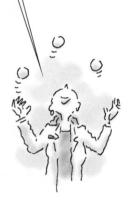

This is confusing! Each drug has at least three names: a chemical name, a generic name, and a trade name.

# Where drugs come from

Traditionally, drugs were derived from *natural* sources, such as:

- plants
- animals
- minerals.

Today, however, laboratory researchers use traditional knowledge, along with chemical science, to develop *synthetic* drug sources. One advantage of chemically developed drugs is that they're free from the impurities found in natural substances.

In addition, researchers and drug developers can manipulate the molecular structure of substances such as antibiotics so that a slight change in the chemical structure makes the drug effective against different organisms. The first-, second-, third-, and fourth-generation cephalosporins are an example.

## Old-fashioned medicine

The earliest drug concoctions from plants used everything: the leaves, roots, bulb, stem, seeds, buds, and blossoms. Subsequently, harmful substances often found their way into the mixture.

As the understanding of plants as drug sources became more sophisticated, researchers sought to isolate and intensify *active components* while avoiding harmful ones.

## Power plant

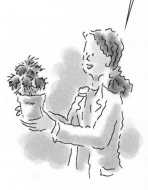

Drugs can be derived from just about any substance on earth.

The active components consist of several types and vary in character and effect:

• *Alkaloids*, the most active component in plants, react with acids to form a salt that can dissolve more readily in body fluids. The names of alkaloids and their salts usually end in "-ine." Examples include atropine, caffeine, and nicotine.

• *Glycosides* are also active components found in plants. Names of glycosides usually end in "-in" such as digoxin.

• *Gums* constitute another group of active components. Gums give products the ability to attract and hold water. Examples include seaweed extractions and seeds with starch.

• *Resins*, of which the chief source is pine tree sap, commonly act as local irritants or as laxatives.

• *Oils*, thick and sometimes greasy liquids, are classified as volatile or fixed. Examples of volatile oils, which readily evaporate, include peppermint, spearmint, and juniper. Fixed oils, which aren't easily evaporated, include castor oil and olive oil.

## Animal magnetism

The body fluids or glands of animals can also be drug sources. The drugs obtained from animal sources include:

• *hormones* such as insulin

• *oils* and *fats* (usually fixed) such as cod-liver oil

• *enzymes*, which are produced by living cells and act as catalysts, such as pancreatin and pepsin

• *vaccines*, which are suspensions of killed, modified, or attenuated microorganisms. (See *Old McDonald had a pharm*, page 4.)

## Mineral springs

Metallic and nonmetallic minerals provide various inorganic materials not available from plants or animals. The mineral sources are used as they occur in nature or are combined with other ingredients. Examples of drugs that contain minerals are iron, iodine, and Epsom salts.

## Down to DNA

Today, most drugs are produced in laboratories and can be:

## Old McDonald had a pharm

In the near future, traditional barnyard animals might also be small, organic pharmaceutical factories. Some animals have already been genetically altered to produce pharmaceuticals, and their products are being tested by the Food and Drug Administration. Here are a few examples of the possibilities:

• a cow that produces milk containing lactoferrin, which can be used to treat human infections

• a goat that produces milk containing antithrombin III, which can help prevent blood clotting in humans

• a sheep that produces milk containing alpha$_1$-antitrypsin, which is used to treat cystic fibrosis.

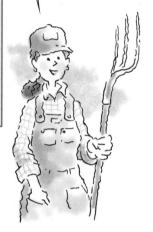

Hmm...farm fresh pharmaceuticals? That's an unusual idea.

• natural (from animal, plant, or mineral sources)
• synthetic.

Examples of drugs produced in the laboratory include thyroid hormone (natural) and ranitidine (synthetic).

Recombinant deoxyribonucleic acid research has led to other chemical sources of organic compounds. For example, the reordering of genetic information has enabled scientists to develop bacteria that produce insulin for humans.

# How drugs are administered

A drug's administration route influences the quantity given and the rate at which the drug is absorbed and distributed. These variables affect the drug's action and the patient's response.

Routes of administration include:

• *buccal, sublingual, translingual:* certain drugs are given buccally (in the pouch between the cheek and gum), sublingually (under the tongue), or translingually (on the tongue) to speed their absorption or to prevent their destruction or transformation in the stomach or small intestine

• *gastric:* this route allows direct instillation of medication into the GI system of patients who can't ingest the drug orally

• *intradermal:* substances are injected into the skin (dermis); this route is used mainly for diagnostic purposes when testing for allergies or tuberculosis

• *intramuscular:* this route allows drugs to be injected directly into various muscle groups at varying tissue depths; it's used to give aqueous suspensions and solutions in oil, immunizations, and medications that aren't available in oral form

## Streaming in

• *intravenous:* the I.V. route allows injection of substances (drugs, fluids, blood or blood products, and diagnostic contrast agents) directly into the bloodstream through a vein; administration can range from a single dose to an ongoing infusion delivered with great precision
• *oral:* this is usually the safest, most convenient, and least expensive route; drugs are administered to patients who are conscious and can swallow
• *rectal and vaginal:* suppositories, ointments, creams, gels, and tablets may be instilled into the rectum or vagina to treat local irritation or infection; some drugs applied to the mucosa of the rectum or vagina can be absorbed systemically
• *respiratory:* drugs that are available as gases can be administered into the respiratory system; drugs given by inhalation are rapidly absorbed, and medications given by such devices as the metered-dose inhaler can be self-administered, or drugs can be administered directly into the lungs through an endotracheal tube in emergency situations
• *subcutaneous (subQ):* with the subQ route, small amounts of a drug are injected beneath the dermis and into the subcutaneous tissue, usually in the patient's upper arm, thigh, or abdomen
• *topical:* this route is used to deliver a drug through the skin or a mucous membrane; it's used for most dermatologic, ophthalmic, otic, and nasal preparations.

Drugs may also be given as specialized infusions injected directly into a specific site in the patient's body, such as an epidural infusion (into the epidural space), intrathecal infusion (into the cerebrospinal fluid), intrapleural infusion (into the pleural cavity), intraperitoneal infusion (into the peritoneal cavity), intraosseous infusion (into the rich vascular network of a long bone), and intra-articular infusion (into a joint).

# New drug development

In the past, drugs were found by trial and error. Now they're developed primarily by systematic scientific research. The Food and Drug Administration (FDA) carefully monitors new drug development, which can take many years to complete.

Only after reviewing extensive animal studies and data on the safety and effectiveness of the proposed drug will the FDA approve an application for an investigational new drug (IND). (See *Phases of new drug development*, page 6.)

## Phases of new drug development

When the Food and Drug Administration (FDA) approves the application for an investigational new drug, the drug must undergo clinical evaluation involving human subjects. This clinical evaluation is divided into four phases:

**Phase I**
The drug is tested on healthy volunteers in phase I.

**Phase II**
Phase II involves trials with people who have the disease for which the drug is thought to be effective.

**Phase III**
Large numbers of patients in medical research centers receive the drug in phase III. This larg-er sampling provides information about infrequent or rare adverse effects. The FDA will approve a new drug application if phase III studies are satisfactory.

**Phase IV**
Phase IV is voluntary and involves postmarket surveillance of the drug's therapeutic effects at the completion of phase III. The pharmaceutical company receives reports from doctors and other health care professionals about the therapeutic results and adverse effects of the drug. Some medications, for example, have been found to be toxic and have been removed from the market after their initial release.

## Exceptions to the rule

Although most INDs undergo all four phases of clinical evaluation mandated by the FDA, some can receive expedited approval. For example, because of the public health threat posed by acquired immunodeficiency syndrome (AIDS), the FDA and drug companies have agreed to shorten the IND approval process for drugs to treat the disease. This allows doctors to give qualified AIDS patients "treatment INDs," which aren't yet approved by the FDA.

Sponsors of drugs that reach phase II or III clinical trials can apply for FDA approval of treatment IND status. When the IND is approved, the sponsor supplies the drug to doctors whose patients meet appropriate criteria.

Despite the extensive testing and development that all drugs go through, serious adverse reactions may occasionally occur, even though they weren't discovered during clinical trials. It's also possible that drug interactions aren't discovered until after clinical trials have concluded and the drug has been approved. The FDA has procedures in place for reporting adverse events and other problems to help track the safety of drugs. (See *Reporting to the FDA.*)

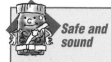
*Safe and sound*

## Reporting to the FDA

The Food and Drug Administration (FDA) compiles and tracks information related to problems associated with drugs under its regulation. Complete a MedWatch form and send it to the FDA if you suspect an FDA-regulated drug is responsible for a patient's:
• death
• life-threatening illness
• prolonged or initial hospitalization
• disability
• congenital anomaly
• need for medical or surgical intervention to prevent a permanent impairment.

# Pharmacokinetics

Kinetics refers to movement. Pharmacokinetics deals with a drug's actions as it moves through the body. Therefore, pharmacokinetics discusses how a drug is:

- absorbed (taken into the body)
- distributed (moved into various tissues)
- metabolized (changed into a form that can be excreted)
- excreted (removed from the body).

    This branch of pharmacology is also concerned with a drug's onset of action, peak concentration level, and duration of action.

Ahhh. I just adore passive transport. It requires no energy. Ooops—time to flip over!

## Absorption

Drug absorption covers a drug's progress from the time it's administered, through its passage to the tissues, until it reaches systemic circulation.

    On a cellular level, drugs are absorbed by several means—primarily through active or passive transport.

### The lazy way

*Passive transport* requires no cellular energy because diffusion allows the drug to move from an area of higher concentration to one of lower concentration. Passive transport occurs when small molecules diffuse across membranes and stops when drug concentration on both sides of the membrane is equal.

### Using muscle

*Active transport* requires cellular energy to move the drug from an area of lower concentration to one of higher concentration. Active transport is used to absorb electrolytes, such as sodium and potassium, as well as some drugs such as levodopa.

### Taking a bite

*Pinocytosis* is a unique form of active transport that occurs when a cell engulfs a drug particle. Pinocytosis is commonly employed to transport fat-soluble vitamins (vitamins A, D, E, and K).

### Watch the speed limit!

If only a few cells separate the active drug from the systemic circulation, absorption will occur rapidly and the drug will quickly reach therapeutic levels in the body. Typically, absorption occurs within seconds or minutes when a drug is administered sublingually, I.V., or by inhalation.

Drugs given under the tongue, I.V., or by inhalation are quickly absorbed.

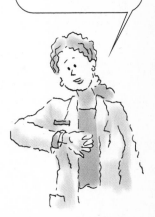

## Not so fast

Absorption occurs at a slower rate when drugs are administered by the oral, I.M., or subQ routes because the complex membrane systems of GI mucosal layers, muscle, and skin delay drug passage.

## At a snail's pace

At the slowest absorption rates, drugs can take several hours or days to reach peak concentration levels. A slow rate usually occurs with rectally administered or sustained-release drugs.

## Not enough time

Other factors can affect how quickly a drug is absorbed. For example, most absorption of oral drugs occurs in the small intestine. If a patient has had large sections of the small intestine surgically removed, drug absorption decreases because of the reduced surface area and the reduced time that the drug is in the intestine.

## Look to the liver

Drugs absorbed by the small intestine are transported to the liver before being circulated to the rest of the body. The liver may metabolize much of the drug before it enters the circulation. This mechanism is referred to as the *first-pass effect*. Liver metabolism may inactivate the drug; if so, the first-pass effect lowers the amount of active drug released into the systemic circulation. Therefore, higher drug dosages must be administered to achieve the desired effect.

## More blood, more absorption

Increased blood flow to an absorption site improves drug absorption, whereas reduced blood flow decreases absorption. More rapid absorption leads to a quicker onset of drug action.

For example, the muscle area selected for I.M. administration can make a difference in the drug absorption rate. Blood flows faster through the deltoid muscle (in the upper arm) than through the gluteal muscle (in the buttocks). The gluteal muscle, however, can accommodate a larger volume of drug than the deltoid muscle.

## Slowed by pain and stress

Pain and stress can decrease the amount of drug absorbed. This may be due to a change in blood flow, reduced movement through the GI tract, or gastric retention triggered by the autonomic nervous system response to pain.

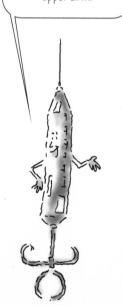

A drug injected into muscle of the buttocks is absorbed more slowly and sometimes more erratically than one injected into the upper arm.

## High fat doesn't help

High-fat meals and solid foods slow the rate at which contents leave the stomach and enter the intestines, delaying intestinal absorption of a drug.

## Dosage form factors

Drug formulation (such as tablets, capsules, liquids, sustained-release formulas, inactive ingredients, and coatings) affects the drug absorption rate and the time needed to reach peak blood concentration levels.

## Absorption increase or decrease?

Combining one drug with another drug, or with food, can cause interactions that increase or decrease drug absorption, depending on the substances involved.

# Distribution

Drug distribution is the process by which the drug is delivered from the systemic circulation to body tissues and fluids. Distribution of an absorbed drug within the body depends on several factors:
- blood flow
- solubility
- protein binding.

## Quick to the heart

After a drug has reached the bloodstream, its distribution in the body depends on blood flow. The drug is quickly distributed to organs with a large supply of blood. These organs include the:
- heart
- liver
- kidneys.

Distribution to other internal organs, skin, fat, and muscle is slower.

## Lucky lipids

The ability of a drug to cross a cell membrane depends on whether the drug is water or lipid (fat) soluble. Lipid-soluble drugs easily cross through cell membranes; water-soluble drugs can't.

Lipid-soluble drugs can also cross the blood-brain barrier and enter the brain.

## Free to work

As a drug travels through the body, it comes in contact with proteins such as the plasma protein albumin. The drug can remain free or bind to the protein. The portion of a drug that's bound to a protein is inactive and can't exert a therapeutic effect. Only the free, or unbound, portion remains active.

A drug is said to be highly protein-bound if more than 80% of the drug is bound to protein.

> Only free drugs, not those bound to protein, can produce a therapeutic effect.

# Metabolism

Drug metabolism, or biotransformation, is the process by which the body changes a drug from its dosage form to a more water-soluble form that can then be excreted. Drugs can be metabolized in several ways:
• Most drugs are metabolized into inactive metabolites (products of metabolism), which are then excreted.
• Other drugs are converted to active metabolites, which are capable of exerting their own pharmacologic action. Active metabolites may undergo further metabolism or may be excreted from the body unchanged.
• Some drugs can be administered as inactive drugs, called *pro-drugs*, which don't become active until they're metabolized.

## Where metabolism happens

The majority of drugs are metabolized by enzymes in the liver; however, metabolism can also occur in the plasma, kidneys, and membranes of the intestines. In contrast, some drugs inhibit or compete for enzyme metabolism, which can cause the accumulation of drugs when they're given together. This accumulation increases the potential for an adverse reaction or drug toxicity.

## Conditional considerations

Certain diseases can reduce metabolism. These include liver diseases such as cirrhosis as well as heart failure, which reduces circulation to the liver.

## Gene machine

Genetics allows some people to metabolize drugs rapidly and others to metabolize them more slowly.

## Stress test

Environment, too, can alter drug metabolism. For example, cigarette smoke may affect the rate of metabolism of some drugs; a stressful situation or event, such as prolonged illness, surgery, or injury, can also change how a person metabolizes drugs.

> If I'm not working right, a drug doesn't get metabolized normally.

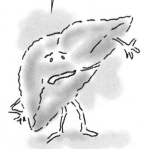

## The age game

Developmental changes can also affect drug metabolism. For instance, infants have immature livers that reduce the rate of metabolism, and elderly patients experience a decline in liver size, blood flow, and enzyme production that also slows metabolism.

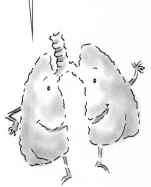

Remember that drugs can go through me, too!

# Excretion

Drug excretion refers to the elimination of drugs from the body. Most drugs are excreted by the kidneys and leave the body through urine. Drugs can also be excreted through the lungs, exocrine (sweat, salivary, or mammary) glands, skin, and intestinal tract.

## Half-life = half the drug

The half-life of a drug is the time it takes for one-half of the drug to be eliminated by the body. Factors that affect a drug's half-life include its rate of absorption, metabolism, and excretion. Knowing how long a drug remains in the body helps determine how frequently it should be administered.

A drug that's given only once is eliminated from the body almost completely after four or five half-lives. A drug that's administered at regular intervals, however, reaches a steady concentration (or steady state) after about four or five half-lives. Steady state occurs when the rate of drug administration equals the rate of drug excretion.

# Onset, peak, and duration

In addition to absorption, distribution, metabolism, and excretion, three other factors play important roles in a drug's pharmacokinetics:
• onset of action
• peak concentration
• duration of action.

## Lights, camera... action!

The onset of action refers to the time interval from when the drug is administered to when its therapeutic effect actually begins. Rate of onset varies depending on the route of administration and other pharmacokinetic properties.

## Peak performance

As the body absorbs more drug, blood concentration levels rise. The peak concentration level is reached when the absorption rate equals the elimination rate. However, the time of peak concentration isn't always the time of peak response.

## Sticking around

The duration of action is the length of time the drug produces its therapeutic effect.

# Pharmacodynamics

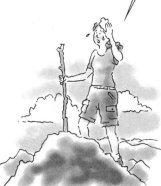

Reaching the peak of concentration can be tough!

Pharmacodynamics is the study of the drug mechanisms that produce biochemical or physiologic changes in the body. The interaction at the cellular level between a drug and cellular components, such as the complex proteins that make up the cell membrane, enzymes, or target receptors, represents drug action. The response resulting from this drug action is the drug effect.

## It's the cell that matters

A drug can modify cell function or rate of function, but it can't impart a new function to a cell or to target tissue. Therefore, the drug effect depends on what the cell is capable of accomplishing.

A drug can alter the target cell's function by:
• modifying the cell's physical or chemical environment
• interacting with a receptor (a specialized location on a cell membrane or inside a cell).

## Agonist drugs

Many drugs work by stimulating or blocking drug receptors. A drug attracted to a receptor displays an affinity for that receptor. When a drug displays an affinity for a receptor and stimulates it, the drug acts as an *agonist*. An agonist binds to the receptor and produces a response. This ability to initiate a response after binding with the receptor is referred to as *intrinsic activity*.

## Antagonist drugs

If a drug has an affinity for a receptor but displays little or no intrinsic activity, it's called an *antagonist*. An antagonist prevents a response from occurring.

## Reversible or irreversible

Antagonists can be competitive or noncompetitive.
• A *competitive antagonist* competes with the agonist for receptor sites. Because this type of antagonist binds reversibly to the receptor site, administering larger doses of an agonist can overcome the antagonist's effects.

• A *noncompetitive antagonist* binds to receptor sites and blocks the effects of the agonist. Administering larger doses of the agonist can't reverse the antagonist's action.

## Regarding receptors

If a drug acts on a variety of receptors, it's said to be nonselective and can cause multiple and widespread effects. In addition, some receptors are classified further by their specific effects. For example, beta receptors typically produce increased heart rate and bronchial relaxation as well as other systemic effects.

Beta receptors, however, can be further divided into $beta_1$ receptors (which act primarily on the heart) and $beta_2$ receptors (which act primarily on smooth muscles and gland cells).

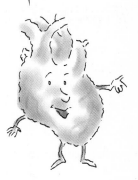

Stimulate beta receptors and I'm likely to speed up.

## Potent power

Drug potency refers to the relative amount of a drug required to produce a desired response. Drug potency is also used to compare two drugs. If drug X produces the same response as drug Y but at a lower dose, then drug X is more potent than drug Y.

As its name implies, a dose-response curve is used to graphically represent the relationship between the dose of a drug and the response it produces. (See *Dose-response curve*, page 14.)

## Maximum effect

On the dose-response curve, a low dose usually corresponds to a low response. At a low dose, a dosage increase produces only a slight increase in response. With further dosage increases, the drug response rises markedly. After a certain point, however, an increase in dose yields little or no increase in response. At this point, the drug is said to have reached maximum effectiveness.

## Margin of safety

Most drugs produce multiple effects. The relationship between a drug's desired therapeutic effects and its adverse effects is called the drug's *therapeutic index*. It's also referred to as its *margin of safety*.

The therapeutic index usually measures the difference between:
• an effective dose for 50% of the patients treated
• the minimal dose at which adverse reactions occur.

I'd say this has a narrow margin of safety. Whoa!

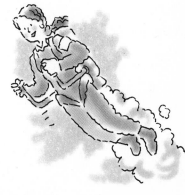

## Narrow index = potential danger

Drugs with a narrow, or low, therapeutic index have a narrow margin of safety. This means that there's a narrow range of safety between an effective dose and a lethal one. On the other hand, a drug with a high therapeutic index has a wide margin of safety and poses less risk of toxic effects.

*Now I get it!*

## Dose-response curve

This graph shows the dose-response curve for two different drugs. As you can see, at low doses of each drug, a dosage increase results in only a small increase in drug response (for example, from point A to point B for drug X). At higher doses, an increase in dosage produces a much greater response (from point B to point C). As the dosage continues to climb, however, an increase in dosage produces very little increase in response (from point C to point D).

This graph also shows that drug X is more potent than drug Y because it produces the same response, but at a lower dose (compare point A to point E).

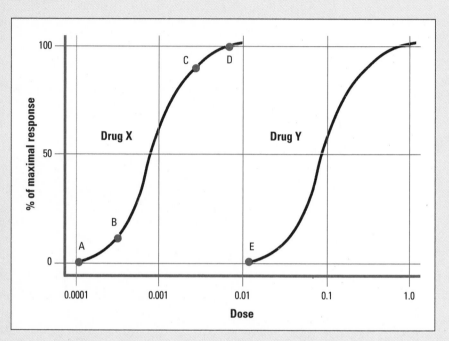

# Pharmacotherapeutics

Pharmacotherapeutics is the use of drugs to treat disease. When choosing a drug to treat a particular condition, health care providers consider not only the drug's effectiveness but also other factors such as the type of therapy the patient will receive.

## Not all therapy is the same

The type of therapy a patient receives depends on the severity, urgency, and prognosis of the patient's condition and can include:
• *acute therapy*, if the patient is critically ill and requires acute intensive therapy
• *empiric therapy*, based on practical experience rather than on pure scientific data
• *maintenance therapy*, for patients with chronic conditions that don't resolve

• *supplemental* or *replacement therapy*, to replenish or substitute for missing substances in the body
• *supportive therapy*, which doesn't treat the cause of the disease but maintains other threatened body systems until the patient's condition resolves
• *palliative therapy*, used for end-stage or terminal diseases to make the patient as comfortable as possible.

## I can only be myself

A patient's overall health as well as other individual factors can alter that patient's response to a drug. Coinciding medical conditions and personal lifestyle characteristics must be considered when selecting drug therapy. (See *Factors affecting a patient's response to a drug.*)

## Decreased response...

In addition, it's important to remember that certain drugs have a tendency to create drug tolerance and drug dependence in patients. *Drug tolerance* occurs when a patient develops a decreased response to a drug over time. The patient then requires larger doses to produce the same response.

## ...and increased desire

Tolerance differs from *drug dependence*, in which a patient displays a physical or psychological need for the drug. Physical dependence produces withdrawal symptoms when the drug is stopped, whereas psychological dependence is based on a desire to continue taking the drug to relieve tension and avoid discomfort.

# Drug interactions

Drug interactions can occur between drugs or between drugs and foods. They can interfere with the results of a laboratory test or produce physical or chemical incompatibilities. The more drugs a patient receives, the greater the chances that a drug interaction will occur.

Potential drug interactions include:
• additive effects
• potentiation
• antagonistic effects
• decreased or increased absorption
• decreased or increased metabolism and excretion.

**Now I get it!**

## Factors affecting a patient's response to a drug

Because no two people are alike physiologically or psychologically, patient response to a drug can vary greatly, depending upon such factors as:
• age
• cardiovascular function
• diet
• disease
• drug interactions
• gender
• GI function
• hepatic function
• infection
• renal function.

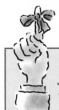

**Memory jogger**

When a drug is said to be *potentiated* by another drug, the results are more *potent*—the drug goes beyond its original potential.

## Adding it all up

*Additive effects* can occur when two drugs with similar actions are administered to a patient. The effects are equivalent to the sum of either drug's effects if it were administered alone in higher doses.

Giving two drugs together, such as two analgesics (pain relievers), has several potential advantages: lower doses of each drug, decreased probability of adverse reactions, and greater pain control than from one drug given alone (most likely because of different mechanisms of action). There's a decreased risk of adverse effects when giving two drugs for the same condition because the patient is given lower doses of each drug—the higher the dose, the greater the risk of adverse effects.

## A synergistic situation

A synergistic effect, also called *potentiation*, occurs when two drugs that produce the same effect are given together and one drug potentiates (enhances the effect of) the other drug. This produces greater effects than when each drug is taken alone.

## Fighting it out

An *antagonistic effect* occurs when the combined response of two drugs is less than the response produced by either drug alone.

## An absorbing problem

Two drugs given together can change the absorption of one or both of the drugs:
• Drugs that change the acidity of the stomach can affect the ability of another drug to dissolve in the stomach.
• Some drugs can interact and form an insoluble compound that can't be absorbed.

Sometimes, an absorption-related drug interaction can be avoided by administering the drugs at least 2 hours apart.

## Bound and determined

After a drug is absorbed, the blood distributes it throughout the body as a free drug or one that's bound to plasma protein.

When two drugs are given together, they can compete for protein-binding sites, leading to an increase in the effects of one drug as that drug is displaced from the protein and becomes a free, unbound drug.

## Toxic waste

Toxic drug levels can occur when a drug's metabolism and excretion are inhibited by another drug. Some drug interactions affect excretion only.

## Back to the lab

Drug interactions can also alter laboratory tests and can produce changes seen on a patient's electrocardiogram.

## Menu planning

Interactions between drugs and food can alter the therapeutic effects of the drug. Food can also alter the rate and amount of drug absorbed from the GI tract, affecting bioavailability—the amount of a drug dose that's made available to the systemic circulation. Drugs can also impair vitamin and mineral absorption.

Some drugs stimulate enzyme production, increasing metabolic rates and the demand for vitamins that are enzyme cofactors (which must unite with the enzyme in order for the enzyme to function). Dangerous interactions can also occur. For instance, when food that contains Vitamin K (such as green, leafy vegetables) is eaten by a person taking warfarin, the drug's anticoagulation properties are decreased and blood clots may form.

Grapefruit can inhibit the metabolism of certain medications, resulting in toxic blood levels; examples include fexofenadine, albendazole, and atorvastatin. Because of all the interactions food can have with drug metabolism, being aware of drug interactions is essential.

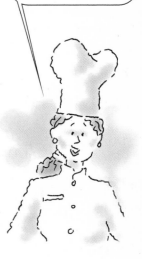

Review a patient's diet carefully—drug interactions with food can reduce absorption or even produce dangerous changes.

# Adverse drug reactions

A drug's desired effect is called the *expected therapeutic response*. An adverse drug reaction (also called a *side effect* or *adverse effect*), on the other hand, is a harmful, undesirable response. Adverse drug reactions can range from mild ones that disappear when the drug is discontinued to debilitating diseases that become chronic. Adverse reactions can appear shortly after starting a new medication but may become less severe with time.

## Dosage dilemma

Adverse drug reactions can be classified as dose-related or patient sensitivity–related. Most adverse drug reactions result from the known pharmacologic effects of a drug and are typically dose-related. These types of reactions can be predicted in most cases.

Dose-related reactions include:
- secondary effects
- hypersusceptibility
- overdose
- iatrogenic effects.

## Extra effects

A drug typically produces not only a major therapeutic effect but also additional, secondary effects that can be harmful or beneficial. For example, morphine used for pain control can lead to two undesirable secondary effects: constipation and respiratory depression. Diphenhydramine used as an antihistamine produces sedation as a secondary effect and is sometimes used as a sleep aid.

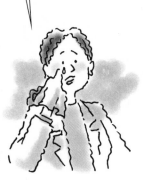

Sensitivity-related adverse reactions are caused by a patient's extreme sensitivity to a drug.

## Enhanced action

A patient can be hypersusceptible to the pharmacologic actions of a drug. Such a patient experiences an excessive therapeutic response or secondary effects even when given the usual therapeutic dose.

Hypersusceptibility typically results from altered pharmacokinetics (absorption, metabolism, and excretion), which leads to higher-than-expected blood concentration levels. Increased receptor sensitivity also can increase the patient's response to therapeutic or adverse effects.

## Oh no—overdose!

A toxic drug reaction can occur when an excessive dose is taken, either intentionally or by accident. The result is an exaggerated response to the drug that can lead to transient changes or more serious reactions, such as respiratory depression, cardiovascular collapse, and even death. To avoid toxic reactions, chronically ill or elderly patients often receive lower drug doses.

## Iatrogenic issues

Some adverse drug reactions, known as iatrogenic effects, can mimic pathologic disorders. For example, such drugs as antineoplastics, aspirin, corticosteroids, and indomethacin commonly cause GI irritation and bleeding. Other examples of iatrogenic effects include induced asthma with propranolol, induced nephritis with methicillin, and induced deafness with gentamicin.

## You're so sensitive

Patient sensitivity–related adverse reactions aren't as common as dose-related reactions. Sensitivity-related reactions result from a patient's unusual and extreme sensitivity to a drug. These adverse reactions arise from a unique tissue response rather than from an exaggerated pharmacologic action. Extreme patient sensitivity can occur as a drug allergy or an idiosyncratic response.

## Friend or foe?

A drug allergy occurs when a patient's immune system identifies a drug, a drug metabolite, or a drug contaminant as a dangerous foreign substance that must be neutralized or destroyed. Previous exposure to the drug or to one with similar chemical characteristics sensitizes the patient's immune system, and subsequent exposure causes an allergic reaction (hypersensitivity).

An allergic reaction not only directly injures cells and tissues but also produces broader systemic damage by initiating cellular release of vasoactive and inflammatory substances.

The allergic reaction can vary in intensity from an immediate, life-threatening anaphylactic reaction with circulatory collapse and swelling of the larynx and bronchioles to a mild reaction with a rash and itching.

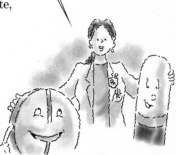

For an allergic reaction to occur, the patient must have received the drug before.

## Idiosyncratic response

Some sensitivity-related adverse reactions don't result from pharmacologic properties of a drug or from an allergy but are specific to the individual patient. These are called *idiosyncratic responses*. Some idiosyncratic responses have a genetic cause.

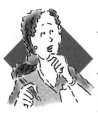

# Quick quiz

**1.** While teaching a patient about drug therapy for diabetes, you review the absorption, distribution, metabolism, and excretion of insulin and oral antidiabetic agents. Which principle of pharmacology are you describing?
A. Pharmacokinetics
B. Pharmacodynamics
C. Pharmacotherapeutics
D. Drug potency

*Answer:* A. Pharmacokinetics discusses the movement of drugs through the body and involves absorption, distribution, metabolism, and excretion.

**2.** Which type of drug therapy is used for a patient who has a chronic condition that can't be cured?
A. Empiric therapy
B. Acute therapy
C. Maintenance therapy
D. Supplemental therapy

*Answer:* C. Maintenance therapy seeks to maintain a certain level of health in patients who have chronic conditions.

**3.** Which branch of pharmacology studies the way drugs work in living organisms?

    A.    Pharmacotherapeutics
    B.    Pharmacokinetics
    C.    Drug interactions
    D.    Pharmacodynamics

*Answer:* D. Pharmacodynamics studies the mechanisms of action of drugs and seeks to understand how drugs work in the body.

## Scoring

☆☆☆  If you answered all three items correctly, excellent! You've absorbed this chapter in a hurry.

☆☆  If you answered two items correctly, terrific! You've reached therapeutic levels of this chapter in a flash.

☆  If you answered fewer than two items correctly, no need for concern. Sometimes food enhances absorption—so grab a quick snack and come back for a review.

# Autonomic nervous system drugs

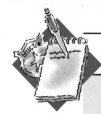

## Just the facts

In this chapter, you'll review:

♦ classes of drugs that affect the autonomic nervous system

♦ uses and varying actions of these drugs

♦ how these drugs are absorbed, distributed, metabolized, and excreted

♦ drug interactions and adverse effects of these drugs.

## Cholinergic drugs

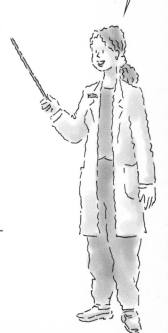

Cholinergic drugs enhance the action of acetylcholine, stimulating the parasympathetic nervous system.

*Cholinergic drugs* promote the action of the neurotransmitter *acetylcholine*. These drugs are also called *parasympathomimetic drugs* because they produce effects that imitate parasympathetic nerve stimulation.

### Mimickers and inhibitors

There are two major classes of cholinergic drugs:

*Cholinergic agonists* mimic the action of the neurotransmitter acetylcholine.

*Anticholinesterase drugs* work by inhibiting the destruction of acetylcholine at the cholinergic receptor sites. (See *How cholinergic drugs work*, page 22.)

## Cholinergic agonists

By directly stimulating cholinergic receptors, cholinergic agonists mimic the action of the neurotransmitter acetylcholine.
They include such drugs as:

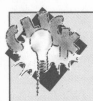

*Now I get it!*

# How cholinergic drugs work

Cholinergic drugs fall into one of two major classes: cholinergic agonists and anticholinesterase drugs. Here's how these drugs achieve their effects.

### Cholinergic agonists

When a neuron in the parasympathetic nervous system is stimulated, the neurotransmitter acetylcholine is released. Acetylcholine crosses the synapse and interacts with receptors in an adjacent neuron. Cholinergic agonists stimulate cholinergic receptors, mimicking the action of acetylcholine.

### Anticholinesterase drugs

After acetylcholine stimulates the cholinergic receptor, it's destroyed by the enzyme acetylcholinesterase. Anticholinesterase drugs inhibit acetylcholinesterase. As a result, acetylcholine isn't broken down and begins to accumulate, leading to prolonged acetylcholine effects.

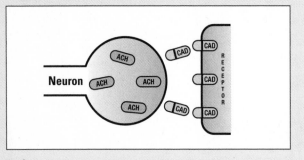

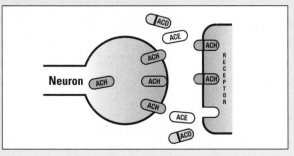

**Key:**

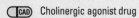

| | | | |
|---|---|---|---|
| **ACH** Acetylcholine | **CAD** Cholinergic agonist drug | **ACE** Acetylcholinesterase | **ACD** Anticholinesterase drug |

- bethanechol
- carbachol
- cevimeline
- pilocarpine.

## Pharmacokinetics (how drugs circulate)

The action and metabolism of cholinergic agonists vary widely and depend on the affinity of the individual drug for muscarinic or nicotinic receptors.

### No I.M. or I.V. injections

Cholinergic agonists rarely are administered by I.M. or I.V. injection because they're almost immediately broken down by cholinesterases in the interstitial spaces between tissues and inside the blood vessels. Moreover, they begin to work rapidly and can cause a cholinergic crisis (a drug overdose resulting in extreme muscle weakness and possibly paralysis of the muscles used in respiration).

## Topically, orally, or under the skin

Cholinergic agonists are usually administered:
- topically, with eye drops
- orally
- by subcutaneous (subQ) injection.
  SubQ injections begin to work more rapidly than oral doses.

### Metabolism and excretion

All cholinergic agonists are metabolized by cholinesterases:
- at the muscarinic and nicotinic receptor sites
- in the plasma (the liquid portion of the blood)
- in the liver.
  All drugs in this class are excreted by the kidneys.

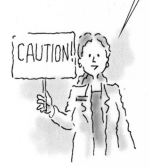

Cholinergic agonists administered by injection are rapidly broken down and could cause a cholinergic crisis.

## Pharmacodynamics (how drugs act)

Cholinergic agonists work by mimicking the action of acetylcholine on the neurons in certain organs of the body called *target organs*. When they combine with receptors on the cell membranes of target organs, they stimulate the muscle and produce:
- salivation
- bradycardia (a slow heart rate)
- dilation of blood vessels
- constriction of the bronchioles
- increased activity of the GI tract
- increased tone and contraction of the bladder muscles
- constriction of the pupils.

## Pharmacotherapeutics (how drugs are used)

Cholinergic agonists are used to:
- treat atonic (weak) bladder conditions and postoperative and postpartum urine retention
- treat GI disorders, such as postoperative abdominal distention and GI atony
- reduce eye pressure in patients with glaucoma and during eye surgery
- treat salivary gland hypofunction caused by radiation therapy or Sjögren's syndrome.

### Drug interactions

Cholinergic agonists have specific interactions with other drugs. Examples include the following:
• Other cholinergic drugs, particularly anticholinesterase drugs (such as ambenonium, edrophonium, neostigmine, physostigmine, and pyridostigmine), boost the effects of cholinergic agonists and increase the risk of toxicity.
• Cholinergic blocking drugs (such as atropine, belladonna, homatropine, methantheline, methscopolamine, propantheline, and scopolamine) reduce the effects of cholinergic drugs.
• Quinidine also reduces the effectiveness of cholinergic agonists. (See *Adverse reactions to cholinergic agonists.*)

## Anticholinesterase drugs

*Anticholinesterase drugs* block the action of the enzyme acetylcholinesterase (which breaks down the neurotransmitter acetylcholine) at cholinergic receptor sites, preventing the breakdown of acetylcholine. As acetylcholine builds up, it continues to stimulate the cholinergic receptors. (See *One day at a time: Recognizing a toxic response.*)

Anticholinesterase drugs are divided into two categories—reversible and irreversible.

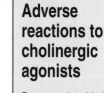

## Adverse reactions to cholinergic agonists

Because they bind with receptors in the parasympathetic nervous system, cholinergic agonists can produce adverse effects in any organ innervated by the parasympathetic nerves.

These adverse effects can include:
• nausea and vomiting
• cramps and diarrhea
• blurred vision
• decreased heart rate and low blood pressure
• shortness of breath
• urinary frequency
• increased salivation and sweating.

*Yea or nay?*

## One day at a time: Recognizing a toxic response

It's difficult to predict adverse reactions to anticholinesterase drugs in a patient with myasthenia gravis because the therapeutic dose varies from day to day. Increased muscle weakness can result from:
• resistance to the drug
• receiving too little of the anticholinesterase
• receiving too much of the anticholinesterase.

**Enter edrophonium**
Deciding whether a patient is experiencing a toxic drug response (too much drug) or a myasthenic crisis (extreme muscle weakness and severe respiratory difficulties) can be difficult. Edrophonium can be used to distinguish between a toxic drug reaction and a myasthenic crisis. When edrophonium is used, suction, oxygen, mechanical ventilation, and emergency drugs, such as atropine, must be readily available in case a cholinergic crisis occurs.

## These you can reverse...

Reversible anticholinesterase drugs have a short duration of action and include:
- ambenonium
- demecarium
- donepezil
- edrophonium
- galantamine
- guanidine
- neostigmine
- physostigmine
- pyridostigmine
- rivastigmine
- tacrine.

## ...these you can't

Irreversible anticholinesterase drugs have long-lasting effects and are used primarily as toxic insecticides and pesticides or as nerve gas in chemical warfare. (Pyridostigmine enhances the effects of antidotes used to counteract nerve agents.) Only one has therapeutic usefulness: echothiophate.

## Pharmacokinetics

Here's a brief rundown of how anticholinesterase drugs move through the body.

### Generally GI

Many of the anticholinesterase drugs are readily absorbed from the GI tract, subcutaneous tissue, and mucous membranes.

Because neostigmine is poorly absorbed from the GI tract, the patient needs a higher dose when taking this drug orally. Because the duration of action for an oral dose is longer, however, the patient doesn't need to take it as frequently. When a rapid effect is needed, neostigmine should be given by the I.M. or I.V. route.

### Distribution

Physostigmine can cross the blood-brain barrier (a protective barrier between the capillaries and brain tissue that prevents harmful substances from entering the brain). Donepezil is highly bound to plasma proteins, tacrine is about 55% bound, rivastigmine is 40% bound, and galantamine is 18% bound.

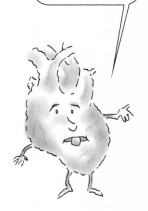

Easy does it. Overstimulation of the parasymphathetic nervous system can send me into cardiac arrest!

### *Metabolism and excretion*

Most anticholinesterase drugs are metabolized by enzymes in the plasma and excreted in urine. Donepezil, galantamine, rivastigmine, and tacrine are metabolized in the liver.

## Pharmacodynamics

Anticholinesterase drugs promote the action of acetylcholine at receptor sites. Depending on the site and the drug's dose and duration of action, they can produce a stimulant or depressant effect on cholinergic receptors.

### From minutes to weeks

Reversible anticholinesterase drugs block the breakdown of acetylcholine for minutes to hours; irreversible anticholinesterase drugs do so for days or weeks.

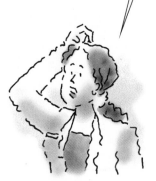

Depending on the dosage, anticholinesterase drugs can produce a stimulant or depressant effect on receptors.

## Pharmacotherapeutics

Anticholinesterase drugs are used for a variety of therapeutic purposes, including:
• to reduce eye pressure in patients with glaucoma and during eye surgery
• to increase bladder tone
• to improve tone and peristalsis (movement) through the GI tract in patients with reduced motility or paralytic ileus (paralysis of the small intestine)
• to promote muscle contractions in patients with myasthenia gravis
• to diagnose myasthenia gravis (neostigmine and edrophonium)
• as an antidote to cholinergic blocking drugs (also called *anticholinergic drugs*), tricyclic antidepressants, belladonna alkaloids, and narcotics
• to treat mild to moderate dementia and enhance cognition in patients with Alzheimer's disease (primarily donepezil, galantamine, rivastigmine, and tacrine).

## Drug interactions

These interactions can occur with anticholinesterase drugs:
• Other cholinergic drugs, particularly cholinergic agonists (such as bethanechol, carbachol, and pilocarpine), increase the risk of a toxic reaction when taken with anticholinesterase drugs.
• Carbamazepine, dexamethasone, rifampin, phenytoin, and phenobarbital may increase donepezil's rate of elimination.
• Aminoglycoside antibiotics, anesthetics, cholinergic blocking drugs (such as atropine, belladonna, propantheline, and scopolamine), magnesium, corticosteroids, and antiarrhythmic drugs

(such as procainamide and quinidine) can reduce the effects of anticholinesterase drugs and can mask early signs of a cholinergic crisis. (See *Adverse reactions to anticholinesterase drugs.*)
• Other medications with cholinergic-blocking properties, such as tricyclic antidepressants, bladder relaxants, and antipsychotics, can also counteract the effects of anticholinesterase drugs.
• The effects of tacrine, donepezil, and galantamine may be increased when these drugs are combined with known inhibitors of cytochrome P-450 enzymes, such as cimetidine and erythromycin.
• Cigarette use increases the clearance of rivastigmine.

# Cholinergic blocking drugs

*Cholinergic blocking drugs* interrupt parasympathetic nerve impulses in the central and autonomic nervous systems. These drugs are also referred to as *anticholinergic drugs* because they prevent acetylcholine from stimulating cholinergic receptors.

## Not all receptors are receptive

Cholinergic blocking drugs don't block all cholinergic receptors, just the muscarinic receptor sites. Muscarinic receptors are cholinergic receptors that are stimulated by the alkaloid muscarine and blocked by atropine.

## First come the belladonna alkaloids

The major cholinergic blocking drugs are the belladonna alkaloids:
• atropine (the prototype cholinergic blocking drug)
• belladonna
• homatropine
• hyoscyamine sulfate
• methscopolamine
• scopolamine.

## Next come their synthetic sisters

Synthetic derivatives of these drugs (the quaternary ammonium drugs) include:
• glycopyrrolate
• propantheline.

## And finally the tertiary and quaternary amines

The tertiary amines include:
• benztropine
• dicyclomine
• oxybutynin

**Warning!**

## Adverse reactions to anticholinesterase drugs

Most of the adverse reactions caused by anticholinesterase drugs result from increased action of acetylcholine at receptor sites.

Adverse reactions associated with these drugs include:
• cardiac arrhythmias
• nausea and vomiting
• diarrhea
• shortness of breath, wheezing, or tightness in the chest
• seizures
• headache
• anorexia
• insomnia
• pruritus
• urinary frequency and nocturia.

- trihexyphenidyl
- tolterodine.

Quaternary amines include one drug, trospium.

Atropine may also be used as an antidote for nerve agents (See the appendix, Vaccines and antidotes for biological and chemical weapons.)

## Let's talk about it later

Because benztropine and trihexyphenidyl are almost exclusively treatments for Parkinson's disease, they're discussed fully in chapter 3, Neurologic and neuromuscular drugs.

## Pharmacokinetics

Here's how cholinergic blockers move through the body.

### Absorption

The belladonna alkaloids are absorbed from the:
- eyes
- GI tract
- mucous membranes
- skin.

The quaternary ammonium drugs and tertiary and quaternary amines are absorbed primarily through the GI tract, although not as readily as the belladonna alkaloids.

## If you want it fast, go I.V.

When administered I.V., cholinergic blockers such as atropine begin to work immediately.

### Distribution

The belladonna alkaloids are distributed more widely throughout the body than the quaternary ammonium derivatives or dicyclomine. The alkaloids readily cross the blood-brain barrier; the other cholinergic blockers don't.

### Metabolism and excretion

The belladonna alkaloids are only slightly to moderately protein-bound. This means that a moderate to high amount of the drug is active and available to produce a therapeutic response. The belladonna alkaloids are metabolized in the liver and excreted by the kidneys as unchanged drug and metabolites.

The quaternary ammonium drugs are a bit more complicated. Hydrolysis is a chemical process whereby a compound cleaved into two or more simpler compounds occurs in the GI tract and the liver; the drugs are excreted in feces and urine. Dicyclomine's

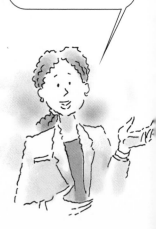

Belladonna alkaloids are less likely to bind with serum proteins, so more drug remains available to produce a therapeutic effect.

metabolism is unknown, but it's excreted equally in feces and urine.

## Pharmacodynamics

Cholinergic blockers can have paradoxical effects on the body, depending on the dosage and the condition being treated.

### Dual duty

Cholinergic blockers can produce a stimulating or depressing effect, depending on the target organ. In the brain, they do both— low drug levels stimulate, and high drug levels depress.

### Conditional considerations

The effects of a drug on your patient are also determined by the patient's disorder. Parkinson's disease, for example, is characterized by low dopamine levels that intensify the stimulating effects of acetylcholine. Cholinergic blockers depress this effect. In other disorders, however, they stimulate the central nervous system.

## Pharmacotherapeutics

Cholinergic blockers are often used to treat GI disorders and complications.
• All cholinergic blockers are used to treat spastic or hyperactive conditions of the GI and urinary tracts because they relax muscles and decrease GI secretions. These drugs may be used to relax the bladder and to treat urinary incontinence. The quaternary ammonium and amine compounds such as propantheline are the drugs of choice for these conditions because they cause fewer adverse reactions than belladonna alkaloids.
• Belladonna alkaloids are used with morphine to treat biliary colic (pain caused by stones in the bile duct).
• Cholinergic blocking drugs are given by injection before such diagnostic procedures as endoscopy and sigmoidoscopy to relax the GI smooth muscle.

### Before surgery

Cholinergic blockers such as atropine are given before surgery to:
• reduce oral, gastric, and respiratory secretions
• prevent a drop in heart rate caused by vagal nerve stimulation during anesthesia.

### Brainy belladonna

The belladonna alkaloids can affect the brain. For example, scopolamine, given with the pain relievers morphine or meperi-

*Now I get it!*

## How atropine speeds the heart rate

To understand how atropine affects the heart, first consider how the heart's electrical conduction system functions.

### Without the drug

When the neurotransmitter acetylcholine is released, the vagus nerve stimulates the sinoatrial (SA) node (the heart's pacemaker) and the atrioventricular (AV) node, which controls conduction between the atria and the ventricles of the heart. This inhibits electrical conduction and causes the heart rate to slow down.

### With the drug

Atropine, a cholinergic blocking drug, competes with acetylcholine for cholinergic receptor sites on the SA and AV nodes. By blocking acetylcholine, atropine speeds up the heart rate.

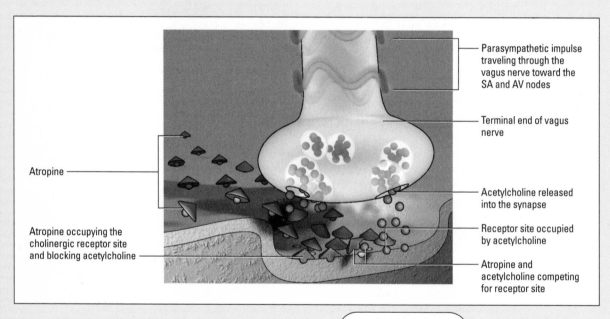

- Atropine
- Atropine occupying the cholinergic receptor site and blocking acetylcholine
- Parasympathetic impulse traveling through the vagus nerve toward the SA and AV nodes
- Terminal end of vagus nerve
- Acetylcholine released into the synapse
- Receptor site occupied by acetylcholine
- Atropine and acetylcholine competing for receptor site

dine, causes drowsiness and amnesia in a patient having surgery. It's also used to treat motion sickness.

Belladonna alkaloids also have important therapeutic effects on the heart. Atropine is the drug of choice to treat:
- symptomatic sinus bradycardia—when the heart beats too slowly, causing low blood pressure or dizziness (see *How atropine speeds the heart rate*)
- arrhythmias resulting from the use of anesthetics, choline esters, or succinylcholine.

*Cholinergic blocking drugs can help me regain my rhythm!*

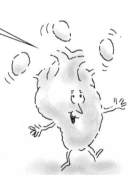

## An eye on the problem

Cholinergic blockers also are used as cycloplegics. That means that they:
- paralyze the ciliary muscles of the eye (used for fine focusing)
- alter the shape of the eye lens.

Moreover, cholinergic blockers act as mydriatics to dilate the pupils, making it easier to measure refractive errors during an eye examination or to perform eye surgery.

## Punishing pesticides

The belladonna alkaloids, particularly atropine and hyoscyamine, are effective antidotes to cholinergic and anticholinesterase drugs. Atropine is the drug of choice to treat poisoning from organophosphate pesticides. Atropine and hyoscyamine also counteract the effects of the neuromuscular blocking drugs by competing for the same receptor sites.

# Drug interactions

Because cholinergic blockers slow the passage of food and drugs through the stomach, drugs remain in prolonged contact with the mucous membranes of the GI tract. This increases the amount of the drug that's absorbed and, therefore, increases the risk of adverse effects.

## Increased effect...

Drugs that increase the effects of cholinergic blockers include:
- disopyramide
- antidyskinetics such as amantadine
- antiemetics and antivertigo drugs, such as buclizine, cyclizine, meclizine, and diphenhydramine
- antipsychotics, such as haloperidol, phenothiazines, and thioxanthenes
- cyclobenzaprine
- orphenadrine
- tricyclic and tetracyclic antidepressants.

## ...or decreased effect

Drugs that decrease the effects of cholinergic blockers include:
- cholinergic agonists such as bethanechol
- anticholinesterase drugs, such as neostigmine and pyridostigmine.

## Mixing it up some more

Other drug interactions can occur:
- The risk of digoxin toxicity increases when digoxin is taken with a cholinergic blocker.

• Opiate-like analgesics further slow the movement of food and drugs through the GI tract when taken with a cholinergic blocker.
• The absorption of nitroglycerin tablets placed under the tongue is reduced when this drug is taken with a cholinergic blocker. (See *Adverse reactions to cholinergic blockers*.)

# Adrenergic drugs

*Adrenergic drugs* are also called *sympathomimetic drugs* because they produce effects similar to those produced by the sympathetic nervous system.

## Classified by chemical...

Adrenergic drugs are classified into two groups based on their chemical structure—catecholamines (naturally occurring as well as synthetic) and noncatecholamines.

## ...or by action

Adrenergic drugs are also classified by how they act. They can be:
• *direct-acting*, in which the drug acts directly on the organ or tissue innervated (supplied with nerves or nerve impulses) by the sympathetic nervous system
• *indirect-acting*, in which the drug triggers the release of a neurotransmitter, usually norepinephrine
• *dual-acting*, in which the drug has both direct and indirect actions. (See *Understanding adrenergics*.)

## Which receptor does it affect?

The therapeutic uses of adrenergics—catecholamines as well as noncatecholamines—depend on which receptors they stimulate and to what degree. Adrenergic drugs can affect:
• alpha-adrenergic receptors
• beta-adrenergic receptors
• dopamine receptors.

## Mimicking norepinephrine and epinephrine

Most adrenergics produce their effects by stimulating alpha receptors and beta receptors. These drugs mimic the action of norepinephrine and epinephrine.

## Doing it like dopamine

Dopaminergic drugs act primarily on receptors in the sympathetic nervous system stimulated by dopamine.

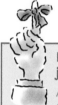

**Memory jogger**

A *direct-acting* drug has a direct effect on a target organ.

An *indirect-acting* drug triggers a neurotransmitter that takes over from there.

A *dual-acting* drug works both ways.

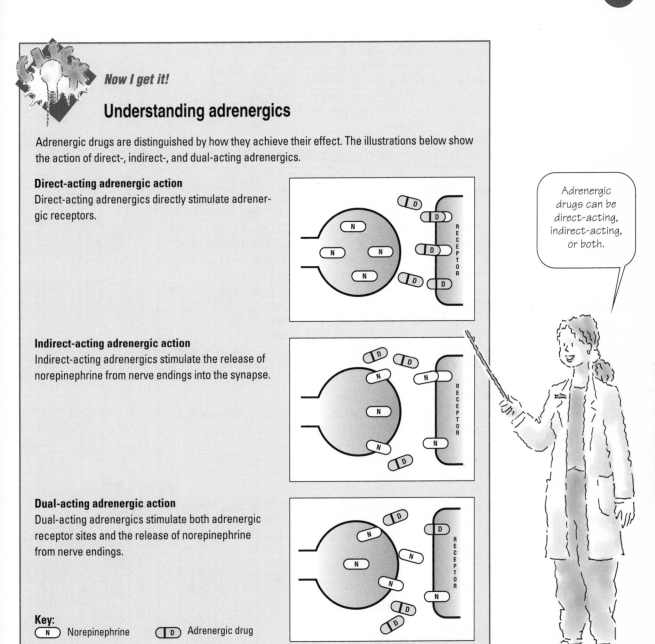

*Now I get it!*

## Understanding adrenergics

Adrenergic drugs are distinguished by how they achieve their effect. The illustrations below show the action of direct-, indirect-, and dual-acting adrenergics.

**Direct-acting adrenergic action**
Direct-acting adrenergics directly stimulate adrenergic receptors.

**Indirect-acting adrenergic action**
Indirect-acting adrenergics stimulate the release of norepinephrine from nerve endings into the synapse.

**Dual-acting adrenergic action**
Dual-acting adrenergics stimulate both adrenergic receptor sites and the release of norepinephrine from nerve endings.

**Key:**
(N) Norepinephrine    (D) Adrenergic drug

Adrenergic drugs can be direct-acting, indirect-acting, or both.

# Catecholamines

Because of their common basic chemical structure, all catecholamines share certain properties—they stimulate the nervous system, constrict peripheral blood vessels, increase heart rate, and dilate the bronchi. They can be manufactured in the body or in a laboratory. Common catecholamines include:

- dobutamine
- dopamine
- epinephrine, epinephrine bitartrate, and epinephrine hydrochloride
- norepinephrine (levarterenol)
- isoproterenol hydrochloride and isoproterenol sulfate.

## Pharmacokinetics

Catecholamines can't be taken orally because they're destroyed by digestive enzymes. In contrast, when these drugs are given sublingually (under the tongue), they're absorbed rapidly through the mucous membranes. Any sublingual drug not completely absorbed is rapidly metabolized by swallowed saliva.

### Subcutaneously slow

SubQ absorption is slowed because catecholamines cause the blood vessels around the injection site to constrict.

I.M. absorption is more rapid because there's less constriction of local blood vessels.

### *Distribution and metabolism*

Catecholamines are widely distributed in the body. They're metabolized and inactivated predominantly in the liver but can also be metabolized in the:

- GI tract
- lungs
- kidneys
- plasma
- other tissues.

### *Excretion*

Catecholamines are excreted primarily in urine; however, a small amount of isoproterenol is excreted in feces and some epinephrine is excreted in breast milk.

## Pharmacodynamics

Catecholamines are primarily direct-acting. When catecholamines combine with alpha receptors or beta receptors, they cause either an excitatory or an inhibitory effect. Typically, activation of alpha receptors generates an excitatory response, except for intestinal relaxation. Activation of beta receptors typically produces an inhibitory response, except in heart cells, where norepinephrine produces excitatory effects.

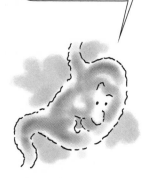

*Catecholamines are ineffective when taken orally because they're destroyed by digestive enzymes.*

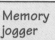

**Memory jogger**

To help you remember the effects of catecholamines on alpha and beta receptors, remember that **A** stands for alpha (and ***activation,*** suggesting an excitatory response), and **B** stands for beta (or ***banished,*** suggesting an inhibitory effect).

## How heartening

The clinical effects of catecholamines depend on the dosage and administration route. Catecholamines are potent inotropes—they make the heart contract more forcefully. As a result, the ventricles empty more completely with each heartbeat, increasing the heart's workload and the amount of oxygen it needs to do this harder work.

Catecholamines increase my workload.

## Rapid rates

Catecholamines also produce a positive chronotropic effect, which means that they cause the heart to beat faster. That happens because the pacemaker cells in the heart's sinoatrial (SA) node depolarize at a faster rate. As catecholamines cause blood vessels to constrict and blood pressure to rise, the heart rate can fall as the body tries to compensate for an excessive rise in blood pressure.

## Fascinating rhythm

Catecholamines can cause the Purkinje fibers (an intricate web of fibers that carry electrical impulses into the ventricles) to fire spontaneously, possibly producing abnormal heart rhythms, such as premature ventricular contractions and fibrillation. Epinephrine is more likely than norepinephrine to produce this spontaneous firing.

## Pharmacotherapeutics

The therapeutic uses of catecholamines depend on the particular receptor that's activated.
- Norepinephrine stimulates alpha receptors almost exclusively.
- Dobutamine and isoproterenol stimulate only beta receptors.
- Epinephrine stimulates both alpha and beta receptors.
- Dopamine activates primarily dopamine receptors.

## Boosting blood pressure

Catecholamines that stimulate alpha receptors are used to treat low blood pressure (hypotension). They generally work best when used to treat hypotension caused by:
- relaxation of the blood vessel (also called a *loss of vasomotor tone*)
- blood loss (such as from hemorrhage).

## Restoring rhythm

Catecholamines that stimulate beta$_1$ receptors are used to treat:
- bradycardia

• heart block (a delay or interruption in the conduction of electrical impulses between the atria and ventricles)
• low cardiac output.

## It's electric

Because they're believed to make the heart more responsive to defibrillation (using an electrical current to terminate a deadly arrhythmia), beta$_1$-adrenergic drugs are used to treat:
• ventricular fibrillation (quivering of the ventricles, resulting in no pulse)
• asystole (no electrical activity in the heart)
• cardiac arrest.

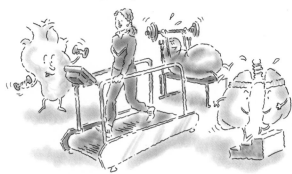

Catecholamines have a wide variety of therapeutic uses. Almost all body systems can feel the impact!

## Better breathing

Catecholamines that exert beta$_2$ activity are used to treat:
• acute or chronic bronchial asthma
• emphysema
• bronchitis
• acute hypersensitivity (allergic) reactions to drugs.

## Kind to the kidneys

Dopamine, which stimulates the dopamine receptors, is used in low doses to improve blood flow to the kidneys by dilating the renal blood vessels.

## Synthetic vs. natural

The effects of natural catecholamines (those produced by the body) differ somewhat from the effects of manufactured catecholamines. Manufactured catecholamines have a short duration of action, which can limit their therapeutic usefulness.

## Drug interactions

Drug interactions involving catecholamines can be serious, resulting in hypotension, hypertension, arrhythmias, seizures, and high blood glucose levels in diabetic patients.
• Alpha-adrenergic blockers, such as phentolamine, can produce hypotension when taken with a catecholamine.
• Beta-adrenergic blockers, such as propranolol, taken with a catecholamine can lead to bronchial constriction.
• Epinephrine may cause hyperglycemia in diabetic patients receiving the drug. These patients may require an increased dose of insulin or oral antidiabetic agents.

**Warning!**

## Adverse reactions to catecholamines

Adverse reactions to catecholamines can include:
- restlessness
- asthmatic episode
- dizziness
- headache
- palpitations
- cardiac arrhythmias
- hypotension
- hypertension and hypertensive crisis
- stroke
- angina
- increased blood glucose levels
- tissue necrosis and sloughing (if a catecholamine given I.V. leaks into surrounding tissue).

- Other adrenergics taken with a catecholamine can produce additive, or double, effects, such as hypertension and arrhythmias, as well as enhance other adverse effects. Increased risk of adverse effects, such as hypertension, may occur when adrenergic drugs are given with other drugs that can cause hypertension.
- Tricyclic antidepressants taken with a catecholamine can lead to hypertension. (See *Adverse reactions to catecholamines*.)

# Noncatecholamines

*Noncatecholamine adrenergic drugs* have a variety of therapeutic uses because of the many effects they can have on the body, including:
- local or systemic constriction of blood vessels (phenylephrine)
- nasal and eye decongestion and dilation of the bronchioles (albuterol, bitolterol, ephedrine, formoterol, isoetharine hydrochloride, isoproterenol, levalbuterol, metaproterenol, pirbuterol, salmeterol, and terbutaline)
- smooth-muscle relaxation (terbutaline).

## Pharmacokinetics

Although these drugs are all excreted in urine, they're absorbed in different ways.

### Absorption and distribution

Absorption of the noncatecholamines depends on the administration route:
• Inhaled drugs, such as albuterol, are absorbed gradually from the bronchi and result in lower drug levels in the body.
• Oral drugs are absorbed well from the GI tract and are distributed widely in body fluids and tissues.
• Some noncatecholamines, such as ephedrine, cross the blood-brain barrier and can be found in high concentrations in the brain and cerebrospinal fluid (fluid that moves through and protects the brain and spinal canal).

### Metabolism

Noncatecholamines are metabolized and inactivated primarily in the liver but also in the lungs, GI tract, and other tissues.

### Excretion

Noncatecholamines and their metabolites are excreted primarily in urine. Some, such as inhaled albuterol, are excreted within 24 hours; others, such as oral albuterol, within 3 days. Acidic urine increases excretion of many noncatecholamines; alkaline urine slows excretion.

## Pharmacodynamics

Noncatecholamines can be direct-acting, indirect-acting, or dual-acting (unlike catecholamines, which are primarily direct-acting).
• Direct-acting noncatecholamines that stimulate alpha receptors include phenylephrine. Those that selectively stimulate beta$_2$ receptors include albuterol, isoetharine, metaproterenol, and terbutaline.
• Dual-acting noncatecholamines include ephedrine.

## Pharmacotherapeutics

Noncatecholamines stimulate the sympathetic nervous system, producing a variety of effects in the body. Phenylephrine, for example, causes vasoconstriction and is used to treat hypotension in cases of severe shock. Terbutaline is used to stop preterm labor.

**Warning!**

## Adverse reactions to noncatecholamines

Adverse reactions to noncate-cholamine drugs may include:
- headache
- restlessness
- anxiety or euphoria
- irritability
- trembling
- drowsiness or insomnia
- light-headedness
- incoherence
- seizures

- hypertension or hypotension
- palpitations
- bradycardia or tachycardia
- irregular heart rhythm
- cardiac arrest
- cerebral hemorrhage
- tingling or coldness in the arms or legs
- pallor or flushing
- angina.

## Drug interactions

Here are a few examples of drugs that interact with noncatechol-amines:

• Anesthetics (general), cyclopropane, and halogenated hydrocarbons can cause arrhythmias. Hypotension can also occur if these drugs are taken with noncatecholamines that exert predominantly beta$_2$ activity, such as terbutaline.

• Monoamine oxidase inhibitors can cause severe hypertension and even death.

• Oxytocic drugs that stimulate the uterus to contract can be inhibited when taken with terbutaline. When taken with other noncatecholamines, oxytocic drugs can cause hypertensive crisis or a stroke.

• Tricyclic antidepressants can cause hypertension and arrhythmias.

• Urine alkalizers, such as acetazolamide and sodium bicarbonate, slow excretion of noncatecholamines, prolonging their duration of action. (See *Adverse reactions to noncatecholamines*.)

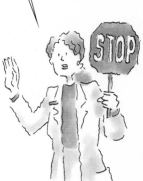

Monoamine oxidase inhibitors interact dangerously with noncatecholamines— possibly resulting in death.

# Adrenergic blocking drugs

*Adrenergic blocking drugs*, also called *sympatholytic drugs*, are used to disrupt sympathetic nervous system function. These drugs work by blocking impulse transmission (and thus sympathetic nervous system stimulation) at adrenergic neurons or adrenergic receptor sites. Their action at these sites can be exerted by:

- interrupting the action of adrenergic (sympathomimetic) drugs
- reducing available norepinephrine
- preventing the action of cholinergic drugs.

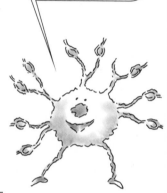

Adrenergic blocking drugs block stimulation of the sympathetic nervous system.

## Classified information

Adrenergic blocking drugs are classified according to their site of action as:

- alpha-adrenergic blockers (or *alpha blockers*)
- beta-adrenergic blockers (or *beta blockers*).

# Alpha-adrenergic blockers

*Alpha-adrenergic blockers* work by interrupting the actions of the catecholamines epinephrine and norepinephrine at alpha receptors. This results in:

- relaxation of the smooth muscle in blood vessels
- increased dilation of blood vessels
- decreased blood pressure.
  Drugs in this class include:
- alfuzosin
- ergoloid mesylates
- phenoxybenzamine
- phentolamine
- prazosin, doxazosin, and terazosin
- tamulosin.

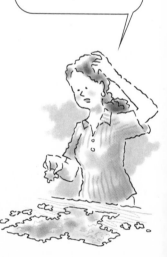

Let's face it—the action of alpha-adrenergic blockers is a bit puzzling.

## A mixed bag

Ergotamine is a mixed alpha agonist and antagonist; at high doses, it acts as an alpha-adrenergic blocker.

## Pharmacokinetics

The action of alpha-adrenergic blockers in the body isn't well understood. Most of these drugs are absorbed erratically when administered orally, and more rapidly and completely when administered sublingually. Alpha-adrenergic blockers vary considerably in their onset of action, peak concentration levels, and duration of action.

## Pharmacodynamics

Alpha-adrenergic blockers work in one of two ways:
• They interfere with or block the synthesis, storage, release, and reuptake of norepinephrine by neurons.
• They antagonize epinephrine, norepinephrine, or adrenergic (sympathomimetic) drugs at alpha receptor sites.

### Not very discriminating

Alpha-adrenergic blockers include drugs that block stimulation of alpha$_1$ receptors and that may block alpha$_2$ receptors.

### Reducing resistance

Alpha-adrenergic blockers occupy alpha receptor sites on the smooth muscle of blood vessels. (See *How alpha-adrenergic blockers affect peripheral blood vessels.*)

This prevents catecholamines from occupying and stimulating the receptor sites. As a result, blood vessels dilate, increasing lo-

*Now I get it!*

## How alpha-adrenergic blockers affect peripheral blood vessels

By occupying alpha receptor sites, alpha-adrenergic blocking drugs cause the blood vessel walls to relax. This leads to dilation of the blood vessels and reduced peripheral vascular resistance (the pressure that blood must overcome as it flows in a vessel).

**One result: Orthostatic hypotension**
These effects can cause <u>orthostatic hypotension</u>, a drop in blood pressure that occurs when changing position from lying down to standing. Redistribution of blood to the dilated blood vessels of the legs causes hypotension.

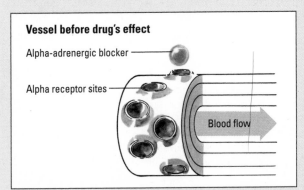

**Vessel before drug's effect**

Alpha-adrenergic blocker

Alpha receptor sites

Blood flow

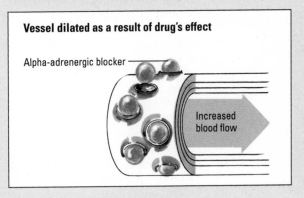

**Vessel dilated as a result of drug's effect**

Alpha-adrenergic blocker

Increased blood flow

cal blood flow to the skin and other organs. The decreased peripheral vascular resistance (resistance to blood flow) helps to decrease blood pressure.

## Sympathetic response?

The therapeutic effect of an alpha-adrenergic blocker depends on the sympathetic tone (the state of partial constriction of blood vessels) in the body before the drug is administered. For instance, when the drug is given with the patient lying down, only a small change in blood pressure occurs. In this position, the sympathetic nerves release very little norepinephrine.

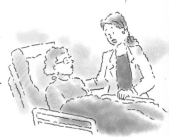

Alpha-adrenergic blockers cause a small change in blood pressure if you're lying down...

## Patient up, pressure down

On the other hand, when a patient stands up, norepinephrine is released to constrict the veins and shoot blood back up to the heart. If the patient receives an alpha-adrenergic blocker, however, the veins can't constrict and blood pools in the legs. Because blood return to the heart is reduced, blood pressure drops. This drop in blood pressure that occurs when a person stands up is called *orthostatic hypotension*.

## Pharmacotherapeutics

Because alpha-adrenergic blockers cause smooth muscles to relax and blood vessels to dilate, they increase local blood flow to the skin and other organs and reduce blood pressure. As a result, they're used to treat:
- benign prostatic hypertrophy
- hypertension
- peripheral vascular disorders (diseases of the blood vessels of the extremities), especially those in which blood vessel spasm causes poor local blood flow, such as Raynaud's disease (intermittent pallor, cyanosis, or redness of fingers), acrocyanosis (symmetrical mottled cyanosis of the hands and feet), and frostbite
- pheochromocytoma (a catecholamine-secreting tumor that causes severe hypertension).

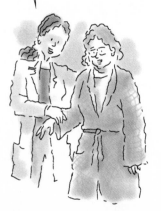

...when you stand, the drug prevents your veins from constricting.

## Drug interactions

Many drugs interact with alpha-adrenergic blockers, producing a synergistic, or exaggerated, effect. The most serious interactions are severe hypotension and vascular collapse.

These interactions can occur when these drugs are taken with ergoloid mesylates and ergotamine:
- Caffeine and macrolide antibiotics can increase the effects of ergotamine.
- Dopamine increases the pressor (rising blood pressure) effect.

**Warning!**

## Adverse reactions to alpha-adrenergic blockers

Most adverse reactions associated with alpha-adrenergic blockers are caused primarily by dilation of the blood vessels. They include:
• orthostatic hypotension or severe rebound hypertension
• bradycardia or tachycardia
• edema
• difficulty breathing
• light-headedness
• flushing
• arrhythmias
• angina
• heart attack
• spasm of blood vessels in the brain
• a shocklike state.

• Nitroglycerin can produce hypotension from excessive dilation of blood vessels.
• Sympathomimetics, including many over-the-counter drugs, can increase the stimulating effects on the heart, possibly resulting in hypotension with rebound hypertension. (See *Adverse reactions to alpha-adrenergic blockers*.)

# Beta-adrenergic blockers

*Beta-adrenergic blockers*, the most widely used adrenergic blockers, prevent stimulation of the sympathetic nervous system by inhibiting the action of catecholamines at beta-adrenergic receptors.

### From not so selective...

Beta-adrenergic blockers can be selective or nonselective. Nonselective beta-adrenergic blockers affect:
• beta$_1$ receptor sites (located mainly in the heart)
• beta$_2$ receptor sites (located in the bronchi, blood vessels, and uterus).

Nonselective beta-adrenergic blockers include carteolol, carvedilol, labetalol, levobunolol, metipranolol, penbutolol, pindolol, sotalol, nadolol, propranolol, and timolol. (Carvedilol and labetalol also block alpha$_1$ receptors.)

---

## ...to highly discriminating

Selective beta-adrenergic blockers primarily affect beta$_1$-adrenergic sites. They include acebutolol, atenolol, betaxolol, bisoprolol, esmolol, and metoprolol.

## The not so beta blockers

Some beta-adrenergic blockers, such as pindolol and acebutolol, have intrinsic sympathetic activity. This means that instead of attaching to beta receptors and blocking them, these beta-adrenergic blockers attach to beta receptors and stimulate them. These drugs are sometimes classified as *partial agonists*.

# Pharmacokinetics

Beta-adrenergic blockers are usually absorbed rapidly and well from the GI tract and are somewhat protein-bound. Food doesn't inhibit—and may even enhance—their absorption. Some beta-adrenergic blockers are absorbed more completely than others.

## Peak by I.V.

The onset of action of beta-adrenergic blockers is primarily dose- and drug-dependent. The time it takes to reach peak concentration levels depends on the administration route. Beta-adrenergic blockers given I.V. reach peak levels much more rapidly than those taken by mouth.

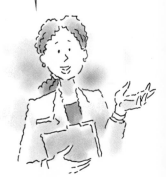

The onset and peak of beta-adrenergic blockers vary widely, depending on the administration route.

### Distribution

Beta-adrenergic blockers are distributed widely in body tissues, with the highest concentrations found in the:
- heart
- liver
- lungs
- saliva.

### Metabolism and excretion

Except for nadolol and atenolol, beta-adrenergic blockers are metabolized in the liver. They're excreted primarily in urine, either unchanged or as metabolites, but can also be excreted in feces, bile and, to some degree, breast milk.

# Pharmacodynamics

Beta-adrenergic blockers have widespread effects in the body because they produce their blocking action not only at adrenergic nerve endings but also in the adrenal medulla.

*Now I get it!*

## How beta-adrenergic blockers work

By occupying beta receptor sites, beta-adrenergic blockers prevent catecholamines (norepinephrine and epinephrine) from occupying these sites and exerting their stimulating effects. This illustration shows the effects of beta-adrenergic blockers on the heart, lungs, and blood vessels.

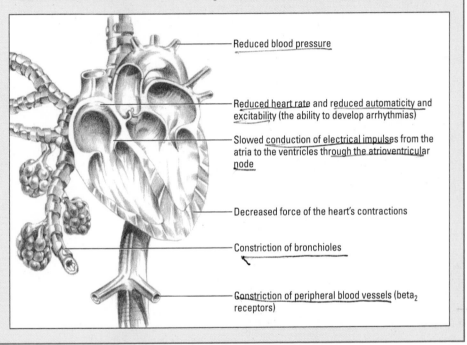

Reduced blood pressure

Reduced heart rate and reduced automaticity and excitability (the ability to develop arrhythmias)

Slowed conduction of electrical impulses from the atria to the ventricles through the atrioventricular node

Decreased force of the heart's contractions

Constriction of bronchioles

Constriction of peripheral blood vessels (beta$_2$ receptors)

## A matter of the heart

Effects on the heart include increased peripheral vascular resistance, decreased blood pressure, decreased force of the heart's contractions, decreased oxygen consumption by the heart, slowed impulse conduction between the atria and ventricles, and decreased cardiac output (the amount of blood the heart pumps each minute). (See *How beta-adrenergic blockers work.*)

## Selective and nonselective effects

Some beta-adrenergic blocker effects depend on whether the drug is classified as selective or nonselective.

Selective beta-adrenergic blockers, which prefer to block beta$_1$-receptor sites, reduce stimulation of the heart. They're often referred to as *cardioselective beta-adrenergic blockers.*

Nonselective beta-adrenergic blockers, which block both beta$_1$- and beta$_2$-receptor sites, not only reduce stimulation of the heart but also cause the bronchioles of the lungs to constrict. For instance, nonselective beta-adrenergic blockers can cause bronchospasm in patients with chronic obstructive lung disease. This adverse effect isn't seen when cardioselective drugs are given at lower doses.

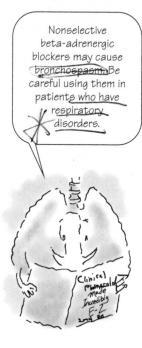

Nonselective beta-adrenergic blockers may cause bronchospasm. Be careful using them in patients who have respiratory disorders.

## Pharmacotherapeutics

Beta-adrenergic blockers are used to treat many conditions and are under investigation for use in many more. As mentioned previously, their clinical usefulness is based largely (but not exclusively) on how they affect the heart. (See *Are beta-adrenergic blockers underused in elderly patients?*)

### Helping the heart

Beta-adrenergic blockers can be prescribed after a heart attack to prevent another heart attack or to treat:
- angina
- heart failure
- hypertension
- cardiomyopathy (a disease of the heart muscle)
- supraventricular arrhythmias (irregular heartbeats that originate in the atria, SA node, or atrioventricular node).

*Yea or nay?*

## Are beta-adrenergic blockers underused in elderly patients?

Research has clearly shown that use of beta-adrenergic blockers after a heart attack reduces the risk of death and another heart attack. However, these drugs aren't being prescribed for elderly patients.

**Study findings**
One study found that only 34% of patients were prescribed a beta-adrenergic blocker after discharge from the hospital following a heart attack. Those least likely to receive a beta-adrenergic blocker included very sick patients, blacks, and the elderly.

**Why?**
The chief investigator of a study that looked at the use of beta-adrenergic blockers in the elderly believes that many doctors fear the adverse effects these drugs may produce in older patients. However, the study suggested that beta-adrenergic blockers are safe for elderly heart attack patients if the lowest effective dose of a selective beta-adrenergic blocker is prescribed.

## Jack of all trades

Beta-adrenergic blockers are also used to treat:
• anxiety
• cardiovascular symptoms associated with thyrotoxicosis (over-production of thyroid hormones)
• essential tremor
• migraine headaches
• open-angle glaucoma
• pheochromocytoma (tumor of the adrenal gland).

## Drug interactions

Many drugs can interact with beta-adrenergic blockers to cause potentially dangerous effects. Some of the most serious effects include cardiac or respiratory depression, arrhythmias, severe bronchospasm, and severe hypotension that can lead to vascular collapse. Other interactions can also occur:
• Increased effects or toxicity can occur when cimetidine, digoxin, or calcium channel blockers (primarily verapamil) are taken with beta-adrenergic blockers.
• Decreased effects can occur when rifampin, antacids, calcium salts, barbiturates, or anti-inflammatories, such as indomethacin and salicylates, are taken with beta-adrenergic blockers.
• Lidocaine toxicity may occur when lidocaine is taken with beta-adrenergic blockers.
• The requirements for insulin and oral antidiabetic drugs can be altered when these drugs are taken with beta-adrenergic blockers.
• The ability of theophylline to produce bronchodilation is impaired by nonselective beta-adrenergic blockers.
• Clonidine taken with a nonselective beta-adrenergic blocker can cause life-threatening hypertension during clonidine withdrawal.
• Sympathomimetics taken with nonselective beta-adrenergic blockers can cause hypertension and reflex bradycardia. (See *Adverse reactions to beta-adrenergic blockers.*)

*Warning!*

## Adverse reactions to beta-adrenergic blockers

Beta-adrenergic blockers generally cause few adverse reactions; those that do occur are drug- or dose-dependent and include:
• hypotension
• bradycardia
• peripheral vascular insufficiency
• atrioventricular block
• heart failure
• fatigue
• bronchospasm
• diarrhea or constipation
• nausea and vomiting
• abdominal discomfort
• anorexia
• flatulence
• rash
• fever with sore throat
• spasm of the larynx
• respiratory distress (allergic response).

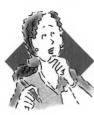

# Quick quiz

1.  During bethanechol therapy, which common adverse reactions should you expect to observe?
    A.  Dry mouth, flushed face, and constipation
    B.  Fasciculations, dysphagia, and respiratory distress
    C.  Nausea, vomiting, diarrhea, and intestinal cramps
    D.  Anorexia, cardiac arrhythmias, fatigue, and bronchospasm

*Answer:*   C. Bethanechol is a cholinergic agonist. Common adverse effects of cholinergic agonists include such GI symptoms as nausea, vomiting, diarrhea, and intestinal cramps.

**2.**    Catecholamines act as potent inotropes. That means that they:
    A.    cause the heart to contract forcefully.
    B.    slow the heart rate.
    C.    lower blood pressure.
    D.    decrease urinary output.

*Answer:*   A. Catecholamines cause the heart to contract forcefully, increasing the heart's workload. They also cause the heart to beat faster and raise blood pressure.

**3.**    Noncatecholamines can interact with monoamine oxidase inhibitors to cause:
    A.    arrhythmias.
    B.    severe hypertension.
    C.    seizures.
    D.    tachycardia.

*Answer:*   B. Noncatecholamines can interact very dangerously with monoamine oxidase inhibitors, causing severe hypertension and even death.

**4.**    Beta-adrenergic blockers have widespread effects because they produce their blocking action in the:
    A.    hypothalamus.
    B.    anterior pituitary gland.
    C.    pituitary gland.
    D.    adrenal medulla.

*Answer:*   D. Beta-adrenergic blockers have widespread effects in the body because they produce their blocking action not only at adrenergic nerve endings but also in the adrenal medulla.

## Scoring

✰✰✰   If you answered all four items correctly, fabulous! You're automatic with the autonomic nervous system.

✰✰   If you answered three items correctly, great! You've had nothing but positive interactions with these drugs.

✰   If you answered fewer than three items correctly, don't worry. Like the nervous system, you have a lot of information to coordinate. Just review the chapter and try again.

# Neurologic and neuromuscular drugs

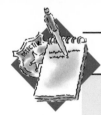

## Just the facts

In this chapter, you'll review:

♦ classes of drugs used to treat neurologic and neuromuscular disorders

♦ uses and varying actions of these drugs

♦ how these drugs are absorbed, distributed, metabolized, and excreted

♦ drug interactions and adverse effects of these drugs.

## Skeletal muscle relaxants

*Skeletal muscle relaxants* relieve musculoskeletal pain or spasm and severe musculoskeletal spasticity (stiff, awkward movements). They're used to treat acute, painful musculoskeletal conditions and the muscle spasticity associated with multiple sclerosis (MS) (a progressive demyelination of the white matter of the brain and spinal cord that causes widespread neurologic dysfunction), cerebral palsy (a motor function disorder caused by neurologic damage), stroke (reduced oxygen supply to the brain, resulting in neurologic deficits), and spinal cord injuries that can result in paralysis or death.

This chapter discusses the two main classes of skeletal muscle relaxants—*centrally acting* and *direct-acting*—as well as other muscle relaxants.

### Cycling problems

Exposure to severe cold, lack of blood flow to a muscle, or overexertion can send sensory impulses from the posterior sensory nerve fibers to the spinal cord and the higher levels of the central nervous system (CNS). These sensory impulses can cause a reflex (involuntary) muscle contraction or spasm from trauma, epilepsy, hypocalcemia (low calcium levels), or muscle disorders.

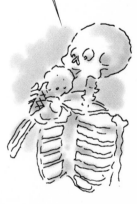

Ahhh. It's so nice to be able to relax!

The muscle contraction further stimulates the sensory receptors to a more intense contraction, establishing a cycle. Centrally acting muscle relaxants are believed to break this cycle by acting as CNS depressants.

# Centrally acting skeletal muscle relaxants

*Centrally acting skeletal muscle relaxants,* which act on the CNS, are used to treat acute spasms caused by such conditions as:
- anxiety
- inflammation
- pain
- trauma.

## For intermittent or chronic spasms

A patient with intermittent or chronic spasms may receive tizanidine.

## For acute spasms

A patient with acute muscle spasms may receive one of these drugs:
- carisoprodol
- chlorzoxazone
- cyclobenzaprine
- metaxalone
- methocarbamol
- orphenadrine
- tizanidine.

## Pharmacokinetics (how drugs circulate)

There's still a lot we don't know about how centrally acting skeletal muscle relaxants circulate within the body. In general, these drugs are absorbed from the GI tract, widely distributed in the body, metabolized in the liver, and excreted by the kidneys.

## Cyclobenzaprine sticks around

When these drugs are administered orally, it can take from 30 minutes to 1 hour for effects to be achieved. The duration of action of most of these drugs varies from 4 to 6 hours; cyclobenzaprine has the longest duration of action, at 12 to 25 hours.

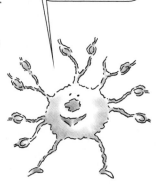

Spasticity can be caused by a cyclical pattern of impulses...

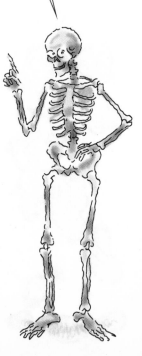

...and skeletal muscle relaxants help to break the pattern.

## Pharmacodynamics (how drugs act)

The centrally acting drugs don't relax skeletal muscles directly or depress neuronal conduction, neuromuscular transmission, or muscle excitability. Although their precise mechanism of action is unknown, these drugs are known to be CNS depressants. Their muscle relaxant effects may be related to their sedative effects.

## Pharmacotherapeutics (how drugs are used)

Patients receive centrally acting skeletal muscle relaxants to treat acute, painful musculoskeletal conditions. They're usually prescribed along with rest and physical therapy.

## Drug interactions

The centrally acting skeletal muscle relaxants interact with other CNS depressants (including alcohol, narcotics, barbiturates, anticonvulsants, tricyclic antidepressants, kava kava, and antianxiety drugs), causing increased sedation, impaired motor function, and respiratory depression. In addition, some of these drugs have other interactions:
• Cyclobenzaprine interacts with monoamine oxidase inhibitors (MAOIs) and can result in a high body temperature, excitation, and seizures.
• Cyclobenzaprine can decrease the antihypertensive effects of the blood pressure–lowering drugs guanethidine and clonidine.
• Orphenadrine and cyclobenzaprine sometimes enhance the effects of cholinergic-blocking drugs.
• Methocarbamol can antagonize the cholinergic effects of the anticholinesterase drugs used to treat myasthenia gravis.
• Orphenadrine can reduce the effects of phenothiazines.
• Orphenadrine and propoxyphene taken together can cause additive CNS effects, including mental confusion, anxiety, and tremors. (See *Adverse reactions to centrally acting skeletal muscle relaxants*, page 52.)
• Tizanidine combined with diuretics, central alpha-adrenergic agonists, or antihypertensives may increase hypotensive drug effects. Concurrent use of tizanidine with CNS depressants may cause additive CNS depression. Hormonal contraceptives may reduce the clearance of tizanidine, necessitating a dosage reduction.

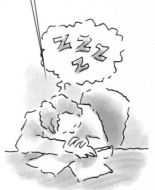

Centrally acting skeletal muscle relaxants (and plenty of rest) are used to treat painful musculoskeletal conditions.

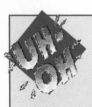

## Adverse reactions to centrally acting skeletal muscle relaxants

A patient can develop physical and psychological dependence after long-term use of these drugs. Abruptly stopping any of these drugs can cause severe withdrawal symptoms. Other adverse reactions can also occur.

**Common reactions**
- Dizziness
- Drowsiness

**Occasional reactions**
- Abdominal distress

- Ataxia
- Constipation
- Diarrhea
- Heartburn
- Nausea and vomiting

**Severe reactions**
- Allergic reactions
- Arrhythmias
- Bradycardia

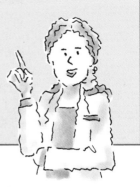

# Direct-acting skeletal muscle relaxants

*Dantrolene* is the most common direct-acting skeletal muscle relaxant. Although dantrolene has a similar therapeutic effect to the centrally acting drugs, it works through a different mechanism of action. Because its major effect is on the muscles, dantrolene has a lower incidence of adverse CNS effects; high therapeutic doses, however, are toxic to the liver.

Common adverse effects of dantrolene include drowsiness, dizziness, malaise, fatigue, and weakness. More serious adverse effects include seizures and hepatitis. (See *Dantrolene.*)

## In the head

Dantrolene seems most effective for spasticity of cerebral origin. Because it produces muscle weakness, dantrolene is of questionable benefit in patients with borderline strength.

## Pharmacokinetics

Although the peak drug concentration of dantrolene usually occurs within about 5 hours after it's ingested, the patient may not notice the therapeutic benefit for a week or more.

### Absorption

Dantrolene is absorbed poorly from the GI tract and is highly plasma protein–bound. This means that only a small portion of the drug is available to produce a therapeutic effect.

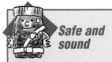

**Safe and sound**

## Dantrolene

Because of the risk of liver damage with long-term use of dantrolene, baseline liver function tests should be obtained and therapy should be discontinued if benefits aren't seen in 45 days.

### Metabolism and excretion

Dantrolene is metabolized by the liver and excreted in urine. Its elimination half-life in healthy adults is about 9 hours. Because dantrolene is metabolized in the liver, its half-life may be prolonged in patients with impaired liver function.

## Pharmacodynamics

Dantrolene is chemically and pharmacologically unrelated to the other skeletal muscle relaxants.

Dantrolene works by acting on the muscle itself. It interferes with calcium ion release from the sarcoplasmic reticulum and weakens the force of contractions. At therapeutic concentrations, dantrolene has little effect on cardiac or intestinal smooth muscle.

## Pharmacotherapeutics

Dantrolene helps manage all types of spasticity but is most effective in patients with:
- cerebral palsy
- MS
- spinal cord injury
- stroke.

Dantrolene is also used to treat and prevent malignant hyperthermia. This rare but potentially fatal complication of anesthesia is characterized by skeletal muscle rigidity and high fever. (See *How dantrolene reduces muscle rigidity*.)

## Drug interactions

- CNS depressants can increase the depressive effects of dantrolene, resulting in sedation, lack of coordination, and respiratory depression.
- Estrogens, when given with dantrolene, can increase the risk of liver toxicity.
- I.V. verapamil, when given with dantrolene, may result in cardiovascular collapse; these drugs shouldn't be administered concurrently.
- Alcohol may increase CNS depression when given with dantrolene.
- Sun exposure may cause photosensitivity.

**Now I get it!**

## How dantrolene reduces muscle rigidity

Dantrolene appears to decrease the number of calcium ions released from the sarcoplasmic reticulum (a structure in muscle cells that plays a role in muscle contraction and relaxation by releasing and storing calcium). The lower the calcium level in the muscle plasma or myoplasm, the less energy produced when calcium prompts the muscle's actin and myosin filaments (responsible for muscle contraction) to interact. Less energy means a weaker muscle contraction.

**Reducing rigidity, halting hyperthermia**

By promoting muscle relaxation, dantrolene prevents or reduces the rigidity that contributes to the life-threatening body temperatures of malignant hyperthermia.

# Other skeletal muscle relaxants

Two other drugs used as skeletal muscle relaxants are baclofen and diazepam. Diazepam, however, is primarily an antianxiety drug. (See *Diazepam as a skeletal muscle relaxant*, page 54.)

## Diazepam as a skeletal muscle relaxant

Diazepam is a benzodiazepine drug that's used to treat acute muscle spasms as well as spasticity caused by chronic disorders. Other uses of diazepam include treating anxiety, alcohol withdrawal, and seizures. It seems to work by promoting the inhibitory effect of the neurotransmitter gamma-aminobutyric acid on muscle contraction.

### The negatives: Sedation and tolerance

Diazepam can be used alone or with other drugs to treat spasticity, especially in patients with spinal cord lesions and, occasionally, in patients with cerebral palsy. It's also helpful in patients with painful, continuous muscle spasms who aren't too susceptible to the drug's sedative effects. Unfortunately, diazepam's use is limited by its central nervous system effects and the tolerance that develops with prolonged use.

## Pharmacokinetics

Baclofen and diazepam are absorbed rapidly from the GI tract. Baclofen is distributed widely (with only small amounts crossing the blood-brain barrier), undergoes minimal liver metabolism, and is excreted primarily unchanged in urine.

Diazepam is metabolized in the liver and mostly excreted in the urine, with a small amount excreted in the feces.

### Slow to a stop

It can take from hours to weeks before the patient notices the beneficial effects of baclofen. The elimination half-life of baclofen is 2½ to 4 hours. Abrupt withdrawal of the drug can cause hallucinations, seizures, and worsening of spasticity.

## Pharmacodynamics

It isn't known exactly how baclofen or diazepam works. Diazepam probably depresses the CNS at the limbic and subcortical levels of the brain. It suppresses the spread of seizure activity in the cortex, thalamus, and limbic areas.

Baclofen is chemically similar to the neurotransmitter gamma-aminobutyric acid (GABA) and probably acts in the spinal cord. It reduces nerve impulses from the spinal cord to skeletal muscle, decreasing the number and severity of muscle spasms and reducing associated pain.

### A choice drug

Because baclofen produces less sedation than diazepam and less peripheral muscle weakness than dantrolene, it's the drug of choice to treat spasticity.

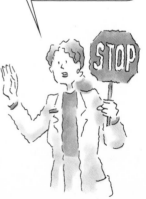

Stopping baclofen treatment abruptly could result in seizures!

## Pharmacotherapeutics

Baclofen's primary clinical use is for paraplegic or quadriplegic patients with spinal cord lesions, most commonly caused by MS or trauma. For these patients, baclofen significantly reduces the number and severity of painful flexor spasms. However, it doesn't improve stiff gait, manual dexterity, or residual muscle function.

Baclofen may be administered intrathecally for patients who are unresponsive to oral baclofen or who experience intolerable adverse reactions. After a positive response to a bolus dose, an implantable port for chronic therapy is inserted.

Diazepam relieves anxiety, muscle spasms, and seizures, and it induces calmness and sleep.

## Drug interactions

Baclofen has few drug interactions:
• The most significant drug interaction is an increase in CNS depression when baclofen is administered with other CNS depressants, including alcohol.
• Analgesia can be prolonged when fentanyl and baclofen are administered together.
• Lithium carbonate and baclofen taken together can aggravate hyperkinesia (an abnormal increase in motor function or activity).
• Tricyclic antidepressants and baclofen taken together can increase muscle relaxation.
• Baclofen may increase blood glucose levels, resulting in the need for increased doses of oral antidiabetic agents and insulin.

Intrathecal baclofen shouldn't be discontinued abruptly because doing so has resulted in high fever, altered mental status, exaggerated rebound spasticity, and muscle rigidity that, in rare cases, has progressed to rhabdomyolysis, multiple organ system failure, and death. (See *Adverse reactions to baclofen*.)

**Warning!**

## Adverse reactions to baclofen

**Most common**
• Transient drowsiness

**Less common**
• Nausea
• Fatigue
• Vertigo
• Hypotonia
• Muscle weakness
• Depression
• Headache

# Neuromuscular blocking drugs

*Neuromuscular blocking drugs* relax skeletal muscles by disrupting the transmission of nerve impulses at the motor end plate (the branching terminals of a motor nerve axon). (See *Motor end plate*, page 56.)

Neuromuscular blockers have three major clinical indications:

   to relax skeletal muscles during surgery

   to reduce the intensity of muscle spasms in drug- or electrically induced seizures

**Now I get it!**

## Motor end plate

The motor nerve axon divides to form branching terminals called *motor end plates*. These are enfolded in muscle fibers, but separated from the fibers by the synaptic cleft.

**Competing with contraction**

A stimulus to the nerve causes the release of acetylcholine into the synaptic cleft. There, acetylcholine occupies receptor sites on the muscle cell membrane, depolarizing the membrane and causing muscle contraction. Neuromuscular blocking agents act at the motor end plate by competing with acetylcholine for the receptor sites or by blocking depolarization.

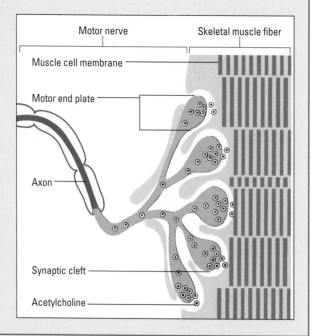

to manage patients who are fighting the use of a ventilator to help with breathing.

## Two main classifications

There are two main classes of natural and synthetic drugs used as neuromuscular blockers—nondepolarizing and depolarizing.

# Nondepolarizing blocking drugs

*Nondepolarizing blocking drugs*, also called *competitive* or *stabilizing drugs*, are derived from curare alkaloids and synthetically similar compounds. They include:
- atracurium
- cisatracurium
- pancuronium
- rocuronium
- vecuronium.

## Pharmacokinetics

Because nondepolarizing blockers are absorbed poorly from the GI tract, they're administered parenterally. The I.V. route is preferred because the action is more predictable.

### Distribution

These drugs are distributed rapidly throughout the body.

### Metabolism and excretion

A variable but large proportion of the nondepolarizing drugs is excreted unchanged in urine. Some drugs, such as atracurium, pancuronium, and vecuronium, are partially metabolized in the liver.

## Pharmacodynamics

Nondepolarizing blockers compete with acetylcholine at the cholinergic receptor sites of the skeletal muscle membrane. This blocks acetylcholine's neurotransmitter action, preventing the muscle from contracting.

The effect can be counteracted by anticholinesterase drugs, such as neostigmine and pyridostigmine, which inhibit the action of acetylcholinesterase, the enzyme that destroys acetylcholine.

### From weakness to paralysis

The initial muscle weakness produced by these drugs quickly changes to a flaccid (loss of muscle tone) paralysis that affects the muscles in a specific sequence. The first muscles to exhibit flaccid paralysis are those of the eyes, face, and neck. Next, the limb, abdomen, and trunk muscles become flaccid. Lastly, the intercostal muscles (between the ribs) and diaphragm (the breathing muscle) are paralyzed. Recovery from the paralysis usually occurs in the reverse order.

### Conscious and aware

Because these drugs don't cross the blood-brain barrier, the patient remains conscious and can feel pain. Even though the patient is paralyzed, he's aware of what's happening to him and can experience extreme anxiety but can't communicate his feelings. For this reason, an analgesic or antianxiety drug should be administered along with a neuromuscular blocker. (See *Using a neuromuscular blocker safely*.)

> Paralysis from neuromuscular blocking drugs proceeds in a specific sequence. Recovery is all about reverse!

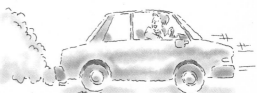

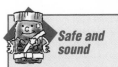

**Safe and sound**

## Using a neuromuscular blocker safely

When using a neuromuscular blocker, remember these important points to keep the patient safe:

• Emergency respiratory support equipment (endotracheal equipment, ventilator, oxygen, atropine, edrophonium, epinephrine, and neostigmine) should be immediately available.

• Drug-induced neuromuscular blockade may be reversed with an anticholinesterase (such as neostigmine or edrophonium), which is usually given with an anticholinergic, such as atropine.

• Sedatives or general anesthetics should be administered before neuromuscular blockers.

## Pharmacotherapeutics

Nondepolarizing blockers are used for intermediate or prolonged muscle relaxation to:
- ease the passage of an endotracheal (ET) tube
- decrease the amount of anesthetic required during surgery
- facilitate realignment of broken bones and dislocated joints
- paralyze patients who need ventilatory support but who fight the ET tube and ventilation
- prevent muscle injury during electroconvulsive therapy (ECT) (passing an electric current through the brain to treat depression) by reducing the intensity of muscle spasms.

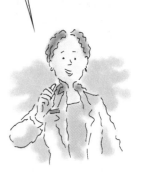

Remember: the effect of these drugs can be frightening for the patient.

## Drug interactions

These drugs alter the effects of nondepolarizing neuromuscular blockers:
- Aminoglycoside antibiotics and anesthetics potentiate or exaggerate the neuromuscular blockade.
- Drugs that alter the serum levels of the electrolytes calcium, magnesium, or potassium also alter the effects of the nondepolarizing blockers.
- The anticholinesterases (neostigmine, pyridostigmine, and edrophonium) antagonize nondepolarizing blockers and are used as antidotes to them.
- Drugs that can increase the intensity and duration of paralysis when taken with a nondepolarizing blocker include inhalation anesthetics, aminoglycosides, clindamycin, polymyxin, verapamil, quinine derivatives, ketamine, lithium, nitrates, thiazide diuretics, tetracyclines, and magnesium salts.
- Drugs that can cause decreased neuromuscular blockade when taken with a nondepolarizing blocker include carbamazepine, hydantoins, ranitidine, and theophylline. (See *Adverse reactions to nondepolarizing blockers.*)
- Concurrent use of corticosteroids may result in prolonged muscle weakness.

# Depolarizing blocking drugs

*Succinylcholine* is the only therapeutic depolarizing blocking drug. Although it's similar to the nondepolarizing blockers in its therapeutic effect, its mechanism of action differs. Succinylcholine acts like acetylcholine, but it isn't inactivated by cholinesterase. It's the drug of choice when short-term muscle relaxation is needed.

*Warning!*

## Adverse reactions to nondepolarizing blockers

**To all drugs in this class**
- Apnea
- Hypotension
- Skin reactions
- Bronchospasm
- Excessive bronchial and salivary secretions

**To pancuronium**
- Tachycardia
- Cardiac arrhythmias
- Hypertension

## Pharmacokinetics

Because succinylcholine is absorbed poorly from the GI tract, the preferred administration route is I.V.; the I.M. route can be used, if necessary.

### Metabolism and excretion

Succinylcholine is hydrolyzed in the liver and plasma by the enzyme pseudocholinesterase, producing a metabolite with a nondepolarizing blocking action. Succinylcholine is excreted by the kidneys, with a small amount excreted unchanged.

## Pharmacodynamics

After administration, succinylcholine is rapidly metabolized, but at a slower rate than acetylcholine. As a result, succinylcholine remains attached to receptor sites on the skeletal muscle membrane for a longer period of time. This prevents repolarization of the motor end plate and results in muscle paralysis.

## Pharmacotherapeutics

Succinylcholine is the drug of choice for short-term muscle relaxation, such as during intubation and ECT.

## Drug interactions

The action of succinylcholine is potentiated by a number of anesthetics and antibiotics. In contrast to their interaction with nondepolarizing blockers, anticholinesterases increase succinylcholine blockade. (See *Adverse reactions to succinylcholine*.)

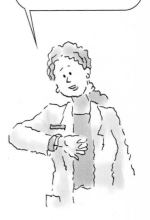

Because succinylcholine is administered I.V. or I.M., it has a very fast onset.

# Antiparkinsonian drugs

Drug therapy is an important part of the treatment for Parkinson's disease, a progressive neurologic disorder characterized by four cardinal features:
- muscle rigidity (inflexibility)
- akinesia (loss of muscle movement)
- tremors at rest
- disturbances of posture and balance.

## A defect in the dopamine pathway...

Parkinson's disease affects the extrapyramidal system, which influences movement. The extrapyramidal system includes the corpus striatum, globus pallidus, and substantia nigra of the brain.

---

**Warning!**

## Adverse reactions to succinylcholine

The primary adverse drug reactions to succinylcholine are:
- prolonged apnea
- hypotension.

### Genetics increases the risk

The risks associated with succinylcholine increase with certain genetic predispositions, such as a low pseudocholinesterase level and the tendency to develop malignant hyperthermia.

In Parkinson's disease, a dopamine deficiency occurs in the basal ganglia, the dopamine-releasing pathway that connects the substantia nigra to the corpus striatum.

## ...causes an imbalance of neurotransmitters

Reduction of dopamine in the corpus striatum upsets the normal balance between two neurotransmitters, acetylcholine and dopamine. This results in a relative excess of acetylcholine. The excessive excitation caused by cholinergic activity creates the movement disorders that characterize Parkinson's disease.

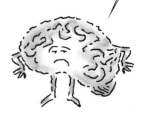

A deficiency of dopamine isn't good news... it prevents me from performing normally.

## Other causes

Parkinson's disease can also result from drugs, encephalitis, neurotoxins, trauma, arteriosclerosis, or other neurologic disorders and environmental factors.

## Goals of drug therapy

The goals of drug therapy are to provide relief of symptoms and to maintain the patient's independence and mobility.

Drug therapy for Parkinson's disease is aimed at correcting the imbalance of neurotransmitters by:
• inhibiting cholinergic effects (with anticholinergic drugs)
• enhancing the effects of dopamine (with dopaminergic drugs).

# Anticholinergic drugs

*Anticholinergic drugs* are sometimes called *parasympatholytic drugs* because they inhibit the action of acetylcholine at special receptors in the parasympathetic nervous system.

## Two classes

Anticholinergics used to treat Parkinson's disease are classified in two chemical categories according to their chemical structure:
• synthetic tertiary amines, such as benztropine, biperiden hydrochloride, biperiden lactate, procyclidine, and trihexyphenidyl
• antihistamines (such as diphenhydramine) that have anticholinergic properties, which are effective in treating the symptoms of Parkinson's disease.

### Pharmacokinetics

Typically, anticholinergic drugs are well absorbed from the GI tract and cross the blood-brain barrier to their action site in the brain. Most are metabolized in the liver, at least partially, and are excreted by the kidneys as metabolites and unchanged drug. The exact distribution of these drugs is unknown.

## Up to 24 hours

Benztropine is a long-acting drug with a duration of up to 24 hours in some patients. For most anticholinergics, half-life is undetermined. In addition to the oral route, some anticholinergics can also be given I.M. or I.V.

## Pharmacodynamics

High acetylcholine levels produce an excitatory effect on the CNS, which can cause a parkinsonian tremor. Patients with Parkinson's disease take anticholinergic drugs to inhibit the action of acetylcholine at receptor sites in the CNS and autonomic nervous system, thus reducing the tremor.

## Pharmacotherapeutics

Anticholinergics are used to treat all forms of Parkinson's disease. They're used most commonly in the early stages of Parkinson's disease when symptoms are mild and don't have a major impact on the patient's lifestyle. These drugs effectively control sialorrhea (excessive flow of saliva) and are about 20% effective in reducing the incidence and severity of akinesia and rigidity.

## Together or alone

Anticholinergics can be used alone or with amantadine in the early stages of Parkinson's disease. In addition, anticholinergics can be given with levodopa during the later stages to further relieve symptoms.

## Drug interactions

Interactions can occur when certain medications are taken with anticholinergics:
• Amantadine can cause increased anticholinergic adverse effects.
• Absorption of levodopa can be decreased, which could lead to worsening of parkinsonian signs and symptoms.
• Antipsychotics taken with anticholinergics (such as phenothiazines, thiothixene, haloperidol, and loxapine) decrease the effectiveness of both anticholinergics and antipsychotics. The incidence of anticholinergic adverse effects can also be increased.
• Over-the-counter cough or cold preparations, diet aids, and analeptics (drugs used to stay awake) increase anticholinergic effects.
• Alcohol increases CNS depression. (See *Adverse reactions to anticholinergics*, page 62.)

Anticholinergic drugs can be used to treat Parkinson's disease.

**Warning!**

## Adverse reactions to anticholinergics

Mild, dose-related adverse reactions are seen in 30% to 50% of patients who take anticholinergics. Dry mouth may be a dose-related reaction to trihexyphenidyl.

**Common reactions**
- Confusion
- Restlessness
- Agitation and excitement
- Drowsiness or insomnia
- Tachycardia and palpitations
- Constipation

- Nausea and vomiting
- Urine retention
- Increased intraocular pressure, blurred vision, pupil dilation, and photophobia

**Sensitivity-related reactions**
- Hives
- Allergic rash

**Reactions in patients older than age 60**
- Increased sensitivity to anticholinergics, resulting in confusion, agitation, hallucinations, and possibly psychotic symptoms

# Dopaminergic drugs

*Dopaminergic drugs* include several drugs that are chemically unrelated:
- levodopa, the metabolic precursor to dopamine
- carbidopa-levodopa, a combination drug composed of carbidopa and levodopa
- amantadine, an antiviral drug with dopaminergic activity
- bromocriptine, an ergot-type dopamine agonist
- ropinirole and pramipexole, two non-ergot-type dopamine agonists
- selegiline and rasagiline, type B MAOIs.

## Pharmacokinetics

Like anticholinergic drugs, dopaminergic drugs are absorbed from the GI tract into the bloodstream and are delivered to their action site in the brain.

### Slowing down with food

Absorption of levodopa is slowed and reduced when it's ingested with food. The body absorbs most levodopa, carbidopa-levodopa, pramipexole, or amantadine from the GI tract after oral administration, but only about 28% of bromocriptine. About 73% of an oral dose of selegiline is absorbed. Rasagiline is rapidly absorbed into the bloodstream.

### Distribution

Levodopa is widely distributed in body tissues, including the GI tract, liver, pancreas, kidneys, salivary glands, and skin. Carbidopa-levodopa and pramipexole are also widely distributed. Amantadine is distributed in saliva, nasal secretions, and breast milk. Bromocriptine and rasagiline are highly protein-bound. The distribution of selegiline is unknown.

### Metabolism and excretion

Dopaminergic drugs are metabolized extensively in various areas of the body and eliminated by the liver, the kidneys, or both.
• Large amounts of levodopa are metabolized in the stomach and during the first pass through the liver. The drug is metabolized extensively to various compounds that are excreted by the kidneys.
• Carbidopa isn't metabolized extensively. The kidneys excrete approximately one-third of it as unchanged drug within 24 hours.
• Amantadine, ropinirole, and pramipexole are excreted mostly unchanged by the kidneys.
• Almost all of a bromocriptine or rasagiline dose is metabolized by the liver to pharmacologically inactive compounds, which are then eliminated primarily in feces, with only a small amount excreted in urine.
• Selegiline is metabolized to L-amphetamine, L-methamphetamine, and N-desmethyldeprenyl (the major metabolite), which are eliminated in urine.

Absorption of levodopa is slowed and reduced when taken with food.

## Pharmacodynamics

Dopaminergic drugs act in the brain to improve motor function in one of two ways: by increasing the dopamine concentration or by enhancing neurotransmission of dopamine.

### Getting the job done

Levodopa is inactive until it crosses the blood-brain barrier and is converted to dopamine by enzymes in the brain, increasing dopamine concentrations in the basal ganglia. Carbidopa enhances levodopa's effectiveness by blocking the peripheral conversion of levodopa, thus permitting increased amounts of levodopa to be transported to the brain.

The other dopaminergic drugs have various mechanisms of action:
• Amantadine's mechanism of action isn't clear. It's thought to release dopamine from intact neurons, but it may also have non-dopaminergic mechanisms.

- Bromocriptine, ropinirole, and pramipexole stimulate dopamine receptors in the brain, producing effects that are similar to dopamine's.
- Rasagiline has an unknown mechanism of action.
- Selegiline can increase dopaminergic activity by inhibiting type B MAO activity or by other mechanisms.

## Pharmacotherapeutics

The choice of therapy is highly individualized, depending on the patient's symptoms and extent of disability. Patients with mild Parkinson's disease whose main symptom is a tremor are commonly given anticholinergics or amantadine. Selegiline is indicated for extending the duration of levodopa by blocking its breakdown; it has also been used in the early stages of Parkinson's disease because of its neuroprotective properties and potential to slow the progression of the disease.

Dopaminergic drugs are usually used to treat patients with severe Parkinson's disease or those who don't respond to anticholinergics alone. Levodopa is the most effective drug used to treat Parkinson's disease; however, it loses its effectiveness after 3 to 5 years. (See *Levodopa: Pros and cons*.)

*Yea or nay?*

## Levodopa: Pros and cons

Levodopa is commonly used to treat Parkinson's disease; however, its use isn't without controversy. Initially, levodopa is very effective in controlling symptoms. But after several years, the effects of the drug sometimes don't last as long (the wearing-off effect) or lead to sharp fluctuations in symptoms (the on-off phenomenon).

### Early vs. late start
Some doctors feel that levodopa should be started early (when the diagnosis is made) in low doses. Others believe it should be started later in the course of the disease (when symptoms compromise function). Advocates of an early start believe that fluctuations in the patient's response to levodopa stem from the progression of Parkinson's disease and not from the effects of levodopa.

Some doctors are concerned that levodopa accelerates the progression of Parkinson's disease by providing a source of free radicals that contribute to the degeneration of dopaminergic neurons.

## Flurry of fluctuations

When the patient's response to levodopa fluctuates, dosage adjustments and increased frequency of administration may be tried. Alternatively, adjunctive therapy, such as dopamine agonists, selegiline, amantadine, or catechol-O-methyltransferase (COMT) inhibitors, may be added. Controlled-release forms of carbidopa-levodopa may be helpful in managing the wearing-off effect (when levodopa's effects don't last as long as they used to) or delayed-onset motor fluctuations.

## Add carbidopa, reduce levodopa

Levodopa is almost always combined with carbidopa as the standard therapy for Parkinson's disease. When these drugs are given together, the dosage of levodopa can be reduced, decreasing the risk of GI and cardiovascular adverse effects.

## Tapered treatment

The dosage of some dopaminergic drugs, such as amantadine, levodopa, pramipexole, and bromocriptine, must be gradually tapered to avoid precipitating parkinsonian crisis (sudden marked clinical deterioration) and possibly life-threatening complications, including muscle rigidity, elevated body temperature, tachycardia, mental changes, and increased serum creatine kinase (resembling neuroleptic malignant syndrome).

## Drug interactions

There are a number of drug interactions related to dopaminergic drugs, including some that are potentially fatal.
• Levodopa's effectiveness may be reduced when used concurrently with pyridoxine (vitamin $B_6$), phenytoin, benzodiazepines, reserpine, or papaverine.
• MAOIs such as tranylcypromine increase the risk of hypertensive crisis.
• Antipsychotics, such as phenothiazines, thiothixene, haloperidol, and loxapine, can reduce the effectiveness of levodopa.
• Amantadine may potentiate the anticholinergic adverse effects, such as confusion and hallucinations, of anticholinergic drugs and reduce the absorption of levodopa.
• Meperidine taken with selegiline at a higher-than-recommended dose can cause a fatal reaction. (See *Adverse reactions to dopaminergic drugs*, page 66.)

In some patients, levodopa can produce a significant interaction with foods. Dietary amino acids can decrease levodopa's effectiveness by competing with it for absorption from the intestine and slowing its transport to the brain.

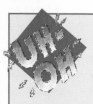

**Warning!**

## Adverse reactions to dopaminergic drugs

**Levodopa**
- Nausea and vomiting
- Orthostatic hypotension
- Anorexia
- Neuroleptic malignant syndrome
- Arrhythmias
- Irritability
- Confusion

**Amantadine**
- Orthostatic hypotension
- Constipation

**Bromocriptine**
- Persistent orthostatic hypotension
- Ventricular tachycardia
- Bradycardia
- Worsening angina

**Rasagiline**
- Hypertensive crisis (if taken with tyramine-containing foods)
- Hallucinations
- Flu syndrome
- Arthralgia
- Depression

**Pramipexole, ropinirole**
- Orthostatic hypotension
- Dizziness
- Confusion
- Insomnia

# COMT inhibitors

COMT inhibitors are used as adjuncts to levodopa-carbidopa therapy in managing patients with Parkinson's disease who experience the wearing-off effect at the end of a dosing interval.

Currently two COMT inhibitors are available:

 tolcapone

 entacapone.

## Pharmacokinetics

Tolcapone and entacapone are rapidly absorbed in the GI tract and have an absolute bioavailability of 65% and 35%, respectively. Both drugs are highly bound to albumin and therefore have limited distribution to the tissues. They're almost completely metabolized in the liver to inactive metabolites and are excreted in urine.

## Pharmacodynamics

Tolcapone and entacapone are selective and reversible inhibitors of COMT, the major metabolizing enzyme for levodopa, in the presence of a decarboxylase inhibitor such as carbidopa. Inhibition of COMT alters the pharmacokinetics of levodopa, leading to sustained plasma levels of this drug. This results in more sustained dopaminergic stimulation in the brain and improvement in signs and symptoms of Parkinson's disease.

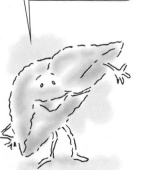

My job is to almost completely metabolize COMT inhibitors. Work, work, work!

## Pharmacotherapeutics

Either tolcapone or entacapone may be added to the carbidopa-levodopa regimen of a patient who experiences wearing-off symptoms at the end of a dosing interval or random "on-off" fluctuations in response to carbidopa-levodopa. COMT inhibitors have no antiparkinsonian effect when used alone and should always be combined with carbidopa-levodopa. The addition of a COMT inhibitor often requires a decrease in the carbidopa-levodopa dosage, particularly for patients receiving a levodopa dose of more than 800 mg.

### Slow and steady

Rapid withdrawal of a COMT inhibitor may lead to parkinsonian crisis and may cause a syndrome of muscle rigidity, high fever, tachycardia, elevated serum creatine kinase, and confusion similar to neuroleptic malignant syndrome. Although tapering schedules haven't been evaluated, a slow tapering of the dosage is suggested.

## Drug interactions

• COMT inhibitors shouldn't be used concurrently with Type A MAOIs but may be used with selegiline.
• Because of MAO inhibition, COMT inhibitors shouldn't be used with linezolid.
• Significant cardiac effects or arrhythmias may result when COMT inhibitors are combined with catecholamine drugs (dopamine, dobutamine, epinephrine, methyldopa, or norepinephrine).
• Use of COMT inhibitors with CNS depressants (benzodiazepines, tricyclic antidepressants, antipsychotics, ethanol, opioid analgesics, and other sedative hypnotics) may cause additive CNS effects.
• Concurrent use of entacapone and bromocriptine may cause fibrotic complications.

### Calling an interference

• Drugs that interfere with glucuronidation (erythromycin, rifampin, cholestyramine, and probenecid) may decrease entacapone elimination.
• Use of COMT inhibitors may increase the risk of orthostatic hypotension in patients receiving dopaminergic therapy.
• Tolcapone shouldn't be initiated in patients with evidence of liver disease or alanine aminotransferase or aspartate aminotransferase values greater than the upper limit of normal. In addition, the patient must be advised of the risks of liver injury and must

**Warning!**

## Adverse reactions to COMT inhibitors

Catechol-O-methyltransferase (COMT) inhibitors may produce acute liver failure, a life-threatening adverse reaction. Consequently, tolcapone should be used only in patients with Parkinson's disease who are experiencing fluctuations in levodopa response and aren't responding to—or aren't appropriate candidates for—other adjunctive therapies. Patients should be advised of the risks of liver injury and provide written informed consent before starting tolcapone.

Liver function tests should be obtained at the start of therapy to provide a baseline and every 2 weeks for the first year of therapy, then every 4 weeks for the next 3 months, and every 8 weeks thereafter.

COMT inhibitors can also produce these adverse reactions.

**Common reactions**
- Nausea
- Dyskinesia
- Diarrhea
- Brown-orange urine discoloration (entacapone)
- Hyperkinesia or hypokinesia

**Less common reactions**
- Orthostatic hypotension
- Syncope
- Dizziness
- Fatigue
- Abdominal pain
- Constipation
- Vomiting
- Dry mouth
- Back pain
- Diaphoresis

give written informed consent before receiving tolcapone. (See *Adverse reactions to COMT inhibitors.*)

# Anticonvulsant drugs

*Anticonvulsant drugs* inhibit neuromuscular transmission and are prescribed for:
- long-term management of chronic epilepsy (recurrent seizures)
- short-term management of acute isolated seizures not caused by epilepsy, such as those occurring after trauma or brain surgery.

In addition, some anticonvulsants are used in the emergency treatment of status epilepticus (a continuous seizure state).

Treatment of epilepsy should begin with a single drug whose dosage is increased until seizures are controlled or adverse reactions become problematic. Generally, a second alternative should be tried as monotherapy before combination therapy is considered. The choice of drug treatment depends on seizure type, drug characteristics, and patient preferences.

## Major classes

Anticonvulsants fall into several major classes:
- hydantoins

- barbiturates
- iminostilbenes
- benzodiazepines
- carboxylic acid derivatives
- 1-(aminomethyl) cyclohexane–acetic acid
- phenyltriazines
- carboxamides
- sulfamate-substituted monosaccharides
- succinimides
- sulfonamides
- pyrrolidines.

# Hydantoins

The two most commonly prescribed anticonvulsants—phenytoin and phenytoin sodium—belong to the *hydantoin* class. Other hydantoins include fosphenytoin and ethotoin.

## Pharmacokinetics

The pharmacokinetics of hydantoins vary from drug to drug.

### Phenytoin fits in slowly

Phenytoin is absorbed slowly after both oral and I.M. administration. It's distributed rapidly to all tissues and is highly (90%) protein-bound. Phenytoin is metabolized in the liver. Inactive metabolites are excreted in bile and then reabsorbed from the GI tract. Eventually, however, they're excreted in urine.

### Fosphenytoin for the short term

Fosphenytoin is indicated for short-term I.M. or I.V. administration. It's widely distributed throughout the body and is highly (90%) protein-bound. Fosphenytoin is metabolized by the liver and excreted in urine.

### Talkin' ethotoin

Ethotoin is readily absorbed from the GI tract and is metabolized by the liver. Extensively protein-bound, ethotoin is excreted in urine, primarily as metabolites.

## Pharmacodynamics

In most cases, the hydantoin anticonvulsants stabilize nerve cells to keep them from getting overexcited. Phenytoin appears to work in the motor cortex of the brain, where it stops the spread of seizure activity. The pharmacodynamics of fosphenytoin and ethotoin are thought to mimic those of phenytoin. Phenytoin may also

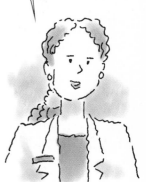

The most commonly prescribed anticonvulsant drugs are phenytoin and phenytoin sodium.

be used as an antiarrhythmic drug to control irregular heart rhythms, with properties similar to those of quinidine or procainamide, although this use is decreasing.

## Pharmacotherapeutics

Because of its effectiveness and relatively low toxicity, phenytoin is the most commonly prescribed anticonvulsant. It's one of the drugs of choice to treat:
• complex partial seizures (also called *psychomotor* or *temporal lobe seizures*)
• tonic-clonic seizures.
    Hydantoins (phenytoin and fosphenytoin) are the long-acting anticonvulsant of choice to treat status epilepticus after initial I.V. benzodiazepines.

### Resistance is futile

Health care providers sometimes prescribe phenytoin and ethotoin in combination with other anticonvulsants for partial and tonic-clonic seizures in patients who are resistant to or intolerant of other anticonvulsants.

## Drug interactions

Hydantoins interact with a number of other drugs. Here are some drug interactions of major to moderate clinical significance:
• Phenytoin's effect is decreased when it's taken with phenobarbital, diazoxide, theophylline, carbamazepine, rifampin, antacids, or sucralfate.
• Phenytoin's effect and potential for toxicity increase when it's taken with cimetidine, disulfiram, fluconazole, isoniazid, omeprazole, sulfonamides, oral anticoagulants, chloramphenicol, valproic acid, or amiodarone.
• Enteral tube feedings may interfere with the absorption of oral phenytoin. Stop feedings for 2 hours before and after phenytoin administration.
• The effect of these drugs is decreased when they're taken with a hydantoin anticonvulsant: oral anticoagulants, antiretrovirals, levodopa, amiodarone, corticosteroids, doxycycline, methadone, metyrapone, quinidine, theophylline, thyroid hormone, hormonal contraceptives, valproic acid, cyclosporine, and carbamazepine. (See *Adverse reactions to hydantoins*.)

## Barbiturates

The long-acting barbiturate phenobarbital was formerly one of the most widely used anticonvulsants. It's now used less frequently

**Warning!**

## Adverse reactions to hydantoins

Adverse reactions to hydantoins include:
• drowsiness
• ataxia
• irritability
• headache
• restlessness
• nystagmus
• dizziness and vertigo
• dysarthria
• nausea and vomiting
• abdominal pain
• anorexia
• depressed atrial and ventricular conduction
• ventricular fibrillation (in toxic states)
• bradycardia, hypotension, and cardiac arrest (with I.V. administration)
• hypersensitivity reactions.

because of its sedative effects. Phenobarbital is sometimes used for long-term treatment of epilepsy and is prescribed selectively to treat status epilepticus if hydantoins are ineffective.

## Other barbiturates

Mephobarbital, also a long-acting barbiturate, is sometimes used as an anticonvulsant. Primidone, which is closely related chemically to the barbiturates, is also used to treat chronic epilepsy.

## Pharmacokinetics

Each barbiturate has a slightly different set of pharmacokinetic properties.

## Phenobarbital for the long haul

Phenobarbital is absorbed slowly but well from the GI tract. Peak plasma levels occur 8 to 12 hours after a single dose. The drug is 20% to 45% bound to serum proteins and to a similar extent to other tissues, including the brain. About 75% of a phenobarbital dose is metabolized by the liver, and 25% is excreted unchanged in urine.

## Mephobarbital moves quickly

Almost one-half of a mephobarbital dose is absorbed from the GI tract and well distributed in body tissues. The drug is bound to tissue and plasma proteins. Mephobarbital undergoes extensive metabolism by the liver; only 1% to 2% is excreted unchanged in urine.

## Primidone and protein

Approximately 60% to 80% of a primidone dose is absorbed from the GI tract and distributed evenly among body tissues. The drug is protein-bound to a small extent in the plasma. Primidone is metabolized by the liver to two active metabolites, phenobarbital and phenylethylmalonamide (PEMA). From 15% to 25% of primidone is excreted unchanged in urine, 15% to 25% is metabolized to phenobarbital, and 50% to 70% is excreted in urine as PEMA. Primidone is also secreted in breast milk.

## Pharmacodynamics

Barbiturates exhibit anticonvulsant action at doses below those that produce hypnotic effects. For this reason, they usually don't produce addiction when used to treat epilepsy. Barbiturates elevate the seizure threshold by decreasing postsynaptic excitation.

## Pharmacotherapeutics

Barbiturates are an effective alternative therapy for:

- partial seizures
- tonic-clonic seizures
- febrile seizures.

Barbiturates can be used alone or with other anticonvulsants. I.V. phenobarbital is also used to treat status epilepticus. The major disadvantage of using phenobarbital for status epilepticus is that it has a delayed onset of action when an immediate response is needed. Barbiturates are ineffective in treating absence seizures.

*Consider this*

Mephobarbital has no advantage over phenobarbital and is used when the patient can't tolerate the adverse effects of phenobarbital. Because of monitoring, costs, and dosing frequency, phenobarbital is usually tried before primidone. Primidone may be effective in patients who fail to respond to phenobarbital.

## Drug interactions

The effects of barbiturates can be reduced when they're taken with rifampin. Here are some other drug interactions:
- The risk of toxicity increases when phenobarbital is taken with CNS depressants, valproic acid, chloramphenicol, felbamate, cimetidine, or phenytoin.
- The metabolism of corticosteroids, digoxin, and estrogens may be enhanced when these drugs are taken with phenobarbital, leading to decreased effects.
- Adverse effects of tricyclic antidepressants increase when they're taken with barbiturates.
- Evening primrose oil may increase anticonvulsant dosage requirements. (See *Adverse reactions to barbiturates.*)

*Reduced effects*

Barbiturate use can decrease the effects of many drugs, including beta-adrenergic blockers, corticosteroids, digoxin, estrogens, doxycycline, oral anticoagulants, hormonal contraceptives, quinidine, phenothiazine, metronidazole, tricyclic antidepressants, theophylline, cyclosporine, carbamazepine, felodipine, and verapamil.

> Because of monitoring, costs, and dosing frequency, phenobarbital is usually tried before primidone.

*Warning!*

## Adverse reactions to barbiturates

Adverse reactions to phenobarbital and mephobarbital include:
- drowsiness, lethargy, and dizziness
- nystagmus, confusion, and ataxia (with large doses)
- laryngospasm, respiratory depression, and hypotension (when administered I.V.).

### The same, plus psychoses

Primidone can cause the same central nervous system and GI adverse reactions as phenobarbital. It can also cause acute psychosis, hair loss, impotence, and osteomalacia.

### As a group

All three barbiturates can produce a hypersensitivity rash, other rashes, lupus erythematosus–like syndrome (an inflammatory disorder), and enlarged lymph nodes.

# Iminostilbenes

*Carbamazepine* is the most commonly used iminostilbene anticonvulsant. It effectively treats:
• partial and generalized tonic-clonic seizures
• mixed seizure types
• complex partial seizures (drug of choice).

## Pharmacokinetics

Carbamazepine is absorbed slowly from the GI tract and is metabolized in the liver by the cytochrome P-450 isoform 3A4 (CYP450) and is excreted in urine. Carbamazepine is distributed rapidly to all tissues; 75% to 90% is bound to plasma proteins. A small amount crosses the placenta, and some is secreted in breast milk. The half-life varies greatly.

## Pharmacodynamics

Carbamazepine's anticonvulsant effect is similar to that of phenytoin. The drug's anticonvulsant action can occur because of its ability to inhibit the spread of seizure activity or neuromuscular transmission in general.

## Pharmacotherapeutics

Carbamazepine is the drug of choice, in adults and children, for treating:
• generalized tonic-clonic seizures
• simple and complex partial seizures.
　　Carbamazepine may worsen absence or myoclonic seizures. However, it relieves pain when used to treat trigeminal neuralgia (tic douloureux, characterized by excruciating facial pain along the trigeminal nerve) and may be useful in treating selective psychiatric disorders.

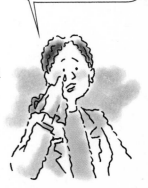

Be aware that (sniff!), even when used as an anticonvulsant, carbamazepine can affect mood and behavior.

## Drug interactions

Carbamazepine can reduce the effects of several drugs, including haloperidol, bupropion, lamotrigine, tricyclic antidepressants, oral anticoagulants, hormonal contraceptives, doxycycline, felbamate, theophylline, protease inhibitors, antipsychotics, and valproic acid. Other drug interactions can also occur:
• Increased carbamazepine levels and toxicity can occur with the use of cimetidine, danazol, diltiazem, erythromycin, isoniazid, selective serotonin reuptake inhibitors, propoxyphene, ketoconazole, valproic acid, and verapamil.

• Lithium and carbamazepine taken together increase the risk of toxic neurologic effects.

## Confusion alert!

Don't confuse Tegretol (a brand name for carbamazepine) with Toradol (a brand name for ketorolac).

• Carbamazepine levels may be decreased when taken with barbiturates, felbamate, or phenytoin. (See *Adverse reactions to carbamazepine*.)

• The herbal remedy plantain may inhibit GI absorption of carbamazepine.

# Benzodiazepines

The four *benzodiazepine drugs* that provide anticonvulsant effects are:

• clonazepam
• clorazepate
• diazepam (parenteral form)
• lorazepam. (See *Sound-alikes: Diazepam and lorazepam*.)

## Only one for ongoing treatment

Only clonazepam is recommended for long-term treatment of epilepsy. Diazepam may be used to treat status epilepticus or, in rectal form, repetitive seizures. Lorazepam I.V. is considered the drug of choice for status epilepticus. Clorazepate is prescribed as an adjunct in treating partial seizures.

*Warning!*

## Adverse reactions to carbamazepine

Occasionally, carbamazepine can result in serious hematologic toxicity. Because carbamazepine is related structurally to the tricyclic antidepressants, it can cause similar toxicities and affect behaviors and emotions.

Hives and Stevens-Johnson syndrome (a potentially fatal inflammatory disease) can also occur. Rash is the most common hypersensitivity response.

*Safe and sound*

## Sound-alikes: Diazepam and lorazepam

Be careful not to confuse the sound-alike drugs diazepam and lorazepam. Both drugs are benzodiazepines that can be used to treat status epilepticus. Lorazepam I.V. is considered the drug of choice. Diazepam provides only short-term effects and isn't recommended for long-term treatment because high serum concentrations are needed to control seizures and long-term use can lead to addiction.

## Pharmacokinetics

The patient can receive benzodiazepines orally, parenterally or, in special situations, rectally (diazepam rectal gel).

### Absorption and distribution

Benzodiazepines are absorbed rapidly and almost completely from the GI tract but are distributed at different rates. Protein binding of benzodiazepines ranges from 85% to 90%.

### Metabolism and excretion

Benzodiazepines are metabolized in the liver to multiple metabolites and are then excreted in urine. They readily cross the placenta and are secreted in breast milk.

## Pharmacodynamics

Benzodiazepines act as:
- anticonvulsants
- antianxiety agents
- sedative-hypnotics
- muscle relaxants.
  Their mechanism of action is poorly understood.

## Pharmacotherapeutics

Each of the benzodiazepines can be used in slightly different ways.

### Absence, atypical, and more

Clonazepam is used to treat the following types of seizures:
- absence (petit mal)
- atypical absence (Lennox-Gastaut syndrome)
- atonic
- myoclonic.

### I.V. or with others

Diazepam isn't recommended for long-term treatment because of its potential for addiction and the high serum concentrations required to control seizures.

I.V. lorazepam is currently considered the benzodiazepine of choice for treating status epilepticus.

I.V. diazepam is used to control status epilepticus. Because diazepam provides only short-term effects of less than 1 hour, the patient must also be given a long-acting anticonvulsant, such as phenytoin or phenobarbital, during diazepam therapy. Diazepam rectal gel is approved

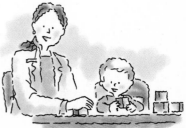

Diazepam can help reduce the incidence of recurrent seizures in children. They can get back to doing what they like to do!

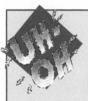

**Warning!**

## Adverse reactions to benzodiazepines

**Most common**
- Drowsiness
- Confusion
- Ataxia
- Weakness
- Dizziness
- Nystagmus
- Vertigo
- Fainting
- Dysarthria

- Headache
- Tremor
- Glassy-eyed appearance

**Less common**
- Depression of the heart and breathing (with high doses and with I.V. diazepam)
- Rash and other acute hypersensitivity reactions

for treatment of repetitive seizures and has reduced the incidence of recurrent seizures in children.

Clorazepate is used with other drugs to treat partial seizures.

## Drug interactions

When benzodiazepines are taken with CNS depressants, sedatives, cimetidine, or hormonal contraceptives, depressant effects are enhanced. This can cause motor skill impairment, respiratory depression, excessive sedation, CNS depression, and even death at high doses. (See *Adverse reactions to benzodiazepines*.)

# Carboxylic acid derivatives

Valproic acid, the most widely used carboxylic acid derivative, is unrelated structurally to the other anticonvulsants. Valproic acid is also available as:
- valproate
- divalproex.

## Pharmacokinetics

Valproate is converted rapidly to valproic acid in the stomach. Divalproex is a precursor of valproic acid and separates into valproic acid in the GI tract. Valproic acid is a hepatic enzyme inhibitor; it's absorbed well, is strongly protein-bound, and is metabolized in the liver. Metabolites and unchanged drug are excreted in urine.

Valproic acid readily crosses the placental barrier and also appears in breast milk.

## Pharmacodynamics

The mechanism of action for valproic acid remains unknown. The drug is thought to increase levels of GABA, an inhibitory neurotransmitter, and to have a direct membrane-stabilizing effect.

## Pharmacotherapeutics

Valproic acid is prescribed for long-term treatment of:
• absence seizures
• myoclonic seizures
• tonic-clonic seizures
• partial seizures.

Valproic acid may also be useful for neonatal seizures.

## Drug interactions

Valproic acid must be used cautiously in children under 2 years old, particularly those receiving multiple anticonvulsants and those with congenital metabolic disorders, severe seizures with mental retardation, or organic brain disease. In these patients, valproic acid carries a risk of potentially fatal liver toxicity (primarily in the first 6 months of treatment).

This risk limits its use as a drug of choice for seizure disorders. However, while it's a risk for all patients, the risk decreases with age. Caution should also be taken with patients with hepatic disease.

### Valproic warnings

These are the most significant drug interactions associated with valproic acid:
• Cimetidine, aspirin, erythromycin, and felbamate may increase levels of valproic acid.
• Carbamazepine, lamotrigine, phenobarbital, primidone, phenytoin, and rifampin may decrease levels of valproic acid.
• Valproic acid may decrease the effects of felbamate, phenobarbital, primidone, benzodiazepines, CNS depressants, warfarin, and zidovudine. (See *Adverse reactions to valproic acid*, page 78.)

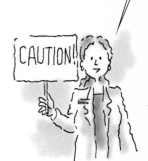

Take caution when giving valproic acid to patients with hepatic disease.

### Warning!

## Adverse reactions to valproic acid

Because rare, but deadly, liver toxicity has occurred with valproic acid, it should be used with caution in patients who have a history of hepatic disease. Children younger than age 2 have a high risk of developing hepatotoxicity.

Most other adverse reactions are tolerable and dose-related.

These include:
• nausea and vomiting
• diarrhea
• constipation
• sedation
• dizziness
• ataxia
• headache
• muscle weakness
• increased blood ammonia level.

# 1- (aminomethyl) cyclohexane–acetic acid

The 1- (aminomethyl) cyclohexane–acetic acid class includes the drug gabapentin, which was designed to be a GABA agonist, although its exact mechanism of action is unknown.

Gabapentin is approved as adjunctive therapy for partial seizures in adults and in children ages 3 and older with epilepsy. It has also been used to treat pain, tremor associated with MS, bipolar disorder, and Parkinson's disease as well as to prevent migraines.

## Pharmacokinetics

Gabapentin is readily absorbed in the GI tract. Because of this active-transport mechanism, the drug's bioavailability may decrease as the dosage increases. Gabapentin isn't metabolized; it's excreted exclusively by the kidneys.

## Pharmacodynamics

Gabapentin's exact mechanism of action is unknown. The drug doesn't appear to act at the GABA receptor, affect GABA uptake, or interfere with GABA transaminase. Instead, gabapentin appears to bind to a carrier protein and act at a unique receptor in the brain, resulting in elevated GABA levels in the brain.

## Pharmacotherapeutics

Gabapentin is used as adjunctive therapy for partial and secondarily generalized seizures in adults and children ages 3 and older. It also seems to be effective as monotherapy although it isn't FDA-approved for that purpose.

## Drug interactions

Like carbamazepine, gabapentin may worsen myoclonic seizures.

Gabapentin doesn't induce or inhibit hepatic enzymes, so it causes very few drug interactions and doesn't affect the metabolism of other anticonvulsants. Antacids and cimetidine may affect gabapentin concentration.

Patients with renal impairment (creatinine clearance less than 60 ml/minute) require a dosage reduction. (See *Adverse reactions to gabapentin.*)

# Phenyltriazines

The phenyltriazine lamotrigine is chemically unrelated to other anticonvulsants. This drug is FDA-approved as adjunctive therapy for adults who have partial seizures and for children older than age 2 who have generalized seizures or Lennox-Gastaut syndrome. It may also be used as monotherapy for partial seizures in adults after a hepatic enzyme–inducing anticonvulsant has been discontinued.

## Pharmacokinetics

Lamotrigine is rapidly and well absorbed. It's metabolized by the liver and excreted by the kidneys. Clearance is increased in the presence of other enzyme-inducing anticonvulsants. Lamotrigine isn't significantly bound to plasma proteins.

## Pharmacodynamics

Lamotrigine's precise mechanism of action is unknown, but the drug is thought to block voltage-sensitive sodium channels, thus inhibiting the release of the excitatory neurotransmitters glutamate and aspartate.

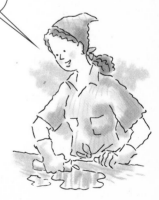

Lamotrigine is rapidly and well absorbed in the body. Wish I could say this sponge was as good at absorption!

### Pharmacotherapeutics

Lamotrigine prevents partial seizure activity. In addition, lamotrigine appears to be effective for many types of generalized seizures. However it can worsen myoclonic seizures.

The drug may also lead to improvement in the patient's mood.

### Drug interactions

• Lamotrigine's effects may be decreased if the drug is given with carbamazepine, phenytoin, phenobarbital, primidone, or acetaminophen.
• Lamotrigine may produce additive effects when combined with folate inhibitors.
• Valproic acid may decrease lamotrigine clearance and increase the steady-state level and effects of lamotrigine. (See *Adverse reactions to lamotrigine.*)

# Carboxamides

Oxcarbazepine, a carboxamide, is chemically similar to carbamazepine but causes less induction of hepatic enzymes. Oxcarbazepine is a prodrug. It's useful as adjunctive therapy or monotherapy for adults with partial seizures and as adjunctive therapy for children with partial seizures.

### Pharmacokinetics

Oxcarbazepine is completely absorbed and extensively metabolized by hepatic enzymes to the 10-monohydroxy metabolite (MHD) that's responsible for its pharmacologic activity. MHD is excreted primarily by the kidneys.

*9 hours in half*

The half-life of MHD is about 9 hours. Unlike carbamazepine, oxcarbazepine doesn't induce its own metabolism.

### Pharmacodynamics

The precise mechanism of action of oxcarbazepine and its metabolite MHD is unknown, but antiseizure activity is thought to occur through blockade of sodium-sensitive channels, which prevents seizure spread in the brain.

*Warning!*

## Adverse reactions to lamotrigine

Adverse reactions to lamotrigine commonly include:
• dizziness
• ataxia
• somnolence
• headache
• diplopia
• nausea
• vomiting
• rash.

Several types of rash, including Stevens-Johnson syndrome, may occur with use of this drug. A generalized, erythematous, morbilliform rash may appear in the first 3 to 4 weeks of therapy; it's usually mild to moderate, but it may be severe.

Lamotrigine now carries a "black box" warning regarding the rash, and the manufacturer recommends discontinuing the drug at the first sign of rash. The risk of rash may be increased by starting at high doses, by rapidly increasing doses, or by using valproate concurrently.

## Pharmacotherapeutics

Oxcarbazepine is FDA-approved as adjunctive therapy for partial seizures in adults and children older than age 4 and as monotherapy for adults.

As with carbamazepine, it's also effective for generalized seizures but may worsen myoclonic and absence seizures.

## Drug interactions

• Carbamazepine, phenytoin, phenobarbital, valproic acid, and verapamil may decrease the levels of oxcarbazepine's active metabolite MHD.

*Pill worries*

• Oxcarbazepine may decrease the effectiveness of hormonal contraceptives and felodipine.
• Dosage reductions are necessary for patients with renal impairment (creatinine clearance less than 30 ml/minute) and those at risk for renal impairment, such as elderly patients. (See *Adverse reactions to oxcarbazepine*.)

> Elderly patients are at risk for renal impairment, so make sure you reduce the dosage of carboxamides in this patient population.

---

**Warning!**

### Adverse reactions to oxcarbazepine

About 20% to 30% of patients who have had an allergic reaction to carbamazepine will experience a hypersensitivity reaction to oxcarbazepine.

**Common reactions**
• Somnolence
• Dizziness
• Diplopia
• Ataxia
• Nausea and vomiting
• Abnormal gait

• Tremor
• Aggravated seizures
• Rectal bleeding

**Less common reactions**
• Agitation
• Confusion
• Hypotension
• Hyponatremia
• Rhinitis
• Speech disorder
• Back pain
• Upper respiratory tract infection

# Sulfamate-substituted monosaccharides

Topiramate, a sulfamate-substituted monosaccharide, is one of the newer anticonvulsants available.

## Pharmacokinetics

Topiramate is absorbed rapidly and is partially metabolized in the liver and excreted mostly unchanged in urine.

## Pharmacodynamics

Topiramate is believed to act by blocking voltage-dependent sodium channels, enhancing activity of the GABA receptors, and antagonizing glutamate receptors.

## Pharmacotherapeutics

Topiramate is approved as adjunctive therapy for partial and primary generalized tonic-clonic seizures in adults and children older than age 2 and for children with Lennox-Gastaut syndrome. It may also prove beneficial for other types of seizures and as monotherapy.

## Drug interactions

• Carbamazepine, phenytoin, and valproic acid may cause decreased topiramate levels.
• Topiramate may decrease the effectiveness of hormonal contraceptives and decrease valproic acid levels.
• CNS depressants may cause additive CNS effect when combined with topiramate.

*50% off*

• For renally impaired patients (creatinine clearance less than 70 ml/minute), the topiramate dosage should be reduced by 50%. (See *Adverse reactions to topiramate.*)

# Succinimides

The succinimides, ethosuximide and methsuximide, are used to manage absence seizures. Ethosuximide is considered the drug of choice for absence seizures.

## Pharmacokinetics

The succinimides are readily absorbed from the GI tract and metabolized in the liver and excreted in urine. Metabolites are be-

**Warning!**

## Adverse reactions to topiramate

Psychomotor slowing, word-finding difficulty, impaired concentration, and memory impairment are common reactions that may require stopping topiramate. Low starting doses and slow dosage titration may minimize these effects.

Other common adverse reactions include:
• drowsiness
• dizziness
• headache
• ataxia
• nervousness
• confusion
• paresthesia
• weight gain
• diplopia.

Serious but infrequent adverse reactions include:
• secondary angle-closure glaucoma
• liver failure
• decreased sweating
• hyperthermia
• heat stroke
• renal calculi.

lieved to be inactive. The elimination half-life of ethosuximide is about 60 hours in adults and 30 hours in children.

## Pharmacodynamics

Ethosuximide's exact mechanism of action is unknown. It's thought to inhibit an enzyme necessary for the formation of gamma-hydroxybutyrate, which has been associated with the induction of absence seizures.

## Pharmacotherapeutics

In addition to being the drug of choice for treating absence seizures, ethosuximide may also be used in combination with valproic acid for hard-to-control absence seizures.

## Drug interactions

Ethosuximide isn't protein-bound, so displacement reactions can't occur. Carbamazepine may induce the metabolism of ethosuximide. Valproic acid may inhibit the metabolism of ethosuximide only if the metabolism is near saturation. (See *Adverse reactions to succinimides*.)

# Sulfonamides

Zonisamide, a sulfonamide, is approved as adjunctive treatment for partial seizures in adults.

## Pharmacokinetics

Zonisamide is absorbed relatively rapidly, with peak concentrations occurring in 2 to 6 hours. Zonisamide is widely distributed and is extensively bound to erythrocytes.

The drug is metabolized by the CYP3A4 enzyme in the liver and is excreted in urine, primarily as the parent drug and the glucuronide metabolite.

## Pharmacodynamics

Zonisamide's precise mechanism of action is unknown, but it's believed to involve stabilization of neuronal membranes and suppression of neuronal hypersensitivity.

## Pharmacotherapeutics

Zonisamide is approved only as adjunctive therapy for partial seizures in adults, but it appears to have a broad spectrum of ac-

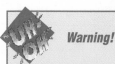

**Warning!**

## Adverse reactions to succinimides

Ethosuximide is generally well tolerated. The most common adverse effects (occurring in up to 40% of patients) are nausea and vomiting. Other common adverse effects include:
• drowsiness and fatigue
• lethargy
• dizziness
• hiccups
• headaches
• mood changes.

Rarely, blood dyscrasias, rashes (including Stevens-Johnson syndrome and erythema multiforme), lupus-like syndrome, and psychotic behaviors can occur.

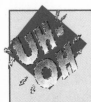

tivity for other types of seizures (infantile spasms; myoclonic, generalized, and atypical absence seizures).

### Drug interactions

• Drugs that induce liver enzymes, such as phenytoin, carbamazepine, and phenobarbital, increase the metabolism and decrease the half-life of zonisamide.

*Serious serum*

• Concurrent use of zonisamide with drugs that inhibit or induce CYP3A4 may increase or decrease the serum concentration of zonisamide. Zonisamide isn't an inducer of CYP3A4, so it's unlikely to affect other drugs metabolized by this system. (See *Adverse reactions to sulfonamides.*)

# Pyrrolidines

Levetiracetam, a pyrrolidine derivative, is a newer antiseizure drug that's chemically unrelated to previously available antiepileptic drugs. It's used as adjunctive therapy to treat certain types of partial and myoclonic seizures.

## Pharmacokinetics

Levetiracetam is administered orally or I.V. Oral administration results in rapid and full absorption with a 100% bioavailability. Peak concentrations occur in about 1 hour. Levetiracetam isn't extensively metabolized; any metabolites that are produced aren't active. The major metabolic pathway is enzymatic hydrolysis, and metabolism doesn't depend on any hepatic cytochrome P450 isoenzymes. Levetiracetam is eliminated by renal excretion. The half-life is about 8 hours and is unaffected by dose, route of administration, or repeated administration.

## Pharmacodynamics

The precise mechanism of action isn't known. The drug's antiepileptic effect doesn't appear to involve known mechanisms relating to inhibitory and excitatory neurotransmission.

## Pharmacotherapeutics

Levetiracetam has several indications for us, including:
• adjunctive therapy for epilepsy in adults and children older than age 4
• adjunctive treatment for myoclonic seizures in adults and children older than age 12
• adjunctive treatment for primary generalized tonic-clonic seizures in adults and children older than age 6.

## Drug interactions

Levetiracetam has no known major drug interactions. (See *Adverse reactions to levetiracetam.*)

**Warning!**

### Adverse reactions to levetiracetam

Common adverse reactions to levetiracetam include:
• drowsiness
• dizziness
• fatigue
• asthenia
• headache
• vomiting.
   Less common adverse reactions include:
• depression
• pharyngitis
• conjunctivitis
• mood swings.

# Antimigraine drugs

Migraine is one of the most common primary headache disorders, affecting an estimated 24 million people in the United States. An episodic disorder, migraine produces a unilateral pain that's commonly described as pounding, pulsating, or throbbing. It may be preceded by an aura. Other common symptoms are sensitivity to light or sound, nausea, vomiting, constipation, and diarrhea.
   Researchers believe that migraine symptoms are caused by cranial vasodilation or the release of vasoactive and proinflammatory substances from nerves in an activated trigeminal system.

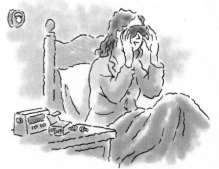

Sensitivity to light may be a symptom of a migraine.

## Attacking aches

Treatment of migraine aims to alter an attack once it's under way (abortive or symptomatic treatment) or to prevent an attack. Choice of therapy depends on the severity, duration, and frequency of the headaches; on the degree of disability that the headache creates in the patient; and on patient characteristics.

Abortive treatments may include analgesics (aspirin and acetaminophen), nonsteroidal anti-inflammatory drugs (NSAIDs), ergotamine, 5-hydroxytryptaminergic (5-HT$_1$)-receptor agonists, and various miscellaneous drugs (such as isometheptene combinations, intranasal butorphanol, metoclopramide, and corticosteroids). Prophylactic therapy includes beta-adrenergic blockers, tricyclic antidepressants, valproic acid, and NSAIDs, to name a few.

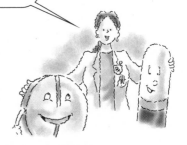

**Memory jogger**

How can you tell if it's a migraine or a headache? Look at the mnemonic PAIN to see if the patient has these key symptoms:

P—pain

A—aura

I—irritated by light

N—nausea.

# 5-HT$_1$- receptor agonists (triptans)

The 5-HT$_1$-receptor agonists, commonly known as the *triptans*, are the treatment of choice for moderate to severe migraine. They include:

- almotriptan
- eletriptan
- frovatriptan
- naratriptan
- rizatriptan
- sumatriptan
- zolmitriptan. (See *Sound-alikes: Sumatriptan and zolmitriptan.*)

> All the triptans come in oral form.

### Pharmacokinetics

When comparing the triptans, the key pharmacokinetic features are onset of action and duration of action. Rizatriptan, sumatriptan, and zolmitriptan have a half-life of approximately 2 hours; almotriptan and eletriptan have a half-life of 3 to 4 hours; naratriptan has a half-life of about 6 hours; and frovatriptan has the longest half-life (25 hours) and the most delayed onset of action.

## Triptan tablets

All of the triptans are available in an oral form. Rizatriptan and zolmitriptan are also available in rapid-dissolve tablets. Zolmitriptan and sumatriptan are available in intransal forms. Sumatriptan is also available as a subcutaneous injection. The injectable form of sumatriptan has the most rapid onset of action of all the triptans.

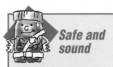

**Safe and sound**

## Sound-alikes: Sumatriptan and zolmitriptan

Don't confuse the sound-alike drugs sumatriptan and zolmitriptan. Both drugs are used to treat acute migraines, but recommended doses are significantly different.

## Pharmacodynamics

Triptans are serotonin $5\text{-}HT_1$-receptor agonists, which constrict the cranial vessels, inhibit neuropeptide release, and reduce the neurogenic inflammatory process transmission along the trigeminal pathway. These actions may abort or provide symptomatic relief for migraines. Aside from relieving pain, triptans are also effective in controlling the nausea and vomiting associated with migraines.

## Pharmacotherapeutics

The choice of a triptan depends on patient preferences for dosage form (if nausea and vomiting are present), presence of recurrent migraines, and formulary restrictions. A patient experiencing nausea and vomiting may prefer injectable or intranasal sumatriptan. Recurrent migraines may respond to triptans with a longer half-life, such as frovatriptan and naratriptan. However, triptans with a longer half-life have a delayed onset of effect. Two newer triptans, almotriptan and eletriptan, have a rapid onset and an intermediate half-life.

## Drug interactions

Triptans have many contraindications and aren't for use in patients with certain conditions. (See *Triptans: Contraindications and cautions*, page 88.)

The safety of treating more than three migraine attacks in a 30-day period with triptans hasn't been established. (See *Adverse reactions to 5-$HT_1$-receptor agonists [triptans]*.)

In addition:
- Triptans shouldn't be administered within 24 hours of another $5\text{-}HT_1$-receptor agonist.
- Ergotamine-containing and ergot-type drugs (such as dihydroergotamine and methysergide) shouldn't be given within 24 hours of a $5\text{-}HT_1$-receptor agonist because prolonged vasospastic reactions may occur.
- Eletriptan shouldn't be used within at least 72 hours of these potent CYP3A4 inhibitors: ketoconazole, itraconazole, nefazodone, clarithromycin, ritonavir, nelfinavir, and any other

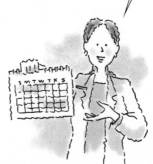

It hasn't been proven yet whether it's safe to treat more than three migraines in a 30-day period with triptans.

*Safe and sound*

# Triptans: Contraindications and cautions

Triptans are contraindicated for patients with ischemic heart disease (such as angina pectoris, history of myocardial infarction, or documented silent ischemia) and in patients who have symptoms or findings consistent with ischemic heart disease, coronary artery vasospasm (including Prinzmetal's variant angina), or other significant underlying cardiovascular conditions.

Triptans shouldn't be prescribed for patients with cerebrovascular syndromes, such as strokes or transient ischemic attacks, or for patients with peripheral vascular disease, including—but not limited to—ischemic bowel disease. Triptans shouldn't be given to patients with uncontrolled hypertension or with hemiplegic or basilar migraines.

In addition, triptans aren't recommended for use in patients who have risk factors for unrecognized coronary artery disease (CAD) (such as hypertension, hypercholesterolemia, smoking, obesity, diabetes, strong family history of CAD, being a female with surgical or physiologic menopause, or being a male over age 40) unless a cardiovascular evaluation indicates that the patient is reasonably free from underlying cardiovascular disease. If a triptan is used in this setting, the first dose should be administered in a doctor's office or other medically staffed and equipped facility.

Also, intermittent, long-term users of triptans and those who have risk factors should undergo periodic cardiac evaluation.

drugs that have demonstrated potent CYP3A4 inhibition, as described in their labeling.

## Wait two weeks

• Almotriptan, rizatriptan, sumatriptan, and zolmitriptan should not be used with, or within 2 weeks of discontinuing, an MAOI.
• Selective serotonin reuptake inhibitors (SSRIs), such as citalopram, fluoxetine, fluvoxamine, paroxetine, and sertraline, have, in rare cases, caused weakness, hyperreflexia, and incoordination when administered with a triptan. (This reaction has also been reported when the appetite suppressant sibutramine is used with a triptan.) Monitor the patient closely if concomitant treatment with a triptan and an SSRI is clinically warranted.
• The bioavailability of frovatriptan is 30% higher in patients taking hormonal contraceptives.
• Propranolol increases the bioavailability of zolmitriptan, rizatriptan, frovatriptan, and eletriptan.

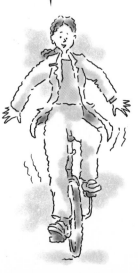

Incoordination can be an adverse effect of mixing SSRIs with triptan.

# Ergotamine preparations

Ergotamine and its derivatives may be used as abortive or symptomatic therapy for migraine.

Some common preparations used for migraine include:
- ergotamine, available in sublingual and oral tablets and suppositories (combined with caffeine)
- dihydroergotamine, available in injectable and intranasal forms.

## Pharmacokinetics

Ergotamine is incompletely absorbed from the GI tract. The intranasal form of dihydroergotamine is rapidly absorbed. Peak plasma concentration, following subcutaneous injection, is within 45 minutes, and 90% of the dose is plasma protein-bound. Ergotamine is metabolized in the liver, and 90% of the metabolites are excreted in bile; traces of unchanged drug are excreted in urine.

## Pharmacodynamics

Ergotamine-derivative antimigraine effects are believed to be due to blockade of neurogenic inflammation. They also act as partial agonists or antagonists at serotonin, dopaminergic, and alpha-adrenergic receptors depending on their site. Ergotamine preparations often need to be prescribed with antiemetic preparations when used for migraine.

Dihydroergotamine, a hydrogenated form of ergotamine, differs mainly in degree of activity. It has less vasoconstrictive action than ergotamine and much less emetic potential.

## Pharmacotherapeutics

Ergotamine preparations are used to prevent or treat vascular headaches, such as migraine, migraine variant, and cluster headaches. Dihydroergotamine is used when rapid control of migraine is desired or when other routes are undesirable.

## Drug interactions

- Propranolol and other beta-adrenergic blocking drugs block the natural pathway for vasodilation in patients receiving ergotamine preparations, resulting in excessive vasoconstriction and cold extremities.

*Warning!*

## Adverse reactions to ergotamine derivatives

Adverse effects of ergotamine derivatives include:
• nausea and vomiting
• numbness
• tingling
• muscle pain
• leg weakness
• itching.
   Prolonged administration of ergotamine derivatives may result in gangrene and rebound headaches. Contraindications to the use of ergotamine preparations include coronary, cerebral, or peripheral vascular disease; hypertension; and liver or kidney disease.

*Vasoconstrictors may increase the risk of high blood pressure.*

*Steady, now...*

• There may be an increased risk of weakness, hyperflexion, and incoordination when using ergotamine preparations with SSRIs.
• Sumatriptan may cause an additive effect, increasing the risk of coronary vasospasm. Don't give any ergotamine preparations and triptans within 24 hours of each other.
• Drugs that inhibit the CYP3A4 enzyme (such as erythromycin, clarithromycin, ritonavir, nelfinavir, indinavir, and azole-derivative antifungal agents) may alter the metabolism of ergotamine, resulting in increased serum concentrations of ergotamine. This increases the risk of vasospasm and cerebral or peripheral ischemia. These drugs shouldn't be used together.
• Vasoconstrictors may cause an additive effect when given with ergotamine preparations, increasing the risk of high blood pressure. (See *Adverse reactions to ergotamine derivatives.*)

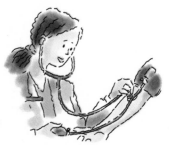

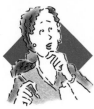

# Quick quiz

**1.** A 15-year-old patient has a tonic-clonic seizure disorder and is prescribed phenytoin. Which term best describes the absorption rate of oral phenytoin?

A. Rapid
B. Intermittent
C. Erratic
D. Slow

*Answer:* D. Phenytoin is absorbed slowly through the GI tract. It's absorbed much more rapidly when administered I.V.

**2.** An 11-year-old patient develops myoclonic seizures. Which potential adverse reaction makes it unlikely that valproate will be prescribed for this patient?

A. Liver toxicity
B. Central nervous system sedation
C. Respiratory depression
D. Renal toxicity

*Answer:* A. When given to children and patients taking other anticonvulsants, valproate carries a risk of fatal liver toxicity.

**3.** A 48-year-old patient has been prescribed trihexyphenidyl for her Parkinson's disease. Which adverse reaction is dose-related?

A. Excessive salivation
B. Dry mouth
C. Bradycardia
D. Nausea

*Answer:* B. Dry mouth may be a dose-related adverse effect of trihexyphenidyl therapy.

**4.** Which antiparkinsonian drug is associated with the on-off phenomenon and the wearing-off effect?

A. Amantadine
B. Benztropine
C. Levodopa
D. Selegiline

*Answer:* C. Levodopa is associated with the on-off phenomenon (sharp fluctuations in symptoms) and the wearing-off effect (shorter duration of the drug's effects) in patients who have taken the drug for many years. Some doctors believe the drug should be given in lower doses or started later in the course of the disorder.

## *Scoring*

☆☆☆ If you answered all four items correctly, marvelous! You're mighty fine with neuromusculars.

☆☆ If you answered three items correctly, congrats! Your knowledge has a rapid onset and long duration.

☆ If you answered fewer than three items correctly, don't worry. Give yourself another dose of the chapter, and recheck the results.

# 4

## Pain medications

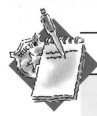

## Just the facts

In this chapter, you'll learn:

♦ classes of drugs used to control pain

♦ uses and varying actions of these drugs

♦ how these drugs are absorbed, distributed, metabolized, and excreted

♦ drug interactions and adverse reactions to these drugs.

## Drugs and pain control

Drugs used to control pain range from mild, over-the-counter (OTC) preparations such as acetaminophen to potent general anesthetics. They include:
• nonopioid analgesics, antipyretics, and nonsteroidal anti-inflammatory drugs (NSAIDs)
• opioid agonist and antagonist drugs
• anesthetic drugs.

## Nonopioid analgesics, antipyretics, and NSAIDs

Nonopioid analgesics, antipyretics, and NSAIDs are a broad group of pain medications. They're discussed together because, in addition to pain control, they also produce antipyretic (fever control) and anti-inflammatory effects. These drugs may be used alone or in combination with other medications. They have a ceiling effect (maximum dose above which there's no added benefit) and don't cause physical dependence.

The drug classes included in this group are:
• salicylates (especially aspirin), which are widely used

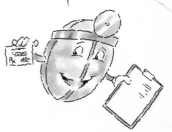

No pain, no gain? Not with me! You'll feel better in no time!

- the para-aminophenol derivative acetaminophen
- NSAIDs
- the urinary tract analgesic phenazopyridine.

# Salicylates

*Salicylates* are among the most commonly used pain medications. They're used regularly to control pain and reduce fever and inflammation.

## Cheap, easy, and reliable

Salicylates usually cost less than other analgesics and are readily available without a prescription. Aspirin is the most commonly used salicylate. Other common salicylates include:
- choline magnesium trisalicylate
- choline salicylate
- diflunisal
- salsalate
- sodium salicylate.

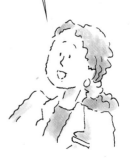

Salicylates are found in many OTC pain and cold preparations.

## Pharmacokinetics (how drugs circulate)

Taken orally, salicylates are absorbed partly in the stomach, but primarily in the upper part of the small intestine. The pure and buffered forms of aspirin are absorbed readily, but sustained-release and enteric-coated salicylate preparations are absorbed more slowly. Food or antacids in the stomach also delay absorption. Salicylates given rectally have a slower, more erratic absorption.

### Distribution, metabolism, and excretion

Salicylates are distributed widely throughout body tissues and fluids, including breast milk. In addition, they easily cross the placental barrier.

The liver extensively metabolizes salicylates into several metabolites. The kidneys excrete the metabolites along with some unchanged drug.

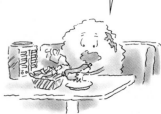

Taking a salicylate with an antacid or food slows absorption.

## Pharmacodynamics (how drugs act)

The different effects of salicylates stem from their separate mechanisms of action. They relieve pain primarily by inhibiting the synthesis of prostaglandin. (Recall that prostaglandin is a chemical mediator that sensitizes nerve cells to pain.) In addition, they may also reduce inflammation by inhibiting the prostaglandin synthesis and release that occurs during inflammation.

## Hot and bothered

Salicylates reduce fever by stimulating the hypothalamus, producing dilation of the peripheral blood vessels and increased sweating. This promotes heat loss through the skin and cooling by evaporation. Also, because prostaglandin E increases body temperature, inhibiting its production lowers a fever.

> Because they relieve muscle ache and reduce temperature, salicylates help treat symptoms of colds and influenza.

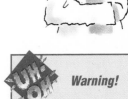

## No clots allowed

One salicylate, aspirin, permanently inhibits platelet aggregation (the clumping of platelets to form a clot) by interfering with the production of a substance called thromboxane $A_2$, necessary for platelet aggregation. Not all salicylates have this effect. For example, choline magnesium doesn't increase bleeding time.

## Pharmacotherapeutics (how drugs are used)

Salicylates are used primarily to relieve pain and reduce fever. However, they don't effectively relieve visceral pain (pain from the organs and smooth muscle) or severe pain from trauma.

## You give me fever...

Salicylates won't reduce a normal body temperature. They can reduce an elevated body temperature, and will relieve headache and muscle ache at the same time.

## What kind of joint is this?

Salicylates can provide considerable relief in 24 hours when they're used to reduce inflammation in rheumatic fever, rheumatoid arthritis, and osteoarthritis.

## Go with the flow

As a result of its anticlotting properties, aspirin can be used to enhance blood flow during myocardial infarction (MI) and to prevent recurrence of MI.

## How low can you go?

No matter what the clinical indication, the main guideline of salicylate therapy is to use the lowest dose that provides relief. This reduces the likelihood of adverse reactions. (See *Adverse reactions to salicylates*.)

## Drug interactions

Because salicylates are highly protein-bound, they can interact with many other protein-bound drugs by displacing those drugs from sites to which they normally bind. This increases the serum

*Warning!*

### Adverse reactions to salicylates

The most common adverse reactions to salicylates include gastric distress, nausea, vomiting, and bleeding tendencies. Other adverse reactions include:
• hearing loss (when taken for prolonged periods)
• diarrhea, thirst, sweating, tinnitus, confusion, dizziness, impaired vision, and hyperventilation (rapid breathing)'
• Reye's syndrome (when given to children with chickenpox or flu-like symptoms).

**Safe and sound**

## Using salicylates safely

Before administering salicylates, be aware of these concerns regarding special populations:

*Children and teenagers:* Don't use aspirin or salicylates to treat flu-like symptoms or chickenpox because of the risk of triggering Reye's syndrome.

*Pregnant women:* Aspirin is classified as pregnancy risk category D, and salicylates are classified as category C. Salicylates appear in breast milk.

*Surgical patients:* Discontinue aspirin, if possible, 1 week before surgery because of the risk of postoperative bleeding.

*Asthmatics:* These patients have an increased risk of sensitivity to aspirin, leading to bronchospasm, urticaria, angioedema, or shock.

concentration of the unbound active drug, causing increased pharmacologic effects (the unbound drug is said to be *potentiated*).

The following drug interactions may occur:

• Oral anticoagulants, heparin, methotrexate, oral antidiabetic agents, and insulin are among the drugs that have an increased effect or risk of toxicity when taken with salicylates.

• Probenecid, sulfinpyrazone, and spironolactone may have a decreased effect when taken with salicylates.

• Corticosteroids may decrease plasma salicylate levels and increase the risk of ulcers.

• Alkalinizing drugs and antacids may reduce salicylate levels.

• The antihypertensive effect of angiotensin-converting enzyme (ACE) inhibitors and beta-adrenergic blockers may be reduced when these drugs are combined with salicylates.

• NSAIDs may have a reduced therapeutic effect and an increased risk of GI effects when taken with salicylates. (See *Using salicylates safely.*)

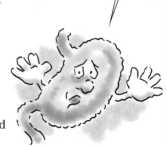

I feel an ulcer coming on... you didn't give me corticosteroids, did you?

# Acetaminophen

Although the class of para-aminophenol derivatives includes two drugs—phenacetin and acetaminophen—only acetaminophen is available in the United States. *Acetaminophen* is an OTC drug that produces analgesic and antipyretic effects. It appears in many products designed to relieve the pain and symptoms associated with colds and influenza.

## Pharmacokinetics

Acetaminophen is absorbed rapidly and completely from the GI tract. It's also absorbed well from the mucous membranes of the rectum.

### Distribution, metabolism, and excretion

Acetaminophen is distributed widely in body fluids and readily crosses the placental barrier. After acetaminophen is metabolized by the liver, it's excreted by the kidneys and, in small amounts, in breast milk.

## Pharmacodynamics

Acetaminophen reduces pain and fever, but unlike salicylates, it doesn't affect inflammation or platelet function. It can cause anticoagulation in the patient taking warfarin.

## Mystery theater

The pain-control effects of acetaminophen aren't well understood. The drug may work in the central nervous system (CNS) by inhibiting prostaglandin synthesis and in the peripheral nervous system in some unknown way. It reduces fever by acting directly on the heat-regulating center in the hypothalamus.

## Pharmacotherapeutics

Acetaminophen is used to reduce fever and relieve headache, muscle ache, and general pain.

## Child's play

Acetaminophen is the drug of choice to treat fever and flulike symptoms in children. Additionally, the American Arthritis Association has indicated that acetaminophen is an effective pain reliever for some types of arthritis.

## Drug interactions

Acetaminophen can produce the following drug interactions:
• The effects of oral anticoagulants and thrombolytic drugs may be slightly increased.
• The risk of liver toxicity is increased when long-term alcohol use, phenytoin, barbiturates, carbamazepine, and isoniazid are combined with acetaminophen.

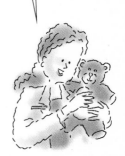

Acetaminophen is the drug of choice to treat fever and flulike symptoms in children.

• The effects of lamotrigine, loop diuretics, and zidovudine may be reduced when these drugs are taken with acetaminophen. (See *Adverse reactions to acetaminophen*.)

# Nonsteroidal anti-inflammatory drugs

As their name suggests, *nonsteroidal anti-inflammatory drugs* (NSAIDs), are typically used to combat inflammation. Their anti-inflammatory action equals that of aspirin. They also have analgesic and antipyretic effects. Unlike aspirin's effects, the effects of NSAIDs on platelet aggregation are temporary.

Picky, picky

There are two types of NSAIDs: selective and nonselective. The nonselective NSAIDs include diclofenac, etodolac, fenoprofen, flurbiprofen, ibuprofen, indomethacin, ketoprofen, ketorolac, meloxicam, nabumetone, naproxen, oxaprozin, piroxicam, and sulindac. The only selective NSAID available on today's market is celecoxib. (See *Risks of using selective NSAIDs.*)

## Pharmacokinetics

All NSAIDs (nonselective and selective) are absorbed in the GI tract. They're mostly metabolized in the liver and excreted primarily by the kidneys.

## Pharmacodynamics

Two isoenzymes of cyclooxygenase, known as COX-1 and COX-2, convert arachidonic acid into prostaglandins. The nonselective

**Warning!**

## Adverse reactions to acetaminophen

Most patients tolerate acetaminophen well. Unlike the salicylates, acetaminophen rarely causes gastric irritation or bleeding tendencies.

Acetaminophen may cause severe liver toxicity, and the total daily dose should be monitored. (The total daily dose shouldn't exceed 4,000 mg/day.)

Other adverse reactions include:
• skin rash
• hypoglycemia
• neutropenia.

*Safe and sound*

### Risks of using selective NSAIDs

Two selective nonsteroidal anti-inflammatory drugs (NSAIDs) were pulled from the market after it was discovered they were associated with an increased risk of heart attack and stroke, leaving celecoxib as the only available drug in its class. Patients considering the use of celecoxib should be carefully screened for a history of cerebrovascular or cardiovascular disease and then closely monitored throughout treatment for signs or symptoms of developing problems.

NSAIDs block both COX-1 and COX-2. Selective NSAIDs block only the COX-2 enzyme.

## Hard to stomach

The prostaglandins produced by COX-1 maintain the stomach lining, while those produced by COX-2 cause inflammation. That's why the nonselective NSAIDs, which inhibit COX-1 along with COX-2, commonly cause GI adverse effects. Selective NSAIDs, however, alleviate pain and inflammation without causing significant GI adverse effects because they inhibit only COX-2.

## Pharmacotherapeutics

NSAIDs are used primarily to decrease inflammation. They're secondarily used to relieve pain, but are seldom prescribed to reduce fever. (See *Using nonselective NSAIDs safely.*)

COX-2 inhibitors are primarily used to relieve pain and to decrease inflammation. These drugs are particularly useful in the treatment of osteoarthritis, rheumatoid arthritis, acute pain, primary dysmenorrhea, and familial adenomatous polyposis.

## Call and response

The following conditions respond favorably to treatment with NSAIDs:
• ankylosing spondylitis (an inflammatory joint disease that first affects the spine)
• moderate to severe rheumatoid arthritis (an inflammatory disease of peripheral joints)

## Adverse reactions to nonselective NSAIDs

Nonselective nonsteroidal anti-inflammatory drugs (NSAIDs) produce similar adverse reactions, including:
• abdominal pain, bleeding, anorexia, diarrhea, nausea, ulcers, and liver toxicity

• drowsiness, headache, dizziness, confusion, tinnitus, vertigo, and depression
• bladder infection, blood in the urine, and kidney necrosis
• hypertension, heart failure, and pedal edema.

## Adverse reactions to COX-2 inhibitors

COX-2 inhibitors can have the following adverse reactions:
• dyspepsia, nausea, and vomiting
• GI ulcers (to a lesser degree than with nonselective NSAIDs)
• hypertension, fluid retention, and peripheral edema
• dizziness and headache.

COX-2 inhibitors are classified as pregnancy risk category C; most appear in breast milk. As a precaution, don't use in breast-feeding women.

• osteoarthritis (a degenerative joint disease) in the hip, shoulder, or other large joints
• osteoarthritis accompanied by inflammation
• acute gouty arthritis (urate deposits in the joints)
• dysmenorrhea (painful menstruation)
• migraine headaches
• bursitis and tendonitis
• mild to moderate pain.

## Drug interactions

A wide variety of drugs can interact with NSAIDs, especially with indomethacin, piroxicam, and sulindac. Because they're highly protein-bound, NSAIDs are likely to interact with other protein-bound drugs. Such drugs as fluconazole, phenobarbital, rifampin, ritonavir, and salicylates affect absorption of NSAIDs, whereas NSAIDs affect the absorption of such drugs as oral anticoagulants, aminoglycosides, ACE inhibitors, beta-adrenergic blockers, digoxin, dilantin, and many others. (See *Adverse reactions to nonselective NSAIDs* and *Adverse reactions to COX-2 inhibitors*.)

Because NSAIDs are metabolized by the liver, drug-drug interactions have been identified for all of them. For example, these drugs decrease the clearance of lithium, which can result in lithium toxicity. They also reduce the antihypertensive effects of ACE inhibitors and diuretics.

# Phenazopyridine hydrochloride

*Phenazopyridine hydrochloride,* an azo dye used in commercial coloring, produces a local analgesic effect on the urinary tract.

### Pharmacokinetics

When taken orally, the liver metabolizes 35% of phenazopyridine. The remainder is excreted unchanged in the urine, causing the patient's urine to turn an orange or red color.

### Pharmacodynamics

Phenazopyridine is taken orally and produces an analgesic effect on the urinary tract usually within 24 to 48 hours after therapy begins.

### Phamacotherapeutics

The drug is used to relieve such symptoms as pain, buring, urgency, and frequency associated with urinary tract infections.

### Drug interactions

There are no listed drug interactions with phenazopyridine. (See *Adverse reactions to phenazopyridine hydrochloride.*)

# Opioid agonist and antagonist drugs

The word *opioid* refers to derivatives of the opium plant or to synthetic drugs that imitate natural narcotics. Opioid agonists (also called *narcotic agonists*) include opium derivatives and synthetic drugs with similar properties. They're used to relieve or decrease pain without causing the person to lose consciousness.

Some opioid agonists may also have antitussive effects that suppress coughing and antidiarrheal actions that can control diarrhea.

*Anta-dote*

Opioid antagonists aren't pain medications. Instead, they block the effects of opioid agonists and are used to reverse adverse drug reactions, such as respiratory and CNS depression, produced by those drugs. Unfortunately, by reversing the analgesic effect, they also cause the patient's pain to recur.

*Having it both ways*

Some opioid analgesics, called *mixed opioid agonist-antagonists*, have agonist and antagonist properties. The agonist component relieves pain, while the antagonist component decreases the risk of toxicity and drug dependence. These mixed opioid agonist-antagonists reduce the risk of respiratory depression and drug abuse.

**Warning!**

## Adverse reactions to phenazopyridine hydrochloride

Phenazopyridine hydrochloride can have certain adverse reactions.
• If the drug accumulates, the patient's skin and sclera may assume a yellow tinge. If this occurs, the drug may need to be discontinued.
• Acute renal or hepatic failure may occur.

*Opioid refers to derivatives of the opium plant or to synthetic drugs that imitate the effects of natural narcotics.*

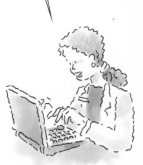

# Opioid agonists

*Opioid agonists* include:
- codeine
- fentanyl
- hydrocodone
- hydromorphone
- levorphanol
- meperidine
- methadone
- morphine sulfate (including morphine sulfate sustained-release tablets and intensified oral solution)
- oxycodone
- oxymorphone
- propoxyphene
- remifentanil
- sufentanil.

## Gold standard

Morphine sulfate is the standard against which the effectiveness and adverse reactions of other pain medications are measured. (See *Using opioid agonists safely.*)

## Pharmacokinetics

A person may receive an opioid agonist by any administration route, although inhalation administration is uncommon. Oral doses are absorbed readily from the GI tract; however, transmucosal and intrathecal opiates are faster-acting.

## Speedy delivery

Opioid agonists administered I.V. provide the most rapid (almost immediate) and reliable pain relief. The subcutaneous (subQ) and I.M. routes may result in delayed absorption, especially in patients with poor circulation.

### Distribution

Opioid agonists are distributed widely throughout body tissues. They have a relatively low plasma protein-binding capacity (30% to 35%).

### Metabolism

Opioid agonists are metabolized extensively in the liver. For example, meperidine is metabolized to normeperidine, a toxic metabolite with a longer half-life than meperidine. This metabolite accumulates in patients with renal failure and may lead to CNS excitation and seizures. Administration of meperidine for more than

**Safe and sound**

## Using opioid agonists safely

Be aware that morphine sulfate ($MSO_4$) can be confused with magnesium sulfate ($MgSO_4$). To avoid confusing the drugs, never use abbreviations.

48 hours increases the risk of neurotoxicity and seizures from buildup of normeperidine.

### Excretion

Metabolites are excreted by the kidneys. A small amount is excreted in stool through the biliary tract.

## Pharmacodynamics

Opioid agonists reduce pain by binding to opiate receptor sites (mu receptors and $N$-methyl-D-aspartate receptors) in the peripheral nervous system and the CNS. When these drugs stimulate the opiate receptors, they mimic the effects of endorphins (naturally occurring opiates that are part of the body's own pain relief system). This receptor-site binding produces the therapeutic effects of analgesia and cough suppression. It also produces adverse reactions, such as respiratory depression and constipation.

### Smooth operator

Opioid agonists, especially morphine, affect the smooth muscle of the GI and genitourinary tracts (the organs of the reproductive and urinary systems). This causes contraction of the bladder and ureters. It also slows intestinal peristalsis (rhythmic contractions that move food along the digestive tract), resulting in constipation, a common adverse effect of opiates.

### Too much of a good thing

These drugs also cause blood vessels to dilate, especially in the face, head, and neck. In addition, they suppress the cough center in the brain, producing antitussive effects and causing constriction of the bronchial muscles. These effects can produce adverse reactions if excessive. For example, if the blood vessels dilate too much, hypotension can occur.

## Pharmacotherapeutics

Opioid agonists are prescribed to relieve severe pain in acute, chronic, and terminal illnesses. They also reduce anxiety before a patient receives anesthesia and are sometimes prescribed to control diarrhea and suppress coughing. (See *How opioid agonists control pain,* page 104.)

Methadone is used for temporary maintenance of narcotic addiction. Other opioids and remifentanil are used for the induction and maintenance of general anesthesia.

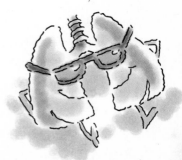

Ahhh. I can breathe easier with morphine.

*Now I get it!*

# How opioid agonists control pain

Opioid agonists, such as meperidine, inhibit pain transmission by mimicking the body's natural pain control mechanisms.

### Where neurons meet
In the dorsal horn of the spinal cord, peripheral pain neurons meet central nervous system (CNS) neurons. At the synapse, the pain neuron releases substance P (a pain neurotransmitter). This agent helps transfer pain impulses to the CNS neurons that carry those impulses to the brain.

### Taking up space
In theory, the spinal interneurons respond to stimulation from the descending neurons of the CNS by releasing endogenous opiates. These opiates bind to the peripheral pain neuron to inhibit release of substance P and to retard the transmission of pain impulses.

### Stopping substance P
Synthetic opiates supplement this pain-blocking effect by binding with free opiate receptors to inhibit the release of substance P. Opiates also alter consciousness of pain, but how this mechanism works remains unknown.

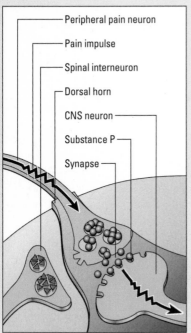

- Peripheral pain neuron
- Pain impulse
- Spinal interneuron
- Dorsal horn
- CNS neuron
- Substance P
- Synapse

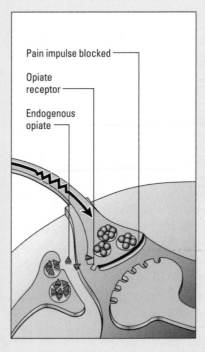

- Pain impulse blocked
- Opiate receptor
- Endogenous opiate

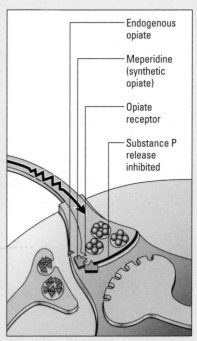

- Endogenous opiate
- Meperidine (synthetic opiate)
- Opiate receptor
- Substance P release inhibited

## Cardio-assistance

Morphine relieves shortness of breath in patients with pulmonary edema (fluid in the lungs) and left-sided heart failure (inability of the heart to pump enough blood to meet the needs of the body). It does this by dilating peripheral blood vessels, keeping more blood in the periphery, and decreasing cardiac preload.

**Warning!**

## Adverse reactions to opioid agonists

One of the most common adverse reactions to opioid agonists is decreased rate and depth of breathing that worsens as the dose of opioid is increased. This may cause periodic, irregular breathing or trigger asthmatic attacks in susceptible patients.

Other adverse reactions include:
• flushing

• orthostatic hypotension
• pupil constriction.
     Adverse reactions to meperidine include:
• tremors
• palpitations
• tachycardia
• delirium
• seizures.

## Drug interactions

• The use of opioid agonists with other drugs that also decrease respirations, such as alcohol, sedatives, hypnotics, and anesthetics, increases the patient's risk of severe respiratory depression.
• Taking tricyclic antidepressants, phenothiazines, or anticholinergics with opioid agonists may cause severe constipation and urine retention.
• Drugs that may affect opioid analgesic activity include amitriptyline, diazepam, phenytoin, protease inhibitors, and rifampin.
• Drugs that may be affected by opioid analgesics include carbamazepine, warfarin, beta-adrenergic blockers, and calcium channel blockers. (See *Adverse reactions to opioid agonists*.)

# Mixed opioid agonist-antagonists

*Mixed opioid agonist-antagonists* attempt to relieve pain while reducing toxic effects and dependency. The mixed opioid agonist-antagonists include:
• buprenorphine
• butorphanol
• nalbuphine
• pentazocine hydrochloride (combined with pentazocine lactate, naloxone, aspirin, or acetaminophen).

## No free ride

Originally, mixed opioid agonist-antagonists appeared to have less abuse potential than the pure opioid agonists. However, butorphanol and pentazocine have reportedly caused dependence. Also,

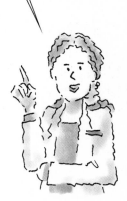

Mixed opioid agonist-antagonists attempt to relieve pain while reducing toxic effects and dependency.

patients with chronic pain who are taking an opioid agonist shouldn't take a mixed opioid agonist-antagonist with it because of the risk of withdrawal symptoms.

## Pharmacokinetics

Absorption of mixed opioid agonist-antagonists occurs rapidly from parenteral sites. These drugs are distributed to most body tissues and also cross the placental barrier. They're metabolized in the liver and excreted primarily by the kidneys, although more than 10% of a butorphanol dose and a small amount of a pentazocine dose are excreted in stool.

## Pharmacodynamics

The exact mechanism of action of the mixed opioid agonist-antagonists isn't known. However, researchers believe that these drugs weakly antagonize the effects of morphine, meperidine, and other opiates at one of the opioid receptor sites, while exerting agonistic effects at other opioid receptor sites.

### No rush to go

Buprenorphine binds with receptors in the CNS, altering perception of and emotional response to pain through an unknown mechanism. It seems to release slowly from binding sites, producing a longer duration of action than the other drugs in this class.

### Don't get emotional

The site of action of butorphanol may be opiate receptors in the limbic system (the part of the brain involved in emotion).

Like pentazocine, butorphanol also acts on pulmonary circulation, increasing pulmonary vascular resistance (the resistance in the blood vessels of the lungs that the right ventricle must pump against). Both drugs also increase blood pressure and the workload of the heart.

## Pharmacotherapeutics

Mixed opioid agonist-antagonists are used as analgesia during childbirth and are also administered postoperatively.

### Independence day

Mixed opioid agonist-antagonists are sometimes prescribed in place of opioid agonists because they have a lower risk of drug dependence. Mixed opioid agonist-antagonists are also less likely to cause respiratory depression and constipation, although they can

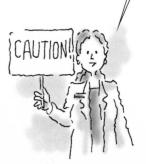

Patients with a history of opioid abuse shouldn't receive mixed opioid agonist-antagonists.

produce some adverse reactions. (See *Adverse reactions to opioid agonist-antagonists.*)

## Drug interactions

Increased CNS depression and an accompanying decrease in respiratory rate and depth may result if mixed opioid agonist-antagonists are administered to patients taking other CNS depressants, such as barbiturates and alcohol.

### Clean and sober?

Patients who abuse opioids shouldn't receive mixed opioid agonist-antagonists because these drugs can cause symptoms of withdrawal.

Mixed opioid agonist-antagonists are listed as pregnancy risk category C drugs; safety and use in breast-feeding women haven't been established.

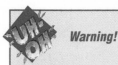

**Warning!**

## Adverse reactions to opioid agonist-antagonists

The most common adverse reactions to opioid agonist-antagonists include nausea, vomiting, light-headedness, sedation, and euphoria.

# Opioid antagonists

*Opioid antagonists* have a greater attraction for opiate receptors than opioids do; however, they don't stimulate those receptors. As a result, opioid antagonists block the effects of opioid drugs, enkephalins, and endorphins.

Opioid antagonists include:
- naloxone
- naltrexone.

## Pharmacokinetics

Naloxone is administered I.M., subQ, or I.V. Naltrexone is administered orally in tablet or liquid form. Both drugs are metabolized by the liver and excreted by the kidneys.

## Pharmacodynamics

Opioid antagonists act by occupying opiate receptor sites, displacing opioids attached to opiate receptors, and preventing opioids from binding at these sites. This process, known as *competitive inhibition,* effectively blocks the effects of opioids.

## Pharmacotherapeutics

Naloxone is the drug of choice for managing an opioid overdose. It reverses respiratory depression and sedation and helps stabilize the patient's vital signs within seconds after administration.

## Managing naltrexone therapy for drug addiction

To prevent acute withdrawal during treatment for opioid addiction, plan to use naltrexone as part of a comprehensive rehabilitation program. Keep in mind the following guidelines:
• Don't give naltrexone until a negative naloxone challenge test is obtained.
• Don't give naltrexone to a patient who's receiving an opioid agonist, addicted to an opioid agonist, or in the acute phase of opioid withdrawal because acute withdrawal symptoms may occur or worsen.
• For a patient who's addicted to a short-acting opioid, such as heroin or meperidine, wait at least 7 days after the last opioid dose before starting naltrexone.
• For a patient who's addicted to a longer-acting opioid, such as methadone, wait at least 10 days after the last opioid dose before starting naltrexone.
• During naltrexone therapy, be alert for signs of opioid withdrawal, such as drug craving, confusion, drowsiness, visual hallucinations, abdominal pain, vomiting, diarrhea, fever, chills, tachypnea, diaphoresis, salivation, lacrimation, runny nose, and mydriasis.

*Warning!*

## Adverse reactions to naloxone and naltrexone

Naloxone and naltrexone produce different adverse reactions.

**Naloxone**
Naloxone may cause nausea, vomiting and, occasionally, hypertension and tachycardia. An unconscious patient returned to consciousness abruptly after naloxone administration may hyperventilate and experience tremors.

**Naltrexone**
Naltrexone can cause a variety of adverse reactions, including:
• edema, hypertension, palpitations, phlebitis, and shortness of breath
• anxiety, depression, disorientation, dizziness, headache, and nervousness
• anorexia, diarrhea or constipation, nausea, thirst, and vomiting
• urinary frequency
• liver toxicity.

Naloxone also reverses the analgesic effects of opioids. Therefore, after naloxone administration, the patient may complain of pain or even experience withdrawal symptoms.

### Kicking the habit

Naltrexone is used along with psychotherapy or counseling to treat drug abuse; however, the recipient must first have gone through a detoxification program. Otherwise, if the patient receives naltrexone while he still has opioids in his body, acute withdrawal symptoms may occur. (See *Managing naltrexone therapy for drug addiction.*)

## Drug interactions

Naloxone produces no significant drug interactions. Naltrexone will cause withdrawal symptoms if given to a patient receiving an opioid agonist or to an opioid addict. (See *Adverse reactions to naloxone and naltrexone.*)

# Anesthetic drugs

*Anesthetic drugs* can be divided into three groups—general anesthetics, local anesthetics, and topical anesthetics.

### Inhale or inject?

General anesthetic drugs are further subdivided into two main types: those given by inhalation and those given intravenously.

# Inhalation anesthetics

Commonly used general anesthetics given by inhalation include:
- desflurane
- enflurane
- halothane
- isoflurane
- nitrous oxide
- sevoflurane.

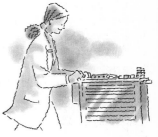

Anesthetic drugs can be general, local, and topical. So many choices!

## Pharmacokinetics

The absorption and elimination rates of an anesthetic are governed by its solubility in blood. *Inhalation anesthetics* enter the blood from the lungs and are distributed to other tissues. Distribution is most rapid to organs with high blood flow, such as the brain, liver, kidneys, and heart. Inhalation anesthetics are eliminated primarily by the lungs; enflurane, halothane, and sevoflurane are also eliminated by the liver. Metabolites are excreted in the urine.

## Pharmacodynamics

Inhalation anesthetics work primarily by depressing the CNS, producing loss of consciousness, loss of responsiveness to sensory stimulation (including pain), and muscle relaxation. They also affect other organ systems.

## Pharmacotherapeutics

Inhalation anesthetics are used for surgery because they offer more precise and rapid control of depth of anesthesia than injection anesthetics do. These anesthetics, which are liquids at room temperature, require a vaporizer and special delivery system for safe use.

Of the inhalation anesthetics available, desflurane, isoflurane, and nitrous oxide are the most commonly used.

*Stop signs*

Inhalation anesthetics are contraindicated in the patient with known hypersensitivity to the drug, a liver disorder, or malignant hyperthermia (a potentially fatal complication of anesthesia characterized by skeletal muscle rigidity and high fever). (See *Unusual but serious reaction* and *Adverse reactions to inhalation anesthetics*, page 110.)

*Safe and sound*

# Unusual but serious reaction

Malignant hyperthermia, characterized by a sudden and often lethal increase in body temperature, is a serious and uncommon reaction to inhalation anesthetics. It occurs in genetically susceptible patients only and may result from a failure in calcium uptake by muscle cells. The skeletal muscle relaxant dantrolene is used to treat this condition.

### Warning!

## Adverse reactions to inhalation anesthetics

The most common adverse reaction to inhalation anesthetics is an exaggerated patient response to a normal dose.

**Waking up**

After surgery, a patient may experience reactions similar to those seen with other central nervous system depressants, including depression of breathing and circulation, confusion, sedation, nausea, vomiting, ataxia, and hypothermia.

**It happens with halothane**

Rarely, liver necrosis develops several days after halothane use and occurs most commonly with multiple drug exposures. Symptoms include rash, fever, jaundice, nausea, vomiting, eosinophilia, and alterations in liver function.

## Drug interactions

The most important drug interactions involving inhalation anesthetics occur with other CNS, cardiac, or respiratory-depressant drugs. Inhalation anesthetics can cause CNS depression, cardiac arrhythmias, or depressed respirations, resulting in compromised patient status.

# Intravenous anesthetics

*Intravenous anesthetics* are typically used when the patient requires general anesthesia for just a short period such as during outpatient surgery. They're also used to promote rapid induction of anesthesia or to supplement inhalation anesthetics.

## Main options

The drugs used as intravenous anesthetics are:
- barbiturates (methohexital, thiopental)
- benzodiazepines (midazolam)
- dissociatives (ketamine)
- hypnotics (etomidate, propofol)
- opiates (fentanyl, sufentanil).

## Pharmacokinetics

Intravenous anesthetics are lipid-soluble and well-distributed throughout the body, crossing the placental barrier and entering breast milk. These drugs are metabolized in the liver and excreted in the urine.

## Pharmacodynamics

Opiates work by occupying sites on specialized receptors scattered throughout the CNS and by modifying the release of neurotransmitters from sensory nerves entering the CNS. Ketamine acts directly on the cortex and limbic system of the brain, producing a profound sense of dissociation from the environment.

*Getting sleepy*

Barbiturates, benzodiazepines, and etomidate seem to enhance responses to the CNS neurotransmitter, gamma-aminobutyric acid. This inhibits the brain's response to stimulation of the reticular activating system, the area of the brain stem that controls alertness. Barbiturates also depress the excitability of CNS neurons.

## Pharmacotherapeutics

Because of the short duration of action of intravenous anesthetics, they're used in brief surgical procedures such as outpatient surgery.

*Going solo*

Barbiturates are used alone in surgery that isn't expected to be painful and as adjuncts to other drugs in more extensive procedures. Benzodiazepines produce sedation and amnesia, but not pain relief.

Etomidate is used to induce anesthesia and to supplement low-potency inhalation anesthetics such as nitrous oxide. The opiates provide pain relief and supplement other anesthetics.

## Drug interactions

I.V. anesthetics, particularly ketamine, can produce a variety of drug interactions.
• Verapamil enhances the anesthetic effects of etomidate, causing respiratory depression and apnea.
• Administering ketamine together with halothane increases the risk of hypotension and reduces cardiac output (the amount of blood pumped by the heart each minute).
• Giving ketamine and nondepolarizing drugs together increases neuromuscular effects, resulting in prolonged respiratory depression.
• Using barbiturates or opioids with ketamine may prolong recovery time after anesthesia.
• Ketamine plus theophylline may promote seizures.

## Adverse reactions to I.V. anesthetics

**Ketamine**
• Prolonged recovery
• Irrational behavior
• Excitement
• Disorientation
• Delirium, hallucinations
• Increased heart rate
• Hypertension

**Propofol**
• Respiratory depression
• Hiccups, coughing, muscle-twitching

**Thiopental**
• Respiratory depression
• Hiccups, coughing, muscle-twitching
• Depressed cardiac function and peripheral dilation

**Etomidate**
• Hiccups, coughing, muscle-twitching

**Fentanyl**
• Central nervous system (CNS) and respiratory depression
• Hypoventilation
• Cardiac arrhythmias

**Midazolam**
• CNS and respiratory depression
• Hypotension
• Dizziness

*Now I get it!*

## Amides and esters

Amide anesthetics are local anesthetics that have nitrogen as part of their molecular makeup. They include:
• bupivacaine
• lidocaine
• mepivacaine
• prilocaine
• ropivacaine.

**Give them oxygen**
Ester anesthetics have oxygen, not nitrogen, as part of their molecular makeup. They include:
• chloroprocaine
• procaine
• tetracaine.

• Ketamine and thyroid hormones may cause hypertension and tachycardia (rapid heart rate). (See *Adverse reactions to I.V. anesthetics.*)

# Local anesthetics

*Local anesthetics* are administered to prevent or relieve pain in a specific area of the body. In addition, these drugs are often used as an alternative to general anesthesia for elderly or debilitated patients.

*Chain gang*

Local anesthetics may be:
• "amide" drugs (with nitrogen in the molecular chain, such as bupivacaine, levobupivacaine, lidocaine, mepivacaine, prilocaine, and ropivacaine)
• "ester" drugs (with oxygen in the molecular chain, such as chloroprocaine, cocaine, procaine, and tetracaine). (See *Amides and esters.*)

## Pharmacokinetics

Absorption of local anesthetics varies widely, but distribution occurs throughout the body. Esters and amides undergo different types of metabolism, but both yield metabolites that are excreted in the urine.

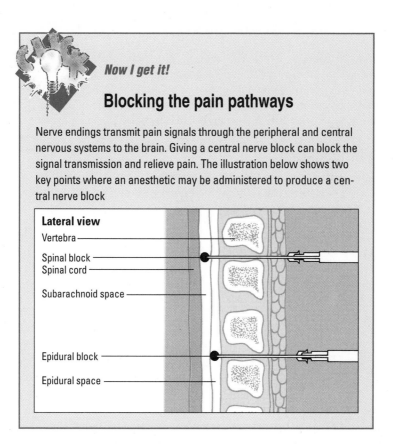

**Now I get it!**

## Blocking the pain pathways

Nerve endings transmit pain signals through the peripheral and central nervous systems to the brain. Giving a central nerve block can block the signal transmission and relieve pain. The illustration below shows two key points where an anesthetic may be administered to produce a central nerve block

**Lateral view**
Vertebra
Spinal block
Spinal cord
Subarachnoid space
Epidural block
Epidural space

## Pharmacodynamics

Local anesthetics block nerve impulses at the point of contact in all kinds of nerves. They accumulate, causing the nerve cell membrane to expand. As the membrane expands, the cell loses its ability to depolarize, which is necessary for impulse transmission. (See *Blocking the pain pathways*.)

## Pharmacotherapeutics

Local anesthetics are used to prevent and relieve pain from medical procedures, disease, or injury. Local anesthetics may also be used for severe pain that topical anesthetics or analgesics can't relieve.

*Staying local*

Local anesthetics are usually preferred to general anesthetics for surgery in an elderly or debilitated patient or a patient with a disorder that affects respiratory function, such as chronic obstructive pulmonary disease and myasthenia gravis.

Tighten up

For some procedures, a local anesthetic is combined with a drug that constricts blood vessels, such as epinephrine. Vasoconstriction helps control local bleeding and reduces absorption of the anesthetic. Reduced absorption prolongs the anesthetic's action at the site and limits its distribution and CNS effects.

## Drug interactions

Local anesthetics produce few significant interactions with other drugs. They can, however, produce adverse reactions. (See *Adverse reactions to local anesthetics.*)

# Topical anesthetics

*Topical anesthetics* are applied directly to intact skin or mucous membranes. All topical anesthetics are used to prevent or relieve minor pain.

All together now

Some injectable local anesthetics, such as lidocaine and tetracaine, are also topically effective. In addition, some topical anesthetics, such as lidocaine, are combined in other products.

## Pharmacokinetics

Topical anesthetics produce little systemic absorption, except for the application of cocaine to mucous membranes. However, systemic absorption may occur if the patient receives frequent or high-dose applications to the eye or large areas of burned or injured skin.

Tetracaine and other esters are metabolized extensively in the blood and to a lesser extent in the liver. Dibucaine, lidocaine, and other amides are metabolized primarily in the liver. Both types of topical anesthetics are excreted in the urine.

## Pharmacodynamics

Benzocaine, butacaine, cocaine, dyclonine, and pramoxine produce topical anesthesia by blocking nerve impulse transmission. They accumulate in the nerve cell membrane, causing it to expand and lose its ability to depolarize, thus blocking impulse transmission. Dibucaine, lidocaine, and tetracaine may also block impulse transmission across the nerve cell membranes.

 *Warning!*

## Adverse reactions to local anesthetics

Dose-related central nervous system (CNS) reactions include anxiety, apprehension, restlessness, nervousness, disorientation, confusion, dizziness, blurred vision, tremors, twitching, shivering, and seizures. Dose-related cardiovascular reactions may include myocardial depression, bradycardia (slow heart rate), arrhythmias, hypotension, cardiovascular collapse, and cardiac arrest.

**All the rest**
Local anesthetic solutions that contain vasoconstrictors such as epinephrine can also produce CNS and cardiovascular reactions, including anxiety, dizziness, headache, restlessness, tremors, palpitations, tachycardia, angina, and hypertension.

## Sensory overload

The aromatic compounds, such as benzyl alcohol and clove oil, appear to stimulate nerve endings. This stimulation causes counterirritation that interferes with pain perception.

## A chilling ending

Ethyl chloride spray superficially freezes the tissue, stimulating the cold-sensation receptors and blocking the nerve endings in the frozen area. Menthol selectively stimulates the sensory nerve endings for cold, causing a cool sensation and some local pain relief.

### Pharmacotherapeutics

Topical anesthetics are used to:
• relieve or prevent pain, especially minor burn pain
• relieve itching and irritation
• anesthetize an area before an injection is given
• numb mucosal surfaces before a tube, such as a urinary catheter, is inserted
• alleviate sore throat or mouth pain when used in a spray or solution.

## All eyes and ears

Tetracaine is also used as a topical anesthetic for the eye. Benzocaine is used with other drugs in several ear preparations.

### Drug interactions

Few interactions with other drugs occur with topical anesthetics because they aren't absorbed well into the systemic circulation. (See *Adverse reactions to topical anesthetics*.)

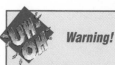

**Warning!**

## Adverse reactions to topical anesthetics

Topical anesthetics can cause several different adverse reactions.
• Benzyl alcohol can cause topical reactions such as skin irritation.
• Refrigerants, such as ethyl chloride, may produce frostbite where they've been applied.
• Topical anesthetics can cause a hypersensitivity reaction, including a rash, itching, hives, swelling of the mouth and throat, and breathing difficulty.

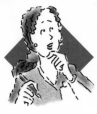

# Quick quiz

**1.** How does the topical anesthetic benzocaine relieve sunburn pain?

    A.    It numbs the skin surface, decreasing the perception of pain.

    B.    It freezes the skin, which prevents nerve impulse transmission.

    C.    It blocks nerve impulse transmission by preventing nerve cell depolarization.

    D.    It stimulates nerve endings, interfering with the perception of pain.

*Answer:*   C. Benzocaine prevents nerve cell depolarization, thus blocking nerve impulse transmission and relieving pain.

**2.** Which adverse reaction is a patient most likely to experience postsurgery after receiving general anesthesia?

    A.    Nausea and vomiting

    B.    Seizures

    C.    Cyanosis

    D.    Fever

*Answer:*   A. After surgery involving general anesthesia, a patient is most likely to experience adverse reactions similar to those produced by other CNS-depressant drugs, including nausea and vomiting.

**3.** Before administering buprenorphine, the nurse asks the patient if he has used opiates. That's because administering a mixed opioid agonist-antagonist to a patient dependent on opioid agonists may cause which reaction?

    A.    Hypersensitivity reaction

    B.    Withdrawal symptoms

    C.    Urinary incontinence

    D.    Respiratory depression

*Answer:*   B. Because they can counteract the effects of opioid agonists, mixed opioid agonist-antagonists can cause withdrawal symptoms in patients dependent on opioid agonists.

**4.** The drug commonly prescribed to treat an opioid overdose is:
A. butorphanol.
B. naloxone.
C. pentazocine.
D. ketamine.

*Answer:* B. Naloxone is the drug of choice for managing opioid overdose.

**5.** What are the most common adverse reactions to aspirin?
A. Increased rate and depth of respirations
B. Confusion, sedation, and hypothermia
C. Dizziness and vision changes
D. Nausea, vomiting, and GI distress

*Answer:* D. Aspirin most commonly produces adverse GI reactions, such as nausea, vomiting, and GI distress.

**6.** Desflurane is which type of anesthetic?
A. Opioid
B. Local
C. Topical
D. General

*Answer:* D. Desflurane is a commonly used general anesthetic that's administered by inhalation.

**7.** Topical anesthetics are used:
A. as an alternative to general anesthesia for elderly or debilitated patients.
B. to numb mucosal surfaces before tube insertion.
C. when anesthesia is needed for only a short period.
D. to promote rapid induction of anesthesia.

*Answer:* B. Topical anesthetics are used to numb mucosal surfaces as well as relieve or prevent pain, relieve itching and irritation, anesthetize an area for an injection, and alleviate sore throat or mouth pain.

## Scoring

☆☆☆   If you answered all seven items correctly, bravo! You're a pain
medication powerhouse.

☆☆   If you answered five or six items correctly, fabulous! For you, this
chapter was painless.

☆   If you answered fewer than five items correctly, hey, don't give
up! Remember: No pain, no gain.

# Cardiovascular drugs

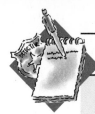

## Just the facts

In this chapter, you'll learn:

♦ classes of drugs used to treat cardiovascular disorders

♦ uses and varying actions of these drugs

♦ how these drugs are absorbed, distributed, metabolized, and excreted

♦ drug interactions and adverse reactions to these drugs.

## Drugs and the cardiovascular system

The heart, arteries, veins, and lymphatics make up the cardiovascular system. These structures transport life-supporting oxygen and nutrients to cells, remove metabolic waste products, and carry hormones from one part of the body to another. Because this system performs such vital functions, a problem with the heart or blood vessels can seriously affect a person's health.

Types of drugs used to improve cardiovascular function include:
- inotropic
- antiarrhythmic
- antianginal
- antihypertensive
- diuretic
- antilipemic.

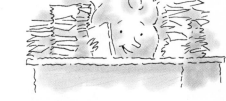

Sometimes it seems like my work is never done!

## Inotropics

Inotropic drugs, such as cardiac glycosides and phosphodiesterase (PDE) inhibitors, increase the force of the heart's contractions. In other words, the drugs have what's known as a *posi-*

*tive inotropic effect.* (Inotropic means affecting the force or energy of muscular contractions.)

Cardiac glycosides also slow the heart rate (called a *negative chronotropic effect*) and slow electrical impulse conduction through the atrioventricular (AV) node (called a *negative dromotropic effect*).

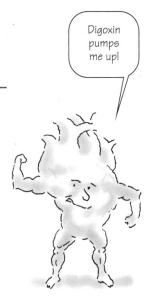

Digoxin pumps me up!

# Cardiac glycosides

*Cardiac glycosides* are a group of drugs derived from digitalis, a substance that occurs naturally in foxglove plants and in certain toads. The most frequently used cardiac glycoside is *digoxin.*

## Pharmacokinetics (how drugs circulate)

The intestinal absorption of digoxin varies greatly; the capsules are absorbed most efficiently, followed by the elixir form, and then tablets. Digoxin is distributed widely throughout the body, with highest concentrations in the heart muscle, liver, and kidneys. Digoxin binds poorly to plasma proteins.

In most patients, a small amount of digoxin is metabolized in the liver and gut by bacteria. This effect varies and may be substantial in some people. Most of the drug is excreted by the kidneys as unchanged drug. (See *Load that dose.*)

## Pharmacodynamics (how drugs act)

Digoxin is used to treat heart failure because it strengthens the contraction of the ventricles by boosting intracellular calcium at the cell membrane, enabling stronger heart contractions.

Digoxin may also enhance the movement of calcium into the myocardial cells and stimulate the release, or block the reuptake, of norepinephrine at the adrenergic nerve terminal.

### Stop that impulse

Digoxin acts on the central nervous system (CNS) to slow the heart rate, thus making it useful for treating supraventricular arrhythmias (abnormal heart rhythms that originate above the bundle branches of the heart's conduction system), such as atrial fibrillation and atrial flutter. It also increases the refractory period (the period when the cells of the conduction system can't conduct an impulse).

## Pharmacotherapeutics (how drugs are used)

In addition to treating heart failure and supraventricular arrhythmias, digoxin is used to treat paroxysmal atrial tachycardia (an ar-

---

## Load that dose

Because digoxin has a long half-life, a loading dose must be given to a patient who requires immediate drug effects, as in supraventricular arrhythmia.

By giving a larger initial dose, a minimum effective concentration of the drug in the blood may be reached faster.

*Note:* Avoid giving a loading dose to a patient with heart failure to avoid toxicity.

rhythmia marked by brief periods of tachycardia that alternate with brief periods of sinus rhythm).

## Drug interactions

Many drugs can interact with digoxin.
• Antacids, barbiturates, cholestyramine resin, kaolin and pectin, neomycin, metoclopramide, rifampin, and sulfasalazine reduce the therapeutic effects of digoxin.
• Calcium preparations, quinidine, verapamil, cyclosporine, tetracycline, clarithromycin, propafenone, amiodarone, spironolactone, hydroxychloroquine, erythromycin, itraconazole, and omeprazole increase the risk of digoxin toxicity.
• Amphotericin B, potassium-wasting diuretics, and steroids taken with digoxin may cause hypokalemia (low potassium levels) and increase the risk of digoxin toxicity.
• Beta-adrenergic blockers and calcium channel blockers taken with digoxin may cause an excessively slow heart rate and arrhythmias.
• Succinylcholine and thyroid preparations increase the risk of arrhythmias when they're taken with digoxin.
• St. John's wort, an herbal preparation, can increase digoxin levels and risk of toxicity.

Digoxin can also produce adverse reactions, mostly involving digoxin toxicity. (See *Recognizing signs and symptoms of digoxin toxicity*, page 122, and *Adverse reactions to cardiac glycosides.*)

*Warning!*

## Adverse reactions to cardiac glycosides

Because cardiac glycosides have a narrow therapeutic index (margin of safety), they may produce digoxin toxicity. To prevent digoxin toxicity, the dosage should be individualized based on the patient's serum digoxin concentration.

Adverse reactions to digoxin include:
• rash
• fever
• eosinophilia
• arrhythmias.

*Safe and sound*

## Recognizing signs and symptoms of digoxin toxicity

Digoxin toxicity usually produces cardiac, gastrointestinal, and neurologic signs and symptoms. To prevent severe or even life-threatening effects, be prepared to recognize the signs and symptoms listed below. Also assess the patient for the most common early indicators of toxicity, which are usually GI-related.

**Cardiac**
- Accelerated junctional rhythms
- Atrial tachycardia with atrioventricular (AV) block
- Second-degree AV block (Wenckebach)
- Sinoatrial arrest or block
- Third-degree AV block (complete)
- Ventricular arrhythmias

**Gastrointestinal**
- Abdominal pain
- Anorexia
- Diarrhea
- Nausea
- Vomiting

**Neurologic**
- Blue-yellow color blindness
- Blurred vision
- Colored dots in vision
- Coma
- Confusion
- Depression
- Disorientation
- Flickering lights
- Headache
- Insomnia
- Irritability
- Lethargy
- Personality changes
- Psychosis
- Restlessness
- Seizures
- White halos on dark objects

# PDE inhibitors

*PDE inhibitors* are typically used for short-term management of heart failure or long-term management in patients awaiting heart transplant surgery. Specific PDE inhibitors are inamrinone and milrinone.

## Pharmacokinetics

Administered I.V., inamrinone is distributed rapidly, metabolized by the liver, and excreted by the kidneys. It's rarely used because secondary thrombocytopenia may occur as an adverse reaction.

Ready for action

Milrinone is also administered I.V. It's distributed rapidly and excreted by the kidneys, primarily as unchanged drug.

**Warning!**

## Adverse reactions to PDE inhibitors

Adverse reactions to phosphodiesterase (PDE) inhibitors are uncommon, but the likelihood increases significantly when a patient is on prolonged therapy.
  Adverse reactions may include:
• arrhythmias

• nausea and vomiting
• headache
• fever
• chest pain
• hypokalemia
• thrombocytopenia (especially
with inamrinone)
• mild increase in heart rate.

## Pharmacodynamics

PDE inhibitors improve cardiac output by strengthening contractions. These drugs are thought to help move calcium into the cardiac cell or to increase calcium storage in the sarcoplasmic reticulum. By directly relaxing vascular smooth muscle, they also decrease peripheral vascular resistance (afterload) and the amount
of blood returning to the heart (preload).

## Pharmacotherapeutics

Inamrinone and milrinone are used to manage heart failure in patients who haven't responded adequately to treatment with cardiac glycosides, diuretics, or vasodilators. Prolonged use of these
drugs may increase the patient's risk of complications and death.
(See *Adverse reactions to PDE inhibitors.*)

## Drug interactions

• PDE inhibitors may interact with disopyramide, causing hypotension.
• Because PDE inhibitors reduce serum potassium levels, taking
them with a potassium-wasting diuretic may lead to hypokalemia.

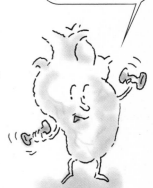

Besides
pumping iron,
cardiac output
can be improved
with PDE
inhibitors.

# Antiarrhythmic drugs

*Antiarrhythmic drugs* are used to treat arrhythmias, disturbances
of the normal heart rhythm.

## Troublemakers

Unfortunately, many antiarrhythmics are also capable of worsening or causing the very arrhythmias they're supposed to treat. The benefits need to be weighed carefully against the risks of antiarrhythmic therapy.

## A touch of class

Antiarrhythmics are categorized into four classes:
- I (which includes classes IA, IB, and IC)
- II
- III
- IV.

Class I antiarrhythmics consist of sodium channel blockers. This is the largest group of antiarrhythmics. Class I agents are frequently subdivided into classes IA, IB, and IC. One drug, adenosine (an AV nodal blocking agent used to treat paroxysmal supraventricular tachycardia), doesn't fall into any of these classes.

The mechanisms of action of antiarrhythmics vary widely, and a few drugs exhibit properties common to more than one class.

# Class IA antiarrhythmics

*Class IA antiarrhythmics* are used to treat a wide variety of atrial and ventricular arrhythmias. Class IA antiarrhythmics include:
- disopyramide
- procainamide
- quinidine (sulfate and gluconate).

## Pharmacokinetics

When administered orally, class IA drugs are rapidly absorbed and metabolized. Because they work so quickly, sustained-release forms of these drugs were developed to help maintain therapeutic levels.

## A shot to the head

These drugs are distributed through all body tissues. Quinidine, however, is the only one that crosses the blood-brain barrier.

All class IA antiarrhythmics are metabolized in the liver and are excreted unchanged by the kidneys. Acidic urine increases the excretion of quinidine.

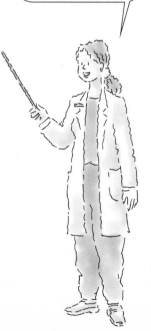

Because class IA antiarrhythmics work so quickly, sustained-release forms of the drugs were created to maintain therapeutic levels.

## Pharmacodynamics

Class IA antiarrhythmics control arrhythmias by altering the myocardial cell membrane and interfering with autonomic nervous system control of pacemaker cells.

### No (para)sympathy

Class IA antiarrhythmics also block parasympathetic stimulation of the sinoatrial (SA) and AV nodes. Because stimulation of the parasympathetic nervous system causes the heart rate to slow down, drugs that block the parasympathetic nervous system increase the conduction rate of the AV node.

### Rhythmic risks

This increase in the conduction rate can produce dangerous increases in the ventricular heart rate if rapid atrial activity is present, as in a patient with atrial fibrillation. In turn, the increased ventricular heart rate can offset the ability of the antiarrhythmics to convert atrial arrhythmias to a regular rhythm.

## Pharmacotherapeutics

Class IA antiarrhythmics are prescribed to treat such arrhythmias as premature ventricular contractions, ventricular tachycardia, atrial fibrillation, atrial flutter, and paroxysmal atrial tachycardia.

## Drug interactions

Class IA antiarrhythmics can interact with other drugs:
• Disopyramide taken with macrolide antibiotics, such as clarithromycin and erythromycin, increases the patient's risk of developing a prolonged QT interval. In turn, this may lead to an increased risk of arrhythmias, especially polymorphic ventricular tachycardia.
• Disopyramide plus verapamil may increase myocardial depression and should be avoided in patients with heart failure.
• Other antiarrhythmics, such as beta-adrenergic blockers, increase the risk of arrhythmias.
• Quinidine plus neuromuscular blockers may cause increased skeletal muscle relaxation.
• Quinidine increases the risk of digoxin toxicity.
• Rifampin, phenytoin, and phenobarbital can reduce the effects of quinidine and disopyramide.

   GI symptoms are a common adverse reaction to class IA antiarrhythmics. (See *Adverse reactions to class IA antiarrhythmics*.)

**Warning!**

## Adverse reactions to class IA antiarrhythmics

Class IA antiarrhythmics, especially quinidine, may produce GI symptoms, such as diarrhea, cramping, nausea, vomiting, anorexia, and a bitter taste.

**Dramatic irony**
Ironically, not only do class IA antiarrhythmics treat arrhythmias, but they can also induce arrhythmias, especially conduction delays that may worsen existing heart blocks.

# Class IB antiarrhythmics

Class IB antiarrhythmics are used for treating acute ventricular arrhythmias. They include:
- lidocaine
- mexiletine.

## Pharmacokinetics

Mexiletine is absorbed from the GI tract after oral administration. Lidocaine is administered I.V. to prevent rapid metabolism by the liver after it enters the hepatic portal circulation.

*All bound up?*

Lidocaine is distributed widely throughout the body, including the brain. Lidocaine and mexiletine are moderately bound to plasma proteins. (Remember, only that portion of a drug that's unbound can produce a response.)

Class IB antiarrhythmics are metabolized in the liver and excreted in urine. Mexiletine also appears in breast milk.

## Pharmacodynamics

Class IB drugs work by blocking the rapid influx of sodium ions during the depolarization phase of the heart's depolarization-repolarization cycle. This decreases the refractory period, which reduces the risk of arrhythmia. (See *How lidocaine works*.)

*Make a IB-line for the ventricle*

Because class IB antiarrhythmics especially affect the Purkinje fibers (fibers in the conducting system of the heart) and myocardial cells in the ventricles, they're used to treat only ventricular arrhythmias.

## Pharmacotherapeutics

Class IB antiarrhythmics are used to treat ventricular ectopic beats, ventricular tachycardia, and ventricular fibrillation.

Class IB antiarrhythmics are usually the drug of choice in acute care because they don't produce immediate serious adverse reactions.

## Drug interactions

Class IB antiarrhythmics may exhibit additive or antagonistic effects when administered with other antiarrhythmics, such as

## Warning!

### Adverse reactions to class IB antiarrhythmics

Adverse reactions to class IB antiarrhythmics include drowsiness, light-headedness, paresthesia, sensory disturbances, hypotension, and bradycardia.

Lidocaine toxicity can cause seizures and respiratory arrest.

Adverse reactions to mexiletine include hypotension, atrioventricular block, bradycardia, confusion, ataxia, and double vision. Mexiletine may also produce nausea and vomiting.

> Think of class IB antiarrhythmics as going straight to the bottom of the heart.

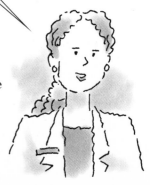

*Now I get it!*

# How lidocaine works

Lidocaine works in injured or ischemic myocardial cells to retard sodium influx and restore cardiac rhythm. Normally, the ventricles contract in response to impulses from the sinoatrial (SA) node. But when tissue damage occurs in the ventricles, ischemic cells can create an ectopic pacemaker, which can trigger ventricular arrhythmias. The illustrations below show how these arrhythmias develop at the cellular level—and how lidocaine suppresses them.

**Ischemic myocardial cell**

Normal myocardial cells permit a limited amount of sodium ions to enter, which leads to controlled depolarization. Ischemic myocardial cells allow a rapid infusion of sodium ions. This causes the cells to depolarize much more quickly than normal and then begin firing spontaneously. The result: a ventricular arrhythmia.

**Ischemic myocardial cell with lidocaine**

By slowing sodium's influx, lidocaine raises the cells' electrical stimulation threshold (EST). The increased EST prolongs depolarization in the ischemic cells and returns control to the SA node, the heart's main pacemaker.

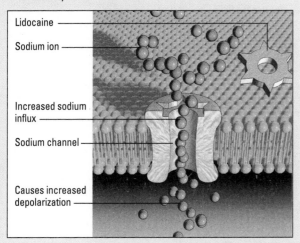

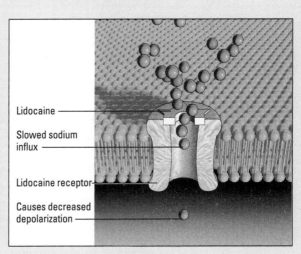

phenytoin, propranolol, procainamide, and quinidine. Other drug interactions include the following:
• Rifampin may reduce the effects of mexiletine.
• Theophylline levels increase when given with mexiletine.
• Use of a beta-adrenergic blocker or disopyramide with mexiletine may reduce the contractility of the heart. (See *Adverse reactions to class IB antiarrhythmics*.)

# Class IC antiarrhythmics

*Class IC antiarrhythmics* are used to treat certain severe, refractory (resistant) ventricular arrhythmias. Class IC antiarrhythmics include:

- flecainide
- moricizine
- propafenone.

## Pharmacokinetics

After oral administration, class IC antiarrhythmics are absorbed well, distributed in varying degrees, and probably metabolized by the liver. They're excreted primarily by the kidneys, except for propafenone, which is excreted primarily in stool.

### More about moricizine

After oral administration, about 38% of moricizine is absorbed. It undergoes extensive metabolism, with less than 1% of a dose excreted unchanged in the urine. Moricizine is highly protein-bound, leaving only a small portion of the drug free to produce its antiarrhythmic effect.

## Pharmacodynamics

Class IC antiarrhythmics primarily slow conduction along the heart's conduction system. Moricizine decreases the fast inward current of sodium ions of the action potential, depressing the depolarization rate and the effective refractory period.

## Pharmacotherapeutics

Like class IB antiarrhythmics, class IC antiarrhythmics are used to treat and prevent life-threatening ventricular arrhythmias. They're also used to treat supraventricular arrhythmias (abnormal heart rhythms that originate above the bundle branches of the heart's conduction system).

Flecainide and propafenone may also be used to prevent paroxysmal supraventricular tachycardia (PSVT) in patients without structural heart disease. Moricizine is used to manage life-threatening ventricular arrhythmias such as sustained ventricular tachycardia.

## Drug interactions

Class IC antiarrhythmics may exhibit additive effects with other antiarrhythmics. Other interactions include the following:

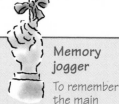

**Memory jogger**

To remember the main differences between what Class IA, Class IB, and Class IC antiarrhythmics do, just think of their names:

Class IA: **A**lters the myocardial cell membrane

Class IB: **B**locks the rapid influx of sodium ions

Class IC: slows **C**onduction

**Warning!**

## Adverse reactions to class IC antiarrhythmics

Class IC antiarrhythmics can produce serious adverse reactions, including the development of new arrhythmias and aggravation of existing arrhythmias. They're avoided in patients with structural heart defects because of a high incidence of mortality.

Because propafenone has beta-blocking properties, it may cause bronchospasm.

**Adverse reactions to moricizine**

The most serious adverse reaction is the appearance of new arrhythmias or the worsening of an existing arrhythmia.

Other cardiovascular adverse reactions include palpitations, shortness of breath, chest pain, heart failure, and cardiac arrest.

GI adverse reactions include abdominal pain, heartburn, nausea, and vomiting.

• When used with digoxin, flecainide and propafenone increase the risk of digoxin toxicity.
• Propafenone increases plasma concentrations of warfarin and increases prothrombin times.
• Quinidine increases the effects of propafenone.
• Cimetidine may increase the plasma level and the risk of toxicity of moricizine.
• Propanolol or digoxin given with moricizine may increase the PR interval on the electrocardiogram.
• Theophylline levels may be reduced in a patient receiving moricizine.
• Ritonavir increases the plasma concentration and the effects of propafenone.
• Propafenone increases the serum concentration and the effects of metoprolol and propranolol. (See *Adverse reactions to class IC antiarrhythmics.*)

# Class II antiarrhythmics

*Class II antiarrhythmics* are composed of beta-adrenergic antagonists, or beta-adrenergic blockers. Beta-adrendergic blockers used as antiarrhythmics include:

- acebutolol (not used very often)
- esmolol
- propranolol.

## Pharmacokinetics

Acebutolol and propranolol are absorbed almost entirely from the GI tract after an oral dose. Esmolol, which can be given only by I.V., is immediately available throughout the body.

**Fat-headed**

Acebutolol and esmolol have low lipid solubility. That means that they can't penetrate the highly fatty cells that act as barriers between the blood and brain, called the blood-brain barrier.

Propranolol has high lipid solubility and readily crosses the blood-brain barrier.

**No leftovers**

Propranolol undergoes significant first-pass effect, leaving only a small portion of these drugs available to reach circulation and be distributed to the body.

Esmolol is metabolized exclusively by red blood cells (RBCs), with only 1% excreted in urine. Propranolol's metabolites are excreted in urine.

## Pharmacodynamics

Class II antiarrhythmics block beta-adrenergic receptor sites in the conduction system of the heart. As a result, the ability of the SA node to fire spontaneously (automaticity) is slowed. The ability of the AV node and other cells to receive and conduct an electrical impulse to nearby cells (conductivity) is also reduced.

Class II antiarrhythmics also reduce the strength of the heart's contractions. When the heart beats less forcefully, it doesn't require as much oxygen to do its work.

## Pharmacotherapeutics

Class II antiarrhythmics slow ventricular rates in patients with atrial flutter, atrial fibrillation, and paroxysmal atrial tachycardia.

## Drug interactions

Class II antiarrhythmics can cause a variety of drug interactions:
- Administering these drugs with phenothiazines and other antihypertensives increases the antihypertensive effect.
- When given with nonsteroidal anti-inflammatory agents, fluid and water retention may occur, decreasing the antihypertensive effect.

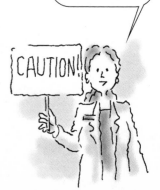

Class II antiarrhythmics can cause hypotension when taken with some drugs.

CAUTION!

• The effects of sympathomimetics may be reduced when taken with class II antiarrhythmics.
• Beta-adrenergic blockers given with verapamil can depress the heart, causing hypotension, bradycardia, AV block, and asystole.
• Beta-adrenergic blockers reduce the effects of sulfonylureas.
• The risk of digoxin toxicity increases when digoxin is taken with esmolol. (See *Adverse reactions to class II antiarrhythmics*.)

# Class III antiarrhythmics

*Class III antiarrhythmics* are used to treat ventricular arrhythmias. The drugs in this class are amiodarone, dofetilide, ibutilide, and sotalol.

## Which class are you in?

Sotalol is a nonselective beta-adrenergic blocker (class II drug) that also has class III properties. Nonselective means that the drug doesn't have a specific affinity for a receptor. Although sotalol is a class II drug, its class III antiarrhythmic effects are more predominant, especially at higher doses. Therefore, it's usually listed as a class III antiarrhythmic.

### Pharmacokinetics

The absorption of these antiarrhythmics varies widely.

## Slow going

After oral administration, amiodarone is absorbed slowly at widely varying rates. The drug is distributed extensively and accumulates in many sites, especially in organs with a rich blood supply and fatty tissue. It's highly protein-bound in plasma, mainly to albumin.

Dofetilide is very well absorbed from the GI tract, with almost 100% overall absorption. Of that, about 70% is bound to plasma proteins. Ibutilide, which is administered only by I.V., has an absorption of 100%. Sotalol's absorption is slow and varies between 60% and 100%, with minimal protein-binding.

### Pharmacodynamics

Although the exact mechanism of action isn't known, class III antiarrhythmics are thought to suppress arrhythmias by converting a unidirectional block to a bidirectional block. Class III antiarrhythmics have little or no effect on depolarization. Rather, these drugs slow repolarization, prolonging the refractory period and duration of the action potential.

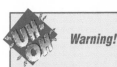

*Warning!*

## Adverse reactions to class II antiarrhythmics

Common adverse reactions include:
• arrhythmias
• bradycardia
• heart failure
• hypotension
• GI reactions, such as nausea, vomiting, and diarrhea
• bronchoconstriction.

## Pharmacotherapeutics

Class III antiarrhythmics are used for life-threatening arrhythmias. Amiodarone is the first-line drug of choice for ventricular tachycardia and ventricular fibrillation.

## Drug interactions

• Amiodarone increases phenytoin, procainamide, and quinidine levels.
• Amiodarone also increases the risk of digoxin toxicity.
• Ibutilide shouldn't be administered within 4 hours of class I or other class III antiarrhythmics because it increases the potential for a prolonged refractory period.
• Dofetilide shouldn't be administered with cimetidine, ketoconazole, megestrol, prochlorperazine, sulfamethoxazole, trimethoprim, or verapamil because of their potential to induce life-threatening arrhythmias.
• Sotalol shouldn't be administered with dolasetron or droperidol because of the increased risk of life-threatening arrhythmias.
• Concomitant use of amiodarone and fluoroquinolones, macrolide antibiotics, and azole antifungals may cause prolongation of the QTc interval, leading to cardiac arrhythmias, including torsades de pointes.

*Pressure plunge*

Severe hypotension may develop from too-rapid I.V. administration of amiodarone. (See *Adverse reactions to class III antiarrhythmics.*)

> When a patient has ventricular tachycardia, I reach for amiodarone.

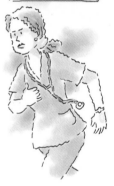

---

*Warning!*

## Adverse reactions to class III antiarrhythmics

Adverse reactions to class III antiarrhythmics, especially amiodarone, vary widely and commonly lead to drug discontinuation. A common adverse effect is aggravation of arrhythmias.

**Adverse reactions to amiodarone...**
Amiodarone may produce hypotension, nausea, and anorexia. Severe pulmonary toxicity occurs in 15% of patients and can be fatal. Vision disturbances and corneal microdeposits may occur.

**... and ibultilide ...**
Ibutilide may cause sustained ventricular tachycardia, prolongation of the QT interval, hypotension, nausea, and headache.

**... and sotalol**
Sotalol may cause atrioventricular block, bradycardia, ventricular arrhythmias, bronchospasm, and hypotension.

# Class IV antiarrhythmics

*Class IV antiarrhythmics* are composed of calcium channel blockers. The calcium channel blockers verapamil and diltiazem are used to treat supraventricular arrhythmias with a rapid ventricular response (rapid heart rate in which the rhythm originates above the ventricles).

For a thorough discussion of calcium channel blockers and how they work, see "Calcium channel blockers," page 138.

# Adenosine

*Adenosine* is an injectable antiarrhythmic indicated for acute treatment of PSVT.

## Pharmacokinetics

After I.V. administration, adenosine is probably distributed rapidly throughout the body. It's metabolized inside RBCs as well as in vascular endothelial cells.

## Pharmacodynamics

Adenosine depresses the pacemaker activity of the SA node, reducing the heart rate and the ability of the AV node to conduct impulses from the atria to the ventricles.

## Pharmacotherapeutics

Adenosine is especially effective against reentry tachycardias (when an impulse depolarizes an area of heart muscle, then returns and repolarizes it) that involve the AV node.

No slouch

Adenosine also effectively resolves PSVT in 90% of cases. It's typically used to treat arrhythmias associated with accessory bypass tracts, as in Wolff-Parkinson-White syndrome (brief periods of rapid heart rate in which the rhythm originates above the ventricle).

## Drug interactions

• Methylxanthines antagonize the effects of adenosine, so larger doses of adenosine may be necessary.
• Dipyridamole and carbamazepine potentiate the effects of adenosine, so smaller doses of adenosine may be necessary.

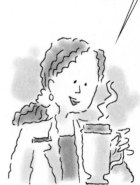

Remember, caffeine antagonizes the effect of adenosine. If the patient is a coffee drinker, larger doses of adenosine may be necessary.

• When adenosine is administered with carbamazepine, there's an increased risk of heart block. (See *Adverse reactions to adenosine.*)

# Antianginal drugs

Although angina's cardinal symptom is chest pain, the drugs used to treat angina aren't typically analgesics.

Instead, *antianginal drugs* treat angina by reducing myocardial oxygen demand (reducing the amount of oxygen the heart needs to do its work), by increasing the supply of oxygen to the heart, or both. (See *How antianginal drugs work.*)

The three classes of antianginal drugs discussed in this section include:

• nitrates (for treating acute angina)
• beta-adrenergic blockers (for long-term prevention of angina)

**Warning!**

## Adverse reactions to adenosine

Common adverse reactions to adenosine include:
• facial flushing
• shortness of breath
• dyspnea
• chest discomfort.

---

*Now I get it!*

## How antianginal drugs work

Angina occurs when the coronary arteries (the heart's primary source of oxygen) supply insufficient oxygen to the myocardium. This increases the heart's workload, increasing heart rate, preload (blood volume in the ventricle at the end of diastole), afterload (pressure in the arteries leading from the ventricle), and force of myocardial contractility.

Antianginal drugs (nitrates, beta-adreneric blockers, and calcium channel blockers) relieve angina by *decreasing* one or more of these four factors. This diagram summarizes how antianginal drugs affect the cardiovascular system.

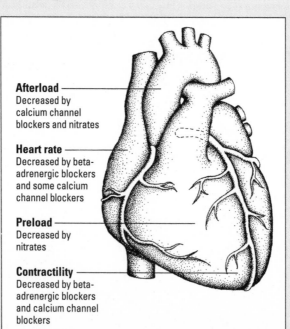

**Afterload**
Decreased by calcium channel blockers and nitrates

**Heart rate**
Decreased by beta-adrenergic blockers and some calcium channel blockers

**Preload**
Decreased by nitrates

**Contractility**
Decreased by beta-adrenergic blockers and calcium channel blockers

• calcium channel blockers (used when other drugs fail to prevent angina).

# Nitrates

*Nitrates* are the drugs of choice for relieving acute angina. Nitrates commonly prescribed to treat angina include:
• amyl nitrite
• isosorbide dinitrate
• isosorbide mononitrate
• nitroglycerin.

## Pharmacokinetics

Nitrates can be administered in a variety of ways.

### All absorbed...

Nitrates given sublingually (under the tongue), buccally (in the pocket of the cheek), as chewable tablets, as lingual aerosols (sprayed onto or under the tongue), or by inhalation (amyl nitrite) are absorbed almost completely because the mucous membranes of the mouth have a rich blood supply.

### ...Half-absorbed...

Swallowed nitrate capsules are absorbed through the mucous membranes of the GI tract, and only about one-half of the dose enters circulation.

Transdermal nitrates (a patch or ointment placed on the skin) are absorbed slowly and in varying amounts, depending on the quantity of drug applied, the location of its application, the surface area of skin used, and circulation to the skin.

### ...Or no absorption required

I.V. nitroglycerin, which doesn't need to be absorbed, goes directly into circulation.

## Pharmacodynamics

Nitrates cause the smooth muscle of the veins and, to a lesser extent, the arteries to relax and dilate. This is what happens:
• When the veins dilate, less blood returns to the heart.
• This, in turn, reduces the amount of blood in the ventricles at the end of diastole, when the ventricles are full. (The volume of blood in the ventricles just before contraction is called preload.)
• By reducing preload, nitrates reduce ventricular size and ventricular wall tension (the left ventricle doesn't have to stretch as

much to pump blood). This, in turn, reduces the oxygen requirements of the heart.

## Don't fight it

The arterioles provide the most resistance to the blood pumped by the left ventricle (called *peripheral vascular resistance*). Nitrates decrease afterload by dilating the arterioles, reducing resistance, easing the heart's workload, and easing the demand for oxygen.

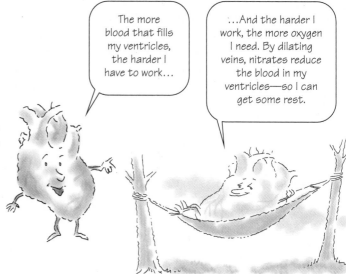

The more blood that fills my ventricles, the harder I have to work...

...And the harder I work, the more oxygen I need. By dilating veins, nitrates reduce the blood in my ventricles—so I can get some rest.

## Pharmacotherapeutics

Nitrates are used to relieve and prevent angina.

## For speedy relief...

The rapidly absorbed nitrates, such as nitroglycerin, are the drugs of choice for relief of acute angina because:
• they have a rapid onset of action
• they're easy to take
• they're inexpensive.

## ...Or prevention

Longer-acting nitrates, such as the daily nitroglycerin transdermal patch, are convenient and can be used to prevent chronic angina. Oral nitrates are also used because they seldom produce serious adverse reactions.

## Drug interactions

• Severe hypotension can result when nitrates interact with alcohol.
• Erectile dysfunction drugs shouldn't be taken within 24 hours of nitrate administration because of possible enhanced hypotensive effects.
• Absorption of sublingual nitrates may be delayed when taken with an anticholinergic drug.
• Marked orthostatic hypotension (a drop in blood pressure when a person stands up) with light-headedness, fainting, or blurred vision may occur when calcium channel blockers, antihypertensives, beta-adrenergic blockers, or phenothiazines and nitrates are used together. (See *Adverse reactions to nitrates*.)

**Warning!**

## Adverse reactions to nitrates

Most adverse reactions to nitrates result from changes in the cardiovascular system. These reactions usually disappear when dosage is reduced.

**The three H's**
Headache is the most common adverse reaction. Hypotension may also occur, accompanied by dizziness and increased heart rate.

# Beta-adrenergic antagonists

*Beta-adrenergic antagonists* (also called *beta blockers*) are used for long-term prevention of angina and are one of the main types of drugs used to treat hypertension. Beta-adrenergic blockers include:
- atenolol
- metoprolol
- nadolol
- propranolol.

## Pharmacokinetics

Metoprolol and propranolol are absorbed almost entirely from the GI tract, whereas less than one-half the dose of atenolol or nadolol is absorbed. These beta-adrenergic blockers are distributed widely. Propranolol is highly protein-bound; the other beta-adrenergic blockers are poorly protein-bound.

*Making an escape*

Propranolol and metoprolol are metabolized in the liver, and their metabolites are excreted in urine. Atenolol and nadolol aren't metabolized and are excreted unchanged in urine and stool.

## Pharmacodynamics

Beta-adrenergic blockers decrease blood pressure and block beta-adrenergic receptor sites in the heart muscle and the conduction system. This decreases the heart rate and reduces the force of the heart's contractions, resulting in a lower demand for oxygen.

## Pharmacotherapeutics

Beta-adrenergic blockers are indicated for long-term prevention of angina. In acute coronary syndrome, metoprolol may be given initially I.V., and then orally. Metoprolol may also be used for heart failure.

Because of their ability to reduce blood pressure, beta-adrenergic blockers are also first-line therapy for treating hypertension.

## Drug interactions

A number of drugs interact with beta-adrenergic blockers.
- Antacids reduce absorption of beta-adrenergic blockers.
- Nonsteroidal anti-inflammatory drugs (NSAIDs) can decrease the hypotensive effects of beta-adrenergic blockers.

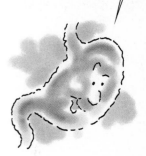

We in the GI tract are like sponges when it comes to metoprolol and propranolol!

**Warning!**

## Adverse reactions to beta-adrenergic blockers

Beta-adrenergic blockers may cause:
• bradycardia
• angina
• fluid retention
• peripheral edema
• heart failure
• arrhythmias, especially atrioventricular block
• hypotension
• dizziness
• nausea and vomiting
• diarrhea
• significant constriction of the bronchioles.

**Quick stop causes concern**
Suddenly stopping a beta-adrenergic blocker may trigger:
• angina
• hypertension
• arrhythmias
• acute myocardial infarction.

• Cardiac glycosides and calcium channel blockers can have negative addictive effects on SA or AV node conduction when administered with a beta-adrenergic blocker.
• Diuretics or other hypotensive agents can potentiate the hypotensive effects of beta-adrenergic blockers.
• Lidocaine toxicity may occur when lidocaine is taken with beta-adrenergic blockers.
• The requirements for insulin and oral antidiabetics can be altered by beta-adrenergic blockers.
• The ability of theophylline to produce bronchodilation is impaired by nonselective beta-adrenergic blockers. (See *Adverse reactions to beta-adrenergic blockers*.)

# Calcium channel blockers

*Calcium channel blockers* are commonly used to prevent angina that doesn't respond to drugs in either of the other antianginal classes. They're the drug of choice to treat Prinzmetal's angina. As mentioned earlier, several of the calcium channel blockers are also used as antiarrhythmics and to treat hypertension. Calcium channel blockers used to treat angina include:
• amlodipine
• diltiazem
• nicardipine
• nifedipine
• verapamil.

*Now I get it!*

## How calcium channel blockers work

Calcium channel blockers increase the myocardial oxygen supply and slow the heart rate. Apparently, the drugs produce these effects by blocking the slow calcium channel. This action inhibits the influx of extracellular calcium ions across both myocardial and vascular smooth muscle cell membranes. Calcium channel blockers achieve this blockade without changing serum calcium concentrations.

**No calcium = dilation**
This calcium blockade causes the coronary arteries (and, to a lesser extent, the peripheral arteries and arterioles) to dilate, decreasing afterload and increasing myocardial oxygen supply.

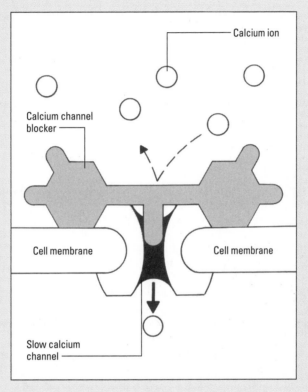

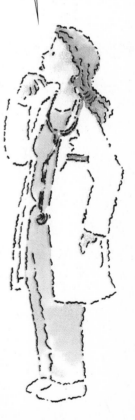

Some calcium channel blockers slow the heart rate but don't change the level of calcium in the blood.

## Pharmacokinetics

When administered orally, calcium channel blockers are absorbed quickly and almost completely. Because of the first-pass effect, however, the bioavailability of these drugs is much lower. The calcium channel blockers are highly bound to plasma proteins.

### Gone without a trace

All calcium channel blockers are metabolized rapidly and almost completely in the liver.

## Pharmacodynamics

Calcium channel blockers prevent the passage of calcium ions across the myocardial cell membrane and vascular smooth-muscle cells. This causes dilation of the coronary and peripheral arteries, which decreases the force of the heart's contractions and reduces the workload of the heart.

## The relaxation response

Also, by preventing arterioles from constricting, calcium channel blockers reduce afterload. Decreasing afterload further decreases the oxygen demands of the heart. (See *How calcium channel blockers work*, page 139.)

## Rate reductions

Some calcium channel blockers (diltiazem and verapamil) also reduce the heart rate by slowing conduction through the SA and AV nodes. A slower heart rate reduces the heart's need for additional oxygen.

### Pharmacotherapeutics

Calcium channel blockers are used for long-term prevention of angina only, not short-term relief of chest pain. Calcium channel blockers are particularly effective for preventing Prinzmetal's angina.

### Drug interactions

- Calcium salts and vitamin D reduce the effectiveness of calcium channel blockers.
- Nondepolarizing blocking drugs may have an enhanced muscle-relaxant effect when taken with calcium channel blockers.
- Verapamil and diltiazem increase the risk of digoxin toxicity, enhance the action of carbamazepine, and may cause myocardial depression. (See *Adverse reactions to calcium channel blockers.*)

# Antihypertensive drugs

*Antihypertensive drugs*, which act to reduce blood pressure, are used to treat hypertension, a disorder characterized by elevation in systolic blood pressure, diastolic blood pressure, or both.

## Know the program

Treatment for hypertension typically begins with a thiazide diuretic or a calcium channel blocker. (For more information, see "Calcium channel blockers," page 138.) The patient may also receive a beta-adrenergic antagonist, angiotensin-converting enzyme (ACE) inhibitor, or an angiotensin II receptor blocker. The choice of

*Warning!*

## Adverse reactions to calcium channel blockers

As with other antianginal drugs, cardiovascular reactions are the most common and serious adverse reactions to calcium channel blockers. These include orthostatic hypotension (a drop in blood pressure when a person stands up), heart failure, and hypotension. Diltiazem and verapamil can cause such arrhythmias as bradycardia, sinus block, and atrioventricular block.

### Others
Other possible adverse reactions include dizziness, headache, flushing, weakness, and persistent peripheral edema.

these drugs depends on whether the patient has a compelling indication, such as heart failure, history of an MI, high risk of coronary artery disease (CAD), diabetes, or chronic kidney disease. (See "Beta-adrenergic antagonists," page 137.)

Other drugs used to treat hypertension include sympatholytic drugs (other than beta-adrenergic blockers), and vasodilators. At times, a combination of drugs may be used.

# Sympatholytic drugs

*Sympatholytic drugs* include several different types of drugs, but all reduce blood pressure by inhibiting or blocking the sympathetic nervous system. They're classified by their site or mechanism of action and include:
• central-acting sympathetic nervous system inhibitors (clonidine and methyldopa)
• alpha-adrenergic blockers (doxazosin, phentolamine, prazosin, and terazosin)
• mixed alpha- and beta-adrenergic blockers (carvedilol and labetalol)
• norepinephrine depletors (guanadrel, guanethidine, and reserpine—these are rarely used).

## Pharmacokinetics

Most sympatholytic drugs are absorbed well from the GI tract, distributed widely, metabolized in the liver, and excreted primarily in urine.

## Pharmacodynamics

All sympatholytic drugs inhibit stimulation of the sympathetic nervous system, causing dilation of the peripheral blood vessels or decreased cardiac output, thereby reducing blood pressure.

## Pharmacotherapeutics

If blood pressure fails to come under control with beta-adrenergic blockers and diuretics, an alpha-adrenergic blocker, such as prazosin, or a mixed alpha- and beta-adrenergic blocker, such as labetalol, may be used. If the patient fails to achieve the desired blood pressure, the physician may add a drug from a different class, substitute a drug in the same class, or increase the drug dosage.

**Warning!**

## Adverse reactions to sympatholytics

**Alpha-adrenergic blockers**
• Hypotension

**Central-acting drugs**
• Depression
• Drowsiness
• Edema
• Liver dysfunction
• Numbness, tingling
• Vertigo

**Guanadrel**
• Difficulty breathing
• Excessive urination
• Fainting
• Orthostatic hypotension

**Guanethidine**
• Decreased heart contrac-
tility
• Diarrhea
• Fluid retention
• Orthostatic hypotension

**Reserpine**
• Abdominal cramps, diarrhea
• Angina
• Blurred vision
• Bradycardia
• Bronchoconstriction
• Decreased libido
• Depression
• Drowsiness
• Weight gain
• Fatigue
• Hypotension

## Drug interactions

Sympatholytic drugs can create these drug interactions:
• Carvedilol taken with antidiabetics may result in increased hypoglycemic effect.
• Carvedilol taken with calcium channel blockers may result in increased conduction disturbances.
• Carvedilol taken with digoxin may result in increased digoxin levels.
• Carvedilol taken with rifampin decreases carvedilol levels.
• Clonidine plus tricyclic antidepressants may increase blood pressure.
• Clonidine taken with CNS depressants may worsen CNS depression.
• Reserpine taken with diuretics or other hypotensive agents can increase the hypotensive effects of reserpine.
• Reserpine taken with cardiac glycosides can lead to cardiac arrhythmias.
   Sympatholytic drugs can also produce significant adverse reactions. (See *Adverse reactions to sympatholytics*.)

# Vasodilating drugs

There are two types of *vasodilating drugs*—direct vasodilators and calcium channel blockers. Both types decrease systolic and diastolic blood pressure.

## Resistance is futile

*Direct vasodilators* act on arteries, veins, or both. They include:
- diazoxide
- hydralazine
- minoxidil
- nitroprusside.

Hydralazine and minoxidil are usually used to treat resistant or refractory hypertension. Diazoxide and nitroprusside are reserved for use in hypertensive crisis.

## No admittance

Calcium channel blockers produce arteriolar relaxation by preventing the entry of calcium into the cells. This prevents the contraction of vascular smooth muscle. (See "Calcium channel blockers," page 138.)

### Pharmacokinetics

Most of these drugs are absorbed rapidly and well-distributed. They're all metabolized in the liver, and most are excreted by the kidneys.

### Pharmacodynamics

The direct vasodilators relax peripheral vascular smooth muscle, causing the blood vessels to dilate. The increased diameter of the blood vessels reduces total peripheral resistance, which lowers blood pressure.

### Pharmacotherapeutics

Vasodilating drugs are rarely used alone to treat hypertension. They're usually combined with other drugs to treat the patient with moderate to severe hypertension (hypertensive crisis).

Calcium channel blockers are occasionally used alone to treat mild to moderate hypertension.

### Drug interactions

- The antihypertensive effects of hydralazine and minoxidil are increased when they're given with other antihypertensive drugs, such as methyldopa or reserpine.
- Vasodilating drugs may produce additive effects when given with nitrates, such as isosorbide dinitrate or nitroglycerin.
- Few other drug interactions occur with vasodilating drugs. (See *Adverse reactions to direct vasodilators.*)

*Warning!*

## Adverse reactions to direct vasodilators

Direct vasodilators commonly produce adverse reactions related to reflex activation of the sympathetic nervous system. As blood pressure falls, the sympathetic nervous system is stimulated, producing compensatory measures, such as vasoconstriction and tachycardia.

Other reactions to sympathetic stimulation include:
- palpitations
- angina
- edema
- breast tenderness
- fatigue
- headache
- rash
- severe pericardial effusion.

# ACE inhibitors

*ACE inhibitors* are typically used when beta-adrenergic blockers or diuretics are ineffective. Commonly prescribed ACE inhibitors include:

- benazepril
- captopril
- enalapril
- enalaprilat
- fosinopril
- lisinopril
- moexipril
- quinapril
- ramipril
- trandolapril.

## Pharmacokinetics

ACE inhibitors are absorbed from the GI tract, distributed to most body tissues, metabolized somewhat in the liver, and excreted by the kidneys. Ramipril is also excreted in stool. Enalaprilat is the only ACE inhibitor that's administered I.V.

## Pharmacodynamics

ACE inhibitors reduce blood pressure by interrupting the renin-angiotensin-aldosterone system. Normally, the kidneys maintain blood pressure by releasing the hormone renin. Renin acts on the plasma protein angiotensinogen to form angiotensin I. Angiotensin I is then converted to angiotensin II. Angiotensin II, a potent vasoconstrictor, increases peripheral resistance and promotes the excretion of aldosterone. Aldosterone, in turn, promotes the retention of sodium and water, increasing the volume of blood the heart needs to pump.

### Conversion diversion

ACE inhibitors prevent the conversion of angiotensin I to angiotensin II. As angiotensin II is reduced, arterioles dilate, reducing peripheral vascular resistance.

### Less water, less work

By reducing aldosterone secretion, ACE inhibitors promote the excretion of sodium and water, which reduces the amount of blood the heart needs to pump, thereby lowering blood pressure.

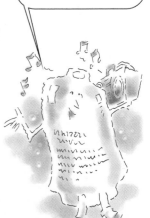

Enalaprilat is the only one I deal with. And that's the way, uh-huh, uh-huh I like it, uh-huh, uh-huh!

## Pharmacotherapeutics

ACE inhibitors may be used alone or with another drug, such as a thiazide diuretic, to treat hypertension. Certain ACE inhibitors—such as captopril, enalapril, fosinopril, lisinopril, quinapril, ramipril, and trandolapril—may also be used to treat patients with heart failure or following MI. Such situations include:

• left ventricular systolic failure (unless contraindicated or intolerant)

• left ventricular systolic dysfunction without symptoms of heart failure

• reducing mortality following acute MI (especially in patients with prior myocardial injury)

• preventing or delaying the development of left ventricular dilation and overt heart failure in patients with left ventricular dysfunction (recent or remote)

• possible production of complementary effects (combined with beta-blockade)

• history of or present fluid retention (combined with diuretics).

Ramipril is also indicated to prevent major cardiovascular events in patients with a history of vascular disease or diabetes. It's also used to reduce overall cardiovascular risk, including death, nonfatal MI, nonfatal stroke, and complications of diabetes. Captopril is also indicated for the long-term treatment of diabetic neuropathy.

## Drug interactions

ACE inhibitors can cause several different types of interactions with other cardiovascular drugs. All ACE inhibitors enhance the hypotensive effects of diuretics and other antihypertensives such as beta-adrenergic blockers. They can also increase serum lithium levels, possibly resulting in lithium toxicity.

When ACE inhibitors are used with potassium-sparing diuretics, potassium supplements, or potassium-containing salt substitutes, hyperkalemia may occur.

### Individual items

ACE inhibitors interact with many other medications, prescription as well as over-the-counter (OTC). For example, patients taking ACE inhibitors should avoid taking all NSAIDs. Besides decreasing the antihypertensive effect of ACE inhibitors, NSAIDs may alter renal function. Also, antacids may impair the absorption of fosinopril, and quinapril may reduce the absorption of tetracycline.

A patient taking ACE inhibitors shouldn't take prescriptions or OTC medications or herbal products without first consulting his physician. (See *Adverse reactions to ACE inhibitors*.)

**Warning!**

## Adverse reactions to ACE inhibitors

Angiotensin-converting enzyme (ACE) inhibitors can produce these adverse reactions:

• headache and fatigue

• dry, nonproductive, persistent cough

• angioedema

• GI reactions

• increased serum potassium concentrations

• tickling in the throat

• transient elevations of blood urea nitrogen and serum creatinine levels (indicators of kidney function).

**Caused by captopril**

Captopril may cause protein in the urine, reduced neutrophils and granulocytes (a type of white blood cells), rash, loss of taste, hypotension, or a severe allergic reaction.

# Angiotensin II receptor blockers

Angiotensin II receptor blockers (ARBs) lower blood pressure by blocking the vasoconstrictive effects of angiotensin II. Specific drugs include:
- candesartan cilexetil
- eprosartan
- irbesartan
- losartan
- olmesartan
- telmisartan
- valsartan.

## Pharmacokinetics

ARBs have varying pharmacokinetic properties and all are highly bound to plasma proteins.

## Pharmacodynamics

ARBs act by interfering with the renin-angiotensin-aldosterone system. Specifically, these drugs block the binding of angiotensin II to the $AT_1$ receptor. This prevents angiotensin II from exerting its vasoconstricting properties and from promoting the excretion of aldosterone. Both of these actions result in lowered blood pressure.

ARBs don't inhibit the conversion of angiotensin I to angiotensin II, nor do they cause a breakdown in bradykinin (a vasodilator).

## Pharmacotherapeutics

ARBs may be used alone or in combination with other drugs such as a diuretic. Valsartan may also be used as an alternative to an ACE inhibitor or for the management of heart failure. Because irbesartan and losartan protect the renal system, they're often prescribed for patients with type 2 diabetes. Losartan is also used to reduce the risk of stroke in high-risk patients with hypertension and left ventricular hypertrophy. (See *Adverse reactions to ARBs.*)

## Drug interactions

ARBs can interact with other drugs in various ways.
- When losartan is taken with fluconazole, an increased blood level of losartan may result, leading to hypotension.
- NSAIDs reduce the antihypertensive effects of ARBs.
- Rifampin may increase metabolism of losartan and decrease its antihypertensive effect.

**Warning!**

## Adverse reactions to ARBs

Adverse reactions to angiotensin II receptor blockers (ARBs) include:
- headache and fatigue
- cough and tickling in the throat
- angioedema
- GI reactions
- increased serum potassium level
- transient elevations of blood urea nitrogen and serum creatinine levels.

• Candesartan may increase blood levels of lithium, leading to lithium toxicity.
• When digoxin is taken with telmisartan, an increased blood level of digoxin may occur, possibly leading to digoxin toxicity.
• Potassium supplements may increase the risk of hyperkalemia when used with ARBs.

# Antilipemic drugs

*Antilipemic drugs* are used to lower abnormally high blood levels of lipids, such as cholesterol, triglycerides, and phospholipids. The risk of developing CAD increases when serum lipid levels are elevated. Drugs are used in combination with lifestyle changes (such as proper diet, weight loss, and exercise) and treatment of an underlying disorder causing the lipid abnormality to help lower lipid levels.

The classes of antilipemic drugs include:
• bile-sequestering drugs
• fibric acid derivatives
• 3-hydroxy-3-methylglutaryl coenzyme A (HMG-CoA) reductase inhibitors
• nicotinic acid
• cholesterol absorption inhibitors.

## Bile-sequestering drugs

The *bile-sequestering drugs* are cholestyramine, colestipol, and colesevelam. These drugs are resins that remove excess bile acids from the fat deposits under the skin.

### Pharmacokinetics

Bile-sequestering drugs aren't absorbed from the GI tract. Instead, they remain in the intestine, where they combine with bile acids for about 5 hours. Eventually, they're excreted in stool.

### Pharmacodynamics

The bile-sequestering drugs lower blood levels of low-density lipoproteins (LDLs). These drugs combine with bile acids in the intestines to form an insoluble compound that's then excreted in stool. The decreasing level of bile acid in the gallbladder triggers the liver to synthesize more bile acids from their precursor, cholesterol.

## Getting out of storage

As cholesterol leaves the bloodstream and other storage areas to replace the lost bile acids, blood cholesterol levels decrease. Because the small intestine needs bile acids to emulsify lipids and form chylomicrons, absorption of all lipids and lipid-soluble drugs decreases until the bile acids are replaced.

### Pharmacotherapeutics

Bile-sequestering drugs are the drugs of choice for treating type IIa hyperlipoproteinemia (familial hypercholesterolemia) when the patient can't lower his LDL levels through diet alone. Patients whose blood cholesterol levels place them at a severe risk of CAD will most likely require one of these drugs in addition to dietary changes.

### Drug interactions

Bile-sequestering drugs produce the following drug interactions:
• They may bind with acidic drugs in the GI tract, decreasing their absorption and effectiveness. Acidic drugs likely to be affected include barbiturates, phenytoin, penicillins, cephalosporins, thyroid hormones, thyroid derivatives, and digoxin.
• Bile-sequestering drugs may decrease absorption of propranolol, tetracycline, furosemide, penicillin G, hydrochlorothiazide and gemfibrozil.
• Bile-sequestering drugs may reduce absorption of lipid-soluble vitamins, such as vitamins A, D, E, and K. Poor absorption of vitamin K can affect prothrombin times significantly, increasing the risk of bleeding. (See *Adverse reactions to bile-sequestering drugs.*)

**Warning!**

## Adverse reactions to bile-sequestering drugs

Short-term adverse reactions to these drugs are relatively mild. More severe reactions can result from long-term use. Adverse GI effects with long-term therapy include severe fecal impaction, vomiting, diarrhea, and hemorrhoid irritation.

Rarely, peptic ulcers and bleeding, gallstones, and inflammation of the gallbladder may occur.

# Fibric acid derivatives

*Fibric acid* is produced by several fungi. Two derivatives of this acid are fenofibrate and gemfibrozil. These drugs are used to reduce high triglyceride levels and, to a lesser extent, high LDL levels.

### Pharmacokinetics

Fenofibrate and gemfibrozil are absorbed readily from the GI tract and are highly protein-bound. Fenofibrate is hydrolyzed while gemfibrozil undergoes extensive metabolism in the liver. Both drugs are excreted in the urine.

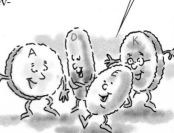

Slow us down? Never! Just don't give us bile-sequestering drugs!

## Pharmacodynamics

Although the exact mechanism of action for these drugs isn't known, researchers believe that fibric acid derivatives may:
- reduce cholesterol production early in its formation
- mobilize cholesterol from the tissues
- increase cholesterol excretion
- decrease synthesis and secretion of lipoproteins
- decrease synthesis of triglycerides.

### Power in the blood

Gemfibrozil produces two other effects:
- It increases high-density lipoprotein (HDL) levels in the blood (remember, this is "good" cholesterol).
- It increases the serum's capacity to dissolve additional cholesterol.

## Pharmacotherapeutics

Fibric acid drugs are used primarily to reduce triglyceride levels, especially very-low-density triglycerides, and secondarily to reduce blood cholesterol levels. They're typically used to treat patients with types II, III, IV, and mild type V hyperlipoproteinemia.

## Drug interactions

- Fibric acid drugs may displace acidic drugs, such as barbiturates, phenytoin, thyroid derivatives, and cardiac glycosides.
- The risk of bleeding increases when fibric acid derivatives are taken with oral anticoagulants.
- Fibric acid derivatives can lead to adverse GI effects.
- The hypoglycemic effects of repaglinide may be increased and prolonged if taken with gemfibrozil.
- Use of fibric acid derivatives and HMG-CoA reductase inhibitors may increase the risk of rhabdomyolysis.

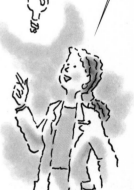

Ah-ha! So, gemfibrozil not only reduces triglycerides but also increases high-density lipoprotein levels and the blood's ability to dissolve cholesterol.

# HMG-CoA reductase inhibitors

*HMG-CoA reductase inhibitors* (also known as the *statins*) lower lipid levels by interfering with cholesterol synthesis. These drugs include atorvastatin, fluvastatin, lovastatin, pravastatin, rosuvastatin, and simvastatin.

## Pharmacokinetics

Each drug has slightly different pharmacokinetic properties. With the exception of pravastatin, all are highly bound to plasma proteins and undergo extensive first-pass metabolism. However, plasma levels don't correlate with the drugs' abilities to lower cholesterol.

## Pharmacodynamics

HMG-CoA reductase inhibitors inhibit the enzyme responsible for the conversion of HMG-CoA to mevalonate, an early step in the synthesis of cholesterol.

## Pharmacotherapeutics

Statins are used primarily to reduce LDL cholesterol and total blood cholesterol levels. These agents also produce a mild increase in HDL cholesterol levels.

Statins are used to treat primary hypercholesterolemia (types IIa and IIb). Because of their effect on LDL and total cholesterol, these drugs are also used to reduce the risk of CAD and to prevent MI or stroke in patients with high cholesterol levels.

## Drug interactions

• Taking a statin drug with amiodarone, clarithromycin, cyclosporine, erythromycin, fluconazole, gemfibrozil, itraconazole, ketoconazole, or niacin increases the risk of myopathy or rhabdomyolysis (a potentially fatal breakdown of skeletal muscle, causing renal failure).
• Lovastatin, rosuvastatin and simvastatin may increase the risk of bleeding when administered with warfarin.
• All of these drugs should be administered 1 hour before or 4 hours after the administration of bile-sequestering drugs (cholestyramine, colesevelam, and colestipol). (See *Adverse reactions to HMG-CoA reductase inhibitors.*)

# Nicotinic acid

Also known as *niacin*, nicotinic acid is a water-soluble vitamin that decreases cholesterol, triglyceride, and apolipoprotein B-100 levels and increases the HDL level. The drug is available in immediate-release and extended-release tablets.

**Warning!**

## Adverse reactions to HMG-CoA reductase inhibitors

HMG-CoA reductase inhibitors may alter liver function studies, increasing aspartate aminotransferase, alanine aminotransferase, alkaline phosphatase, and bilirubin levels. Other hepatic effects may include pancreatitis, hepatitis, and cirrhosis.

Myalgia is the most common musculoskeletal effect, although arthralgia and muscle cramps may also occur. Myopathy and rhabdomyolysis are rare, but potentially severe, reactions that may occur with these drugs.

Possible adverse GI reactions include nausea, vomiting, diarrhea, abdominal pain, flatulence, and constipation.

## Pharmacokinetics

Nicotinic acid is rapidly and extensively absorbed following oral administration. It's moderately bound to plasma proteins; its overall binding ranges from 60% to 70%. The drug undergoes rapid metabolism by the liver to active and inactive metabolites. About 75% of the drug is excreted in urine.

## Pharmacodynamics

The mechanism of action by which nicotinic acid lowers triglyceride and apolipoprotein levels is unknown. However, it may work by inhibiting hepatic synthesis of lipoproteins that contain apolipoprotein B-100, promoting lipoprotein lipase activity, reducing free fatty acid mobilization from adipose tissue, and increasing fecal elimination of sterols.

## Pharmacotherapeutics

Nicotinic acid is usually used in combination with other drugs to lower triglyceride levels in patients with type IV or V hyperlipidemia who are at high risk for pancreatitis and to lower cholesterol and LDL levels in patients with hypercholesterolemia. It may also be used with other antilipemics to boost HDL levels.

Nicotinic acid is contraindicated in patients who are hypersensitive to nicotinic acid and in those with hepatic dysfunction, active peptic ulcer disease, or arterial bleeding.

## Drug interactions

• Together, nicotinic acid and an HMG-CoA reductase inhibitor may increase the risk of myopathy or rhabdomyolysis.
• Bile-sequestering drugs (cholestyramine, colesevelam, and colestipol) can bind with nicotinic acid and decrease its effectiveness.
• When given with nicotinic acid, kava may increase the risk of hepatotoxicity. (See *Adverse reactions to nicotinic acid*.)

*Warning!*

## Adverse reactions to nicotinic acid

High doses of nicotinic acid may produce vasodilation and cause flushing. Extended-release forms tend to produce less severe vasodilation than immediate-release forms do. To help minimize flushing, administer aspirin 30 minutes before nicotinic acid, or give the extended-release form at night.

Nicotinic acid can cause hepatotoxicity; the risk of this adverse reaction is greater with extended-release forms.

Other adverse reactions include nausea, vomiting, diarrhea, and epigastric or substernal pain.

# Cholesterol absorption inhibitors

As the name implies, *cholesterol absorption inhibitors* inhibit the absorption of cholesterol and related phytosterols from the intestine. Ezetimibe is the drug in this class.

## Pharmacokinetics

Ezetimibe is rapidly and extensively absorbed following oral administration. It's is readily absorbed and is highly bound to plasma proteins. It's primarily metabolized in the small intestine and excreted by the liver and kidneys.

## Pharmacodynamics

Ezetimibe reduces blood cholesterol levels by inhibiting the absorption of cholesterol by the small intestine. This leads to a decrease in delivery of intestinal cholesterol to the liver, reducing hepatic cholesterol stores and increasing clearance from the blood.

## Pharmacotherapeutics

Ezetimibe may be administered alone or with dietary changes to treat primary hypercholesterolemia and homozygous sitosterolemia (hereditary hyperabsorption of cholesterol and plant sterols). The drug is also used in combination with HMG-CoA reductase inhibitors to treat primary hypercholesterolemia and homozygous familial hypercholesterolemia.

Ezetimibe may also help lower total cholesterol and LDL cholesterol, and increase HDL cholesterol, when maximum-dose HMG-CoA reductase inhibitor therapy has been ineffective.

## Drug interactions

• Ezetimibe administered with cholestyramine may lead to decreased effectiveness of ezetimibe.
• Ezetimibe administered with cyclosporine, fenofibrate, or gemfibrozil leads to increased levels of ezetimibe. (See *Adverse reactions to cholesterol absorption inhibitors.*)

 *Warning!*

## Adverse reactions to cholesterol absorption inhibitors

The most common adverse reactions include:
• fatigue
• abdominal pain and diarrhea
• pharyngitis and sinusitis
• arthralgia
• back pain
• cough.

When these drugs are given with an HMG-CoA reductase inhibitor, the most common adverse reactions are chest pain, dizziness, headache, abdominal pain, diarrhea, pharyngitis, sinusitis, upper respiratory tract infection, arthralgia, back pain, and myalgia.

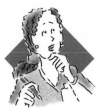

# Quick quiz

**1.** Treatment with fenofibrate, a type of fibric acid derivative, would have to proceed cautiously if the patient is also receiving which drug?

A. Penicillin
B. Thiazide diuretic
C. Digoxin
D. Oral anticoagulant

*Answer:* D. Fibric acid derivatives cause an increased risk of bleeding when given with an oral anticoagulant.

**2.** A patient is taking lovastatin, an HMG-CoA reductase inhibitor. Which parameter should the patient monitor periodically?

A. Liver function test results
B. Electrolyte levels
C. Vision testing
D. Coagulation studies

*Answer:* A. Because increased liver enzyme levels may occur in patients receiving long-term lovastatin therapy, liver function test results should be monitored.

**3.** A patient diagnosed with hypertension is most likely to be prescribed which class of drugs first?

A. Angiotensin II receptor blocker
B. Beta-adrenergic blocker
C. Calcium channel blocker
D. Angiotensin-converting enzyme inhibitor

*Answer:* C. Calcium channel blockers are typically the first treatment for hypertension.

**4.** Nitrates are the drug of choice for relieving acute angina. Nitrates work by:

A. promoting vasodilation, reducing preload, and increasing afterload.
B. promoting vasodilation, reducing preload, and reducing afterload.
C. promoting vasodilation, increasing preload, and increasing afterload.
D. promoting vasodilation, increasing preload, and reducing afterload.

*Answer:* B. Nitrates cause smooth muscle of the veins and arteries to relax and dilate. When veins dilate, less blood returns to the heart, thus reducing preload. Dilation of arterioles decreases resistance, thus decreasing afterload.

## Scoring

★★★ If you answered all four items correctly, A+! You're aces with ACE inhibitors!

★★ If you answered three items correctly, cool! Cardiovascular drugs aren't giving you complications.

★ If you answered fewer than three items correctly, stay mellow. This is a complex chapter, and it might just take another go.

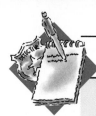

# Hematologic drugs

## Just the facts

In this chapter, you'll learn:

♦ classes of drugs used to treat hematologic disorders

♦ uses and varying actions of these drugs

♦ how these drugs are absorbed, distributed, metabolized, and excreted

♦ drug interactions and adverse reactions to these drugs.

## Drugs and the hematologic system

The hematologic system includes plasma (the liquid component of blood) and blood cells, such as red blood cells (RBCs), white blood cells, and platelets. Types of drugs used to treat disorders of the hematologic system include:
• hematinic
• anticoagulant
• thrombolytic.

## Hematinic drugs

*Hematinic drugs* provide essential building blocks for RBC production. They do so by increasing hemoglobin, the necessary element for oxygen transportation.

### Iron, vitamin $B_{12}$, folic acid

This section discusses hematinic drugs used to treat microcytic and macrocytic anemia—iron, vitamin $B_{12}$, and folic acid.

It also describes the use of erythropoietin agents to treat normocytic anemia.

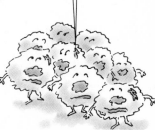

Need some RBCs built? Turn to hematinic drugs.

# Iron

*Iron* preparations are used to treat the most common form of anemia—iron deficiency anemia. Iron preparations discussed in this section include ferrous fumarate, ferrous gluconate, ferrous sulfate, iron dextran, and sodium ferric gluconate complex.

## Pharmacokinetics (how drugs circulate)

Iron is absorbed primarily from the duodenum and upper jejunum of the intestine. Different iron formulations don't vary in absorption, but they do vary in the amount of elemental iron supplied.

### Low iron increases absorption

The amount of iron absorbed depends partially on the body's stores of iron. When body stores are low or RBC production is accelerated, iron absorption may increase by 20% to 30%. On the other hand, when total iron stores are large, the body absorbs only about 5% to 10% of the iron available.

Enteric-coated preparations decrease iron absorption because, in that form, iron isn't released until after it leaves the duodenum. The lymphatic system absorbs the parenteral form after I.M. injections.

### Hemoglobin has it

Iron is transported by the blood and bound to transferrin, its carrier plasma protein. About 30% of the iron is stored primarily as hemosiderin or ferritin in the reticuloendothelial cells of the liver, spleen, and bone marrow. About 66% of the total body iron is contained in hemoglobin. Excess iron is excreted in urine, stool, sweat, and through intestinal cell-sloughing. It appears in breast milk and crosses the placenta.

## Pharmacodynamics (how drugs act)

Although iron has other roles, its most important role is the production of hemoglobin. About 80% of iron in the plasma goes to the bone marrow, where it's used for erythropoiesis (production of RBCs).

## Pharmacotherapeutics (how drugs are used)

Oral iron therapy is the preferred route for preventing or treating iron deficiency anemia. It's used to prevent anemias in children ages 6 months to 2 years because this is a period of rapid growth and development. Pregnant women may need iron supplements to replace the iron used by the developing fetus.

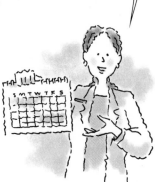

It takes about 6 months for iron therapy to correct iron deficiency anemia.

## Warning!

## Adverse reactions to iron therapy

The most common adverse reactions to iron therapy are gastric irritation and constipation. Iron preparations also darken stool, and liquid preparations can stain the teeth.

The most serious reaction is anaphylaxis, which may occur after administration of parenteral iron. To guard against such a reaction, administer an initial test dose before giving a full-dose infusion.

### Safe and sound

## Testing for parenteral iron sensitivity

Parenteral iron can cause acute hypersensitivity reactions, including anaphylaxis, dyspnea, urticaria, other rashes, pruritus, arthralgia, myalgia, fever, sweating, and allergic purpura. To test for drug sensitivity and prevent serious reactions, always give a test dose of iron dextran before beginning therapy.

Carefully assess the patient's response to the test dose. If no adverse reactions occur within 1 hour, give the total dose. If adverse reactions occur, notify the prescriber immediately. To treat anaphylaxis, keep epinephrine and standard emergency equipment readily available.

## Ironclad options

Parenteral iron therapy is used for patients who can't absorb oral preparations, aren't compliant with oral therapy, or have bowel disorders (such as ulcerative colitis or Crohn's disease). Patients with end-stage renal disease who are receiving hemodialysis may also receive parenteral iron therapy at the end of their dialysis session. While parenteral iron therapy corrects the iron store deficiency quickly, it doesn't correct the anemia any faster than oral preparations would.

Iron preparations available for parenteral administration are iron dextran (given by I.M. injection or slow, continuous I.V. infusion) and iron sucrose. Iron sucrose is used for patients on hemodialysis. (See *Testing for parenteral iron sensitivity*.)

## Drug interactions

Iron absorption is reduced by antacids as well as by such foods as coffee, tea, eggs, and milk. Other drug interactions involving iron include:
• Absorption of tetracyclines (demeclocycline, doxycycline, minocycline, oxytetracycline, and tetracycline), methyldopa, quinolones (ciprofloxacin, levofloxacin, lomefloxacin, moxifloxacin, norfloxacin, ofloxacin, and sparfloxacin), levothyroxine, and penicillamine may be reduced when taken with oral iron preparations.
• Cholestyramine, cimetidine, proton-pump inhibitors, and colestipol may reduce iron absorption in the GI tract. (See *Adverse reactions to iron therapy*.)

Iron absorption was reduced? Oops. Sorry about that.

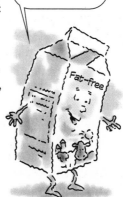

# Vitamin B$_{12}$

*Vitamin B$_{12}$* preparations are used to treat pernicious anemia. Common vitamin B$_{12}$ preparations include cyanocobalamin and hydroxocobalamin.

## Pharmacokinetics

Vitamin B$_{12}$ is available in parenteral, oral, and intranasal forms. For the body to absorb oral forms of vitamin B$_{12}$, the gastric mucosa must secrete a substance called *intrinsic factor.* People who have a deficiency of intrinsic factor develop a special type of anemia known as *vitamin B$_{12}$-deficiency pernicious anemia.*

### Parenteral possibilities

When cyanocobalamin is injected by the I.M. or subcutaneous (subQ) route, it's absorbed and bound to transcobalamin II for transport to the tissues. It then travels via the bloodstream to the liver, where 90% of the body's supply of vitamin B$_{12}$ is stored.

Although hydroxocobalamin is absorbed more slowly from the injection site, its uptake in the liver may be greater than that of cyanocobalamin. Hydroxocobalamin is only administered I.M.

### Most gets lost

With either drug, the liver slowly releases vitamin B$_{12}$ as needed by the body. About 3 to 8 mcg of vitamin B$_{12}$ are excreted in bile each day and then reabsorbed in the ileum. It's also secreted in breast milk during lactation.

Within 48 hours after a vitamin B$_{12}$ injection, 50% to 95% of the dose is excreted unchanged in urine.

## Pharmacodynamics

When vitamin B$_{12}$ is administered, it replaces vitamin B$_{12}$ that the body would normally absorb from the diet. This vitamin is essential for cell growth and replication and for the maintenance of myelin (nerve coverings) throughout the nervous system. Vitamin B$_{12}$ may also be involved in lipid and carbohydrate metabolism.

## Pharmacotherapeutics

Cyanocobalamin and hydroxocobalamin are used to treat pernicious anemia, a megaloblastic anemia characterized by decreased gastric production of hydrochloric acid and intrinsic factor deficiency. Intrinsic factor, a substance normally secreted by the parietal cells of the gastric mucosa, is essential for vitamin B$_{12}$ absorption. Intrinsic factor deficiencies are common in patients who have had total or partial gastrectomies or total ileal resection.

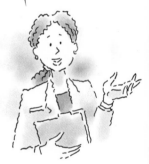

Some patients lack a crucial "intrinsic factor" that allows vitamin B$_{12}$ absorption.

*Warning!*

## Adverse reactions to vitamin B$_{12}$ therapy

No dose-related adverse reactions occur with vitamin B$_{12}$ therapy. However, some rare reactions may occur when vitamin B$_{12}$ is administered parenterally.

**Parenteral problems**
Adverse reactions to parenteral administration can include hypersensitivity reactions that could result in anaphylaxis and death, pulmonary edema, heart failure, peripheral vascular thrombosis, polycythemia vera, hypokalemia, itching, transient rash, hives, and mild diarrhea.

Oral vitamin B$_{12}$ preparations are used to supplement nutritional deficiencies of the vitamin. The parenteral and intranasal formulations are used to treat patients with pernicious anemia.

## Drug interactions

Alcohol, aspirin, neomycin, chloramphenicol, and colchicine may decrease the absorption of oral cyanocobalamin. (See *Adverse reactions to vitamin B$_{12}$ therapy*.)

# Folic acid

*Folic acid* is given to treat megaloblastic anemia due to folic acid deficiency. This type of anemia usually occurs in patients who have tropical or nontropical sprue, although it can also result from poor nutritional intake during pregnancy, infancy, or childhood.

## Pharmacokinetics

Folic acid is absorbed rapidly in the first third of the small intestine, distributed into all body tissues, and metabolized in the liver. Excess folate is excreted unchanged in urine, and small amounts of folic acid are excreted in stool. Folic acid also appears in breast milk. Synthetic folic acid is readily absorbed, even in malabsorption syndromes.

## Pharmacodynamics

Folic acid is an essential component for normal RBC production and growth. A deficiency in folic acid results in megaloblastic anemia and low serum and RBC folate levels.

## Pharmacotherapeutics

Folic acid is used to treat folic acid deficiency. Patients who are pregnant or undergoing treatment for liver disease, hemolytic anemia, alcohol abuse, or skin or renal disorders typically need folic acid supplementation. Serum folic acid levels below 5 ng/ml indicate folic acid deficiency.

Leucovorin is a folic acid derivative used to treat folic acid deficiencies resulting from administration of methotrexate.

## Drug interactions

• Methotrexate, sulfasalazine, hormonal contraceptives, aspirin, triamterene, pentamidine, and trimethoprim reduce the effectiveness of folic acid.
• In large doses, folic acid may counteract the effects of anticonvulsants, such as phenytoin, potentially leading to seizures. (See *Adverse reactions to folic acid*.)

**Warning!**

## Adverse reactions to folic acid

Adverse reactions to folic acid include:
• erythema
• itching
• rash
• anorexia and nausea
• altered sleep patterns
• difficulty concentrating
• irritability
• hyperactivity.

# Erythropoietin agents

*Epoetin alfa* and *darbepoetin alfa* are glycoproteins that stimulate RBC production (erythropoiesis).

## Pharmacokinetics

Epoetin alfa and darbepoetin alfa may be given subQ or I.V. After subQ administration, serum levels of epoetin alfa peak in 5 to 24 hours, while serum levels of darbepoetin alfa peak in 24 to 72 hours.

The circulating half-life of epoetin alfa is also shorter at 4 to 13 hours, compared to 49 hours for darbepoetin alfa. The therapeutic effect of these agents lasts for several days after administration.

## Pharmacodynamics

Epoetin alfa and darbepoetin alfa boost the production of erythropoietin, thus stimulating RBC production in bone marrow. Normally, erythropoietin is formed in the kidneys in response to hypoxia (reduced oxygen) and anemia.

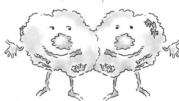

It takes a lot to make an RBC! Folic acid, iron, vitamin $B_{12}$, amino acids, copper, and cobalt are all necessary components...

...And hematinic drugs usually replace one of these missing parts.

Patients with conditions that decrease production of erythropoietin typically develop normocytic anemia. This anemia can usually be corrected after 5 to 6 weeks of treatment with an erythropoietin agent.

## Pharmacotherapeutics

Epoetin alfa is used to:
• treat patients with anemia associated with chronic renal failure
• treat anemia associated with zidovudine therapy in patients with human immunodeficiency virus infection
• treat anemia in cancer patients receiving chemotherapy
• reduce the need for allogenic blood transfusions in surgical patients.

Darbepoetin alfa is used to treat anemia associated with chronic renal failure.

## Drug interactions

No known drug interactions exist with either drug, although they can cause some adverse reactions. (See *Adverse reactions to erythropoietin agents.*)

# Anticoagulant drugs

*Anticoagulant drugs* are used to reduce the ability of the blood to clot. Major categories of anticoagulants include:
• heparin and its derivatives
• oral anticoagulants
• antiplatelet drugs
• direct thrombin inhibitors
• factor Xa inhibitor drugs.

# Heparin

*Heparin,* prepared commercially from animal tissue, is an antithrombolytic agent used to treat and prevent clot formation. Because it doesn't affect the synthesis of clotting factors, heparin can't dissolve already-formed clots.

*Weighty words*

The two types of heparin are unfractionated heparin (UFH) and low-molecular-weight heparin (LMWH). LMWHs, such as dalteparin, enoxaparin, and tinzaparin, were developed to prevent

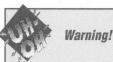

**Warning!**

## Adverse reactions to erythropoietin agents

Hypertension is the most common adverse reaction. Other adverse reactions may include:
• headache
• joint pain
• nausea
• edema
• fatigue
• diarrhea
• vomiting
• chest pain
• skin reactions at the injection site
• weakness
• dizziness.

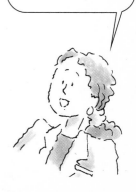

Heparin prevents clots from forming but doesn't dissolve existing clots.

deep vein thrombosis (DVT) (a blood clot in the deep veins, usually of the legs) in surgical patients.

## Pharmacokinetics

Because heparin isn't absorbed well from the GI tract, it must be
administered parenterally. UFH is administered I.V. by continuous
infusion or by subQ injection. LMWHs, because of their prolonged
circulating half-life, can be administered once or twice daily by
subQ injection.

After I.V. administration, the distribution of heparin is immediate; however, distribution isn't as predictable following subQ injection.

**I.M. is out**

Heparin isn't given I.M. because of the risk of localized bleeding.
Heparin is metabolized in the liver, and its metabolites are excreted in urine.

## Pharmacodynamics

Heparin prevents the formation of new thrombi.
Here's how it works:
• Heparin inhibits the formation of thrombin and
fibrin by activating antithrombin III.
• Antithrombin III then inactivates factors IXa, Xa,
XIa, and XIIa in the intrinsic and common pathways.
The end result is prevention of a stable fibrin clot.
• In low doses, heparin increases the activity of antithrombin III against factor Xa and thrombin and inhibits clot formation.
• Much larger doses are necessary to inhibit fibrin
formation after a clot has been formed. This relationship between
dose and effect is the rationale for using low-dose heparin to prevent clotting.
• Whole blood clotting time, thrombin time, and partial thromboplastin time (PTT) are prolonged during heparin therapy. However, these times may be only slightly prolonged with low or ultra-
low preventive doses.

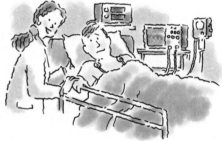

LMWHs help
prevent DVT in
surgical
patients.

## Pharmacotherapeutics

Heparin may be used in a number of clinical situations to prevent
the formation of new clots or the extension of existing clots.
These situations include:
• preventing or treating venous thromboemboli, characterized by
inappropriate or excessive intravascular activation of blood clotting

*Safe and sound*

# Monitoring PTT in heparin therapy

A patient receiving unfractionated heparin (UFH) therapy requires close monitoring of his partial thromboplastin time (PTT). Dosage adjustments, based on the test results, are typically necessary to ensure therapeutic effectiveness without increased risk of bleeding.

Low-molecular-weight heparin (LMWH) therapy doesn't require PTT monitoring. Currently, no laboratory test exists to assess the effectiveness of LMWH therapy.

### Heparin-induced thrombocytopenia

Platelet counts should be monitored in all patients receiving heparin therapy. A patient who develops heparin-induced thrombocytopenia (HIT) should be switched from anticoagulant therapy to argatroban, bivalirudin, or lepirudin. These drugs are direct thrombin inhibitors indicated for use in the patient who needs anticoagulation therapy but has HIT.

- treating disseminated intravascular coagulation, a complication of other diseases, resulting in accelerated clotting
- treating arterial clotting and preventing embolus formation in patients with atrial fibrillation, an arrhythmia in which ineffective atrial contractions cause blood to pool in the atria, increasing the risk of clot formation
- preventing thrombus formation and promoting cardiac circulation in an acute myocardial infarction (MI) by preventing further clot formation at the site of the already formed clot.

## Circulate freely

Heparin can be used to prevent clotting whenever the patient's blood must circulate outside the body through a machine, such as the cardiopulmonary bypass machine or hemodialysis machine, and during blood transfusions. (See *Monitoring PTT in heparin therapy*.)

## You're the one

Heparin is also useful for preventing clotting during intra-abdominal or orthopedic surgery. (These types of surgeries, in many cases, activate the coagulation mechanisms excessively.) In fact, heparin is the drug of choice for orthopedic surgery.

Heparin increases the effects of oral anticoagulants. If a patient is also taking warfarin, watch out for bleeding.

## Drug interactions

• Because heparin acts synergistically with all oral anticoagulants, the risk of bleeding increases when the patient takes both drugs together. The prothrombin time and International Normalized Ratio (INR), used to monitor the effects of oral anticoagulants, may also be prolonged.
• The risk of bleeding increases when the patient takes nonsteroidal anti-inflammatory drugs (NSAIDs), iron dextran, cilostazol, or an antiplatelet drug, such as aspirin, clopidogrel, ticlopidine, or dipyridamole, while receiving heparin.

### Another reason to quit

• Drugs that antagonize or inactivate heparin include antihistamines, cephalosporins, digoxin, neomycin, nicotine, nitroglycerin, penicillins, phenothiazines, quinidine, and tetracycline.
• Nicotine may inactivate heparin; nitroglycerin may inhibit the effects of heparin.
• Administration of protamine sulfate and fresh frozen plasma counteract the effects of heparin. (See *Adverse reactions to heparin.*)

# Oral anticoagulants

The major *oral anticoagulant* used in the United States is the coumarin compound warfarin.

## Pharmacokinetics

Warfarin is absorbed rapidly and almost completely when it's taken orally. It binds extensively to plasma albumin and is metabolized in the liver and excreted in urine. Although warfarin is absorbed quickly, its effects don't occur for about 48 hours, with the full effect taking 3 to 4 days.

Because warfarin is highly plasma-protein-bound and is metabolized by the liver, administration of warfarin with other medications may alter the amount of warfarin in the body. This may increase the risk of bleeding or clotting, depending upon the medications administered.

## Pharmacodynamics

Oral anticoagulants alter the ability of the liver to synthesize vitamin K–dependent clotting factors, including prothrombin and factors VII, IX, and X. However, clotting factors already in the bloodstream continue to coagulate blood until they become depleted, so anticoagulation doesn't begin immediately. (See *Monitoring warfarin levels.*)

## Pharmacotherapeutics

Oral anticoagulants are prescribed to treat or prevent thromboembolism. Patients with this disorder begin taking the medication while still receiving heparin. However, outpatients at high risk for thromboembolism may begin oral anticoagulants without first receiving heparin.

### Deep in the veins

Oral anticoagulants are also the drugs of choice to prevent DVT and for patients with prosthetic heart valves or diseased mitral valves. To decrease the risk of arterial clotting, oral anticoagulants are sometimes combined with an antiplatelet drug, such as aspirin, clopidogrel, or dipyridamole.

## Drug interactions

Many patients who take oral anticoagulants also receive other drugs, placing them at risk for serious drug interactions.
• Many drugs, such as highly protein-bound medications, increase the effects of warfarin, resulting in an increased risk of bleeding. Examples include acetaminophen, allopurinol, amiodarone, cephalosporins, cimetidine, ciprofloxacin, clofibrate, danazol, diazoxide, disulfiram, erythromycin, fluoroquinolones, glucagon, heparin, ibuprofen, isoniazid, ketoprofen, methylthiouracil, metronidazole, miconazole, neomycin, propafenone, propylthiouracil,

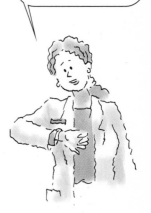

Although oral anticoagulants are absorbed quickly, it can take a couple of days for their full effect to occur.

---

### Monitoring warfarin levels

Patients taking warfarin need close monitoring of prothrombin time and International Normalized Ratios to make sure they are maintaining therapeutic levels of the drug. If laboratory results fall outside the accepted range, warfarin dosage should be adjusted.

quinidine, streptokinase, sulfonamides, tamoxifen, tetracyclines, thiazides, thyroid drugs, tricyclic antidepressants, urokinase, and vitamin E.
• Drugs metabolized by the liver may increase or decrease the effectiveness of warfarin. Examples include barbiturates, carbamazepine, corticosteroids, corticotropin, mercaptopurine, nafcillin, hormonal contraceptives containing estrogen, rifampin, spironolactone, sucralfate, and trazodone.
• The risk of phenytoin toxicity increases when phenytoin is taken with warfarin, and phenytoin may increase or decrease the effects of warfarin.
  Other interactions include the following:
• A diet high in vitamin K reduces the effectiveness of warfarin.
• Chronic alcohol abuse increases the patient's risk of clotting while taking warfarin. Acute alcohol intoxication increases the risk of bleeding.
• Vitamin K and fresh frozen plasma reduce the effects of warfarin. (See *Adverse reactions to oral anticoagulants.*)

# Antiplatelet drugs

*Antiplatelet drugs* are used to prevent arterial thromboembolism, particularly in patients at risk for MI, stroke, and arteriosclerosis (hardening of the arteries).

Aspirin, clopidogrel, dipyridamole, sulfinpyrazone, and ticlopidine are examples of oral antiplatelet drugs. Antiplatelet drugs administered I.V. include abciximab, eptifibatide, and tirofiban.

## Pharmacokinetics

When taken orally, antiplatelet drugs are absorbed very quickly and reach peak concentration in 1 to 2 hours. Aspirin maintains its antiplatelet effect for about 10 days, or as long as platelets normally survive. The effects of clopidogrel last about 5 days. Sulfinpyrazone may require several days of administration before its antiplatelet effects occur.

After I.V. administration, antiplatelet drugs are quickly distributed throughout the body. They're minimally metabolized and excreted unchanged in urine. The effects of these drugs occur within 15 to 20 minutes of administration and last about 6 to 8 hours.

Elderly patients and patients with renal failure may have decreased clearance of antiplatelet drugs, which would prolong the antiplatelet effect.

*Warning!*

## Adverse reactions to oral anticoagulants

The primary adverse reaction to oral anticoagulant therapy is minor bleeding. Severe bleeding can occur, however, with the most common site being the GI tract. Bleeding into the brain may be fatal. Bruises and hematomas may form at arterial puncture sites (for example, after a blood gas sample is drawn). Necrosis or gangrene of the skin and other tissues can occur.

**Quick fix**
The effects of oral anticoagulants can be reversed with phytonadione (vitamin $K_1$).

## Pharmacodynamics

Antiplatelet drugs interfere with platelet activity in different drug-specific and dose-related ways.

• Low doses of aspirin inhibit clot formation by blocking the synthesis of prostaglandin, which in turn prevents formation of the platelet-aggregating substance thromboxane $A_2$.

• Clopidogrel inhibits platelet aggregation by inhibiting platelet-fibrinogen binding.

• I.V. antiplatelet drugs inhibit the glycoprotein IIa-IIIb receptor, which is the major receptor involved in platelet aggregation.

• Dipyridamole may inhibit platelet aggregation because it increases adenosine, a coronary vasodilator and platelet aggregation inhibitor.

• Ticlopidine inhibits the binding of fibrinogen to platelets during the first stage of the clotting cascade.

• Sulfinpyrazone inhibits several platelet functions. It lengthens platelet survival and prolongs the patency of arteriovenous shunts used for hemodialysis. A single dose rapidly inhibits platelet aggregation.

## Pharmacotherapeutics

Antiplatelet drugs have many different uses.

### Managing MIs

Aspirin is used in patients who have had a previous MI or who have unstable angina to reduce the risk of death in patients at high risk for CAD. It's also prescribed to reduce the risk of transient ischemic attacks (TIAs) (temporary reduction in circulation to the brain).

Clopidogrel is used to reduce the risk of stroke or vascular death in patients with a history of a recent MI, stroke, or established peripheral artery disease. Clopidogrel is also used to help treat acute coronary syndromes, especially in patients undergoing percutaneous transluminal coronary angioplasty (PTCA) or coronary artery bypass graft.

Eptifibatide may be used for patients with acute coronary syndrome and for those undergoing percutaneous coronary intervention (PCI). Abciximab may also be used in combination with PCI. Tirofiban may be used to treat acute coronary syndrome.

### Salve for surgery

Dipyridamole is used with a coumarin compound to prevent thrombus formation after cardiac valve replacement. Dipyridamole may be administered with aspirin to prevent blood clots in

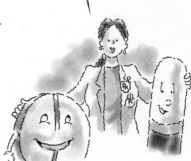

Aspirin can help patients who have had an MI and can also reduce the risk of stroke.

patients who have had coronary artery bypass grafts (bypass surgery) or prosthetic (artificial) heart valves.

## Circumventing stroke

Ticlopidine is used to reduce the risk of thrombotic stroke in high-risk patients, such as those with a history of frequent TIAs or a previous thrombotic stroke.

## Drug interactions

- Antiplatelet medications taken with NSAIDs, heparin, oral anticoagulants, or another antiplatelet medication increase the risk of bleeding.
- Sulfinpyrazone taken with aspirin and oral anticoagulants increases the risk of bleeding.

## Tales of toxicity

- Aspirin increases the risk of toxicity of methotrexate and valproic acid.
- Aspirin and ticlopidine may reduce the effectiveness of sulfinpyrazone to relieve signs and symptoms of gout.
- Antacids may reduce the plasma levels of ticlopidine.

- Cimetidine increases the risk of ticlopidine toxicity and bleeding.

## You just don't know

Because guidelines haven't been established for administrating ticlopidine with heparin, oral anticoagulants, aspirin, or fibrinolytic drugs, these drugs should be discontinued before ticlopidine therapy begins. (See *Adverse reactions to antiplatelet drugs*.)

# Direct thrombin inhibitors

Thrombin inhibitors, including argatroban, bivalirudin, and lepirudin, help prevent the formation of blood clots.

## Pharmacokinetics

Direct thrombin inhibitors are typically administered by continuous I.V. infusion. They may also be given as an intra-coronary bolus during cardiac catheterization. In that case, the drug begins acting in 2 minutes, with a peak response of 15 minutes and a duration of 2 hours. After subQ injection, plasma levels peak in 2 hours; after I.V. administration, levels peak in less than 1 hour.

Effects on PTT become apparent within 4 to 5 hours of administration. In patients with heparin-induced thrombocytopenia, platelet count recovery becomes apparent within 3 days.

Argatroban is metabolized by the liver and excreted primarily in stool. Bivalirudin and lepirudin are metabolized by the liver and kidneys and excreted in urine

## Pharmacodynamics

Direct thrombin inhibitors interfere with blood clotting by directly blocking all thrombin activity. These drugs offer several advantages over heparin: direct thrombin inhibitors act against soluble as well as clot-bound thrombin (thrombin in clots that have already formed); their anticoagulant effects are more predictable than those of heparin; and their actions aren't inhibited by the platelet release reaction.

The binding of the drug to thrombin is reversible.

## Pharmacotherapeutics

Administered by I.V. infusion, argatroban and lepirudin are used to treat heparin-induced thrombocytopenia (HIT). Argatroban may also be given with aspirin to patients with HIT who are undergoing a cardiac procedure, such as PTCA, coronary stent placement, or atherectomy.

Bivalirudin has been approved for use in patients with unstable angina undergoing PTCA, and should be used in conjunction with aspirin therapy.

Patients with liver dysfunction may require a reduced dose of argatroban. Also, the dosage of bivalirudin and lepirudin may need to be reduced in patients with impaired renal function.

Use caution when administering a direct thrombin inhibitor to a patient who has an increased risk of bleeding. Patients at greatest risk for hemorrhage are those with severe hypertension, gastric ulcers, or hematologic disorders associated with increased bleeding. Patients receiving spinal anesthesia or those undergoing a lumbar puncture or having major surgery (especially surgery of the brain, spinal cord, or the eye) also have an increased risk for bleeding.

## Drug interactions

• Hemorrhage can occur as an adverse reaction to direct thrombin inhibitors, so avoid giving these drugs with another drug that may also increase the risk of bleeding.
• Discontinue all parenteral anticoagulants before administering argatroban.
• Administration of argatroban along with warfarin increases the INR.
• If the patient has received heparin, allow time for heparin's effect on PTT to decrease before administering argatroban. (See *Adverse reactions to bivalirudin.*)

**Warning!**

## Adverse reactions to bivalirudin

The major adverse reaction to bivalirudin is bleeding; major hemorrhage occurs infrequently. Other adverse reactions include:
• intracranial hemorrhage
• retroperitoneal hemorrhage
• nausea, vomiting, abdominal cramps, and diarrhea
• headache
• hematoma at I.V. infusion site.

# Factor Xa inhibitor drugs

Factor Xa inhibitor drugs are used to prevent DVT in patients undergoing total hip and knee replacement surgery or surgery to repair a hip fracture. The only factor Xa inhibitor drug used in the United States is fondaparinux.

## Pharmacokinetics

Administered subQ, fondaparinux is absorbed rapidly and completely and is excreted primarily unchanged in urine. Its effects peak within 2 hours of administration and last for about 17 to 24 hours.

## Pharmacodynamics

Fondaparinux binds to antithrombin III and greatly influences the neutralization of factor Xa by antithrombin III. Neutralization of factor Xa interrupts the coagulation cascade, thereby inhibiting clot formation.

## Pharmacotherapeutics

Fondaparinux is used only to prevent the formation of blood clots.

## Drug interactions

Avoid administering fondaparinux with another drug that may increase the risk of bleeding. (See *Adverse reactions to factor Xa inhibitors*.)

# Thrombolytic drugs

*Thrombolytic drugs* are used to dissolve a preexisting clot or thrombus, often in an acute or emergency situation. Some of the thrombolytic drugs currently used include alteplase, reteplase, streptokinase, tenecteplase, and urokinase.

## Pharmacokinetics

After I.V. or intracoronary administration, thrombolytic drugs are distributed immediately throughout the circulation, quickly activating plasminogen (a precursor to plasmin, which dissolves fibrin clots).

*Blood work*

Alteplase, reteplase, tenecteplase, and urokinase are cleared rapidly from circulating plasma, primarily by the liver. Streptokinase is removed rapidly from the circulation by antibodies and the reticuloendothelial system (a body system involved in defending against infection and disposing of products of cell breakdown). These agents don't appear to cross the placental barrier.

## Pharmacodynamics

Thrombolytic drugs convert plasminogen to plasmin, which lyses (dissolves) thrombi, fibrinogen, and other plasma proteins. (See *How alteplase helps restore circulation*, page 172.)

## Pharmacotherapeutics

Thrombolytic drugs have a number of uses. They're used to treat certain thromboembolic disorders (such as acute MI, acute ischemic stroke, and peripheral artery occlusion) and have also

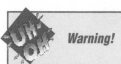

**Warning!**

## Adverse reactions to factor Xa inhibitors

Adverse reactions that can occur with factor Xa inhibitor therapy include:
- bleeding
- nausea
- anemia
- fever
- rash
- constipation
- edema.

Thrombolytic drugs dissolve clots or thrombi in emergency situations.

EMERGENCY

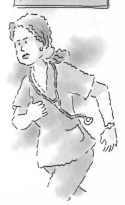

*Now I get it!*

# How alteplase helps restore circulation

When a thrombus forms in an artery, it obstructs the blood supply, causing ischemia and necrosis. Alteplase can dissolve a thrombus in either the coronary or pulmonary artery, restoring the blood supply to the area beyond the blockage.

**Obstructed artery**
A thrombus blocks blood flow through the artery, causing distal ischemia.

**Inside the thrombus**
Alteplase enters the thrombus, which consists of plasminogen bound to fibrin. Alteplase binds to the fibrin-plasminogen complex, converting the inactive plasminogen into active plasmin. This active plasmin digests the fibrin, dissolving the thrombus. As the thrombus dissolves, blood flow resumes.

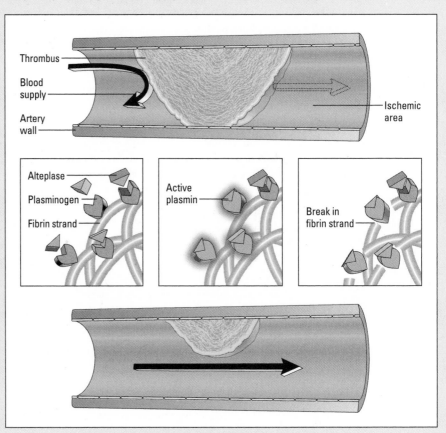

been used to dissolve thrombi in arteriovenous cannulas (used in dialysis) and I.V. catheters to reestablish blood flow.

## The sooner the better

Thrombolytic drugs are the drugs of choice to break down newly formed thrombi. They seem most effective when administered within 6 hours of the symptoms onset.

## Acute MI and others

In addition, each drug has specific uses.
• Alteplase is used to treat acute MI, pulmonary embolism, acute ischemic stroke, peripheral artery occlusion, and to restore patency to clotted grafts and I.V. access devices.
• Streptokinase is used to treat acute MI, pulmonary embolus, and DVT.
• Reteplase and tenecteplase are used to treat acute MI.
• Urokinase is used to treat pulmonary embolism and coronary artery thrombosis and for catheter clearance.

## Drug interactions

• Thrombolytic drugs interact with heparin, oral anticoagulants, antiplatelet drugs, and NSAIDs to increase the patient's risk of bleeding.
• Aminocaproic acid inhibits streptokinase and can be used to reverse its fibrinolytic effects. (See *Adverse reactions to thrombolytic drugs.*)

**Warning!**

### Adverse reactions to thrombolytic drugs

The major reactions associated with thrombolytic drugs are bleeding and allergic responses, especially with streptokinase.

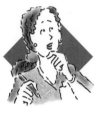

# Quick quiz

**1.** A patient is given heparin to treat thrombophlebitis. If the patient starts to bleed excessively during heparin therapy, which drug is likely to be prescribed to reverse its effects?
    A. Vitamin K
    B. Factor VIII
    C. Argatroban
    D. Protamine sulfate

*Answer:* D. Protamine sulfate reverses the effects of heparin.

**2.** Why is heparin administered concurrently with warfarin?
    A. Warfarin's therapeutic effects don't occur until clotting factors are depleted.
    B. Heparin activates warfarin.
    C. Warfarin and heparin have a synergistic effect.
    D. Heparin helps the body absorb warfarin.

*Answer:* A. Heparin is administered concurrently with warfarin because warfarin is ineffective until clotting factors are depleted.

**3.**   How soon after cyanocobalamin (vitamin B$_{12}$) therapy is begun can a patient expect to feel better?
  A.   24 hours
  B.   72 hours
  C.   1 week
  D.   2 weeks

*Answer:*   A. The effects of cyanocobalamin can be felt 24 hours after initiation of treatment.

## Scoring

☆☆☆   If you answered all three items correctly, far out! You're hip to hematologic drugs.

☆☆   If you answered two items correctly, that's great! You've caught the wave of anticoagulants.

☆   If you answered fewer than two items correctly, play it cool. You just might need some time to get the blood flowing.

That was really informative. I wonder what we'll read about next.

# Respiratory drugs

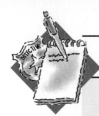

## Just the facts

In this chapter, you'll learn:

♦ classes of drugs used to treat respiratory disorders

♦ uses and varying actions of these drugs

♦ how these drugs are absorbed, distributed, metabolized, and excreted

♦ drug interactions and adverse reactions to these drugs.

## Drugs and the respiratory system

The respiratory system, extending from the nose to the pulmonary capillaries, performs the essential function of gas exchange between the body and its environment. In other words, it takes in oxygen and expels carbon dioxide.

*Breathe easy*

Drugs used to improve respiratory symptoms are available in inhalation and systemic formulations. These drugs include:

- beta$_2$-adrenergic agonists
- anticholinergics
- corticosteroids
- leukotriene modifiers
- mast cell stabilizers
- methylxanthines
- monoclonal antibodies
- expectorants
- antitussives
- mucolytics
- decongestants.

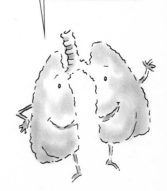

I've got an important job—gas exchange—and sometimes I need a little help from respiratory drugs to get it done.

# Beta₂-adrenergic agonists

*Beta₂-adrenergic agonists* are used to treat symptoms associated with asthma and chronic obstructive pulmonary disease (COPD). Drugs in this class can be either short-acting or long-acting.

## Short-acting beta₂-adrenergic agonists

Short-acting beta₂-adrenergic agonists include:
- albuterol (systemic, inhalation)
- levalbuterol (inhalation)
- metaproterenol (inhalation)
- pirbuterol (inhalation)
- terbutaline (systemic).

## Long-acting beta₂-adrenergic agonists

Long-acting beta₂-adrenergic agonists include:
- formoterol (inhalation)
- salmeterol (inhalation).

### Pharmacokinetics (how drugs circulate)

Beta₂-adrenergic agonists are minimally absorbed from the GI tract; inhaled forms exert their effects locally. After inhalation, beta₂-adrenergic agonists appear to be absorbed over several hours from the respiratory tract. These drugs don't cross the blood-brain barrier; they're extensively metabolized in the liver to inactive compounds and rapidly excreted in urine and stool.

### Pharmacodynamics (how drugs act)

Beta₂-adrenergic agonists increase levels of cyclic adenosine monophosphate by stimulating the beta₂-adrenergic receptors in the smooth muscle, resulting in bronchodilation. These drugs may lose their selectivity at higher doses, which can increase the risk of toxicity. Inhaled forms are preferred because they act locally in the lungs, resulting in fewer adverse reactions than systemically absorbed forms.

### Pharmacotherapeutics (how drugs are used)

Short-acting inhaled beta₂-adrenergic agonists are the drugs of choice for fast relief of symptoms in the patient with asthma. They're generally used as needed for asthma (including exercise-induced asthma) and COPD. A patient with COPD may use them around-the-clock on a specified schedule. However, excessive use of a short-acting beta₂-adrenergic agonist

Short-acting inhaled beta₂-adrenergic agonists provide relief that's fast!

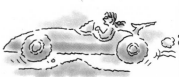

### Safe and sound

## Problems with long-acting beta₂-adrenergic agonists

If a patient is taking a long-acting beta₂-adrenergic agonist, make sure that he's using it only as part of a combination therapy with other medications such as inhaled corticosteroids. Patients who use long-acting beta₂-adrenergic agonists as their only means of asthma control are at serious risk for adverse effects, including death.

### Warning!

## Adverse reactions to beta₂-adrenergic agonists

Adverse reactions to short-acting beta₂-adrenergic agonists include:

• paradoxical bronchospasm
• tachycardia
• palpitations
• tremors
• dry mouth.

  Adverse reactions to long-acting beta₂-adrenergic agonists include:

• bronchospasm
• tachycardia
• palpitations
• hypertension
• tremors.

may indicate poor asthma control, requiring reassessment of the patient's therapeutic regimen.

## A good combination

Long-acting beta₂-adrenergic agonists tend to be used with anti-inflammatory agents, namely inhaled corticosteroids, to help control asthma. (See *Problems with long-acting beta₂-adrenergic agonists.*) They're especially useful for the patient with nocturnal asthmatic symptoms. These drugs must be administered on a schedule. They aren't used to relieve acute symptoms because their onset of action isn't fast enough. They also don't affect the chronic inflammation associated with asthma.

### Drug interactions

Interactions are uncommon when using the inhaled forms. Beta-adrenergic blockers decrease the bronchodilating effects of beta₂-adrenergic agonists. They should be used together cautiously. (See *Adverse reactions to beta₂-adrenergic agonists.*)

# Anticholinergics

Inhaled ipratropium, an *anticholinergic*, is a bronchodilator used primarily in the patient suffering from COPD, but it may also be used as an adjunct to beta₂-adrenergic agonists.

## Ipratropium

*Ipratropium* is the most common anticholinergic used for respiratory disorders.

## Pharmacokinetics

Anticholinergics are minimally absorbed from the GI tract; they come in inhaled forms that exert their effects locally.

## Pharmacodynamics

Ipratropium inhibits muscarinic receptors, which results in bronchodilation. This drug works by blocking the parasympathetic nervous system, rather than stimulating the sympathetic nervous system.

## Pharmacotherapeutics

Anticholinergics are used to relieve symptoms in the patient with COPD. They're less effective in long-term management of the patient with asthma; however, they may be used as adjunctive therapy (usually in combination with a short-acting beta$_2$-adrenergic agonist on a scheduled basis).

## Drug interactions

Interactions are uncommon when using the inhaled forms. Ipratropium should be used cautiously with antimuscarinic drugs and other anticholinergics. (See *Adverse reactions to anticholinergics*.)

*Warning!*

### Adverse reactions to anticholinergics

The most common adverse reactions to anticholinergics include:
• nervousness
• tachycardia
• nausea and vomiting
• paradoxical bronchospasm (with excessive use)
• dry mouth.

# Corticosteroids

*Corticosteroids* are anti-inflammatory drugs available in inhaled and systemic forms for the short- and long-term control of asthma symptoms. Many products with differing potencies are available.

Inhaled corticosteroids include:
• beclomethasone dipropionate
• budesonide
• flunisolide
• fluticasone
• triamcinolone acetonide.

Oral corticosteroids include:
• prednisolone
• prednisone.

I.V. corticosteroids include:
• hydrocortisone sodium succinate
• methylprednisolone sodium succinate.

*Safe and sound*

## Corticosteroids

These special populations may require special care when taking corticosteroids:
• *Children:* Growth should be monitored, especially when they're taking systemic drugs or higher doses of inhaled drugs.
• *Elderly patients:* May benefit from receiving drugs that prevent osteoporosis, such as alendronate during therapy with corticosteroids, especially if they're taking higher doses of inhaled or systemic steroids.

• *Patients with diabetes:* May require closer monitoring of their blood glucose levels while on steroids.
• *Breast-feeding women:* Corticosteroid levels are negligible in the breast milk of mothers who take less than 20 mg/day of oral prednisone. The amount found in breast milk can be minimized if the woman waits at least 4 hours after taking prednisone to breast-feed her infant.

## Pharmacokinetics

Oral prednisone is readily absorbed and extensively metabolized in the liver to the active metabolite prednisolone. The I.V. form has a rapid onset. Inhaled drugs are minimally absorbed, although absorption increases as the dosage is increased.

## Pharmacodynamics

Corticosteroids work by inhibiting the production of cytokines, leukotrienes, and prostaglandins; the recruitment of eosinophils; and the release of other inflammatory mediators. They also affect other areas in the body, which can cause long-term adverse reactions. (See *Corticosteroids.*)

## Pharmacotherapeutics

Corticosteroids are the most effective drugs available for the long-term treatment and prevention of acute asthma attacks.

### Inhalation for prevention

Inhaled corticosteroids are the preferred drugs for preventing future attacks in the patient with mild to severe asthma. Use of inhaled corticosteroids reduces the need for systemic steroids in many cases, thus reducing the patient's risk of developing serious long-term adverse reactions.

### Systemic for the serious

Systemic forms are usually reserved for moderate to severe attacks, but they're also used in the patient with milder asthma that

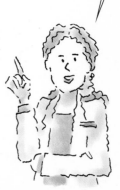

Corticosteroids are the most effective drugs for the long-term treatment and prevention of acute asthma attacks.

fails to respond to other measures. Systemic corticosteroids should be used at the lowest effective dosage and for the shortest period possible to avoid adverse reactions.

## Drug interactions

Interactions are uncommon when using inhaled forms.
• Hormonal contraceptives, ketoconazole, and macrolide antibiotics may increase the activity of corticosteroids in general, resulting in the need to decrease the steroid dosage.
• Barbiturates, cholestyramine, rifampin, and phenytoin may decrease the effectiveness of corticosteroids, resulting in the need to increase the steroid dosage. (See *Adverse reactions to inhaled corticosteroids.*)

# Leukotriene modifiers

*Leukotriene modifiers* are used for the prevention and long-term control of mild asthma.
    Leukotriene receptor antagonists include:
• montelukast
• zafirlukast.
    Leukotriene formation inhibitors include:
• zileuton.

## Pharmacokinetics

Montelukast is rapidly absorbed. Zafirlukast's absorption is decreased by food, so it should be given 1 hour before or 2 hours after meals.
    All of the leukotriene modifiers are highly protein-bound (more than 90%).

### Metabolism and excretion

Zafirlukast is extensively metabolized in the liver by the cytochrome P450 2C9 (CYP2C9) enzyme into inactive metabolites and excreted primarily in stool. In general, this class of drugs is metabolized, induced, or inhibited by the cytochrome P450 enzyme system, which is important for establishing drug interactions.

### Caution required

Zileuton is contraindicated in the patient with active liver disease. Closely monitor the patient with liver impairment who's taking zafirlukast for adverse reactions; he may require a dosage adjustment. This doesn't apply for montelukast.

*Warning!*

## Adverse reactions to inhaled corticosteroids

Adverse reactions to inhaled corticosteroids may include:
• mouth irritation
• oral candidiasis
• upper respiratory tract infection.
    To reduce the risk of adverse reactions from inhaled steroids, the patient should use the lowest possible dosage to maintain control, administer doses using a spacer, and rinse out his mouth after administration.

## Pharmacodynamics

Leukotrienes are substances released from mast cells, eosinophils, and basophils that can cause smooth-muscle contraction of the airways, increased permeability of the vasculature, increased secretions, and activation of other inflammatory mediators.

Leukotrienes may be inhibited by two different mechanisms. The leukotriene receptor antagonists zafirlukast and montelukast prevent the D4 and E4 leukotrienes from interacting with their receptors, thereby blocking their action. The leukotriene formation inhibitor zileuton inhibits the production of 5-lipoxygenase, thereby preventing the formation of leukotrienes.

## Pharmacotherapeutics

Leukotriene modifiers are primarily used to prevent and control asthma attacks in the patient with mild to moderate disease. Montelukast is also indicated for the treatment of allergic rhinitis.

## Drug interactions

- Zafirlukast inhibits CYP2C9 and thus could increase the risk of toxicity if used with phenytoin or warfarin.
- Zafirlukast and zileuton inhibit CYP3A4 and thus could increase the risk of toxicity if used with amlodipine, atorvastatin, carbamazepine, clarithromycin, cyclosporine, erythromycin, hormonal contraceptives, itraconazole, ketoconazole, lovastatin, nelfinavir, nifedipine, ritonavir, sertraline, simvastatin, or warfarin.
- Zileuton inhibits CYP1A2 and thus could increase the risk of toxicity if used with amitriptyline, clozapine, desipramine, fluvoxamine, imipramine, theophylline, or warfarin.

Talkin' toxicity

- Zafirlukast, zileuton, and montelukast are metabolized by CYP2C9 and thus could increase the risk of toxicity if used with amiodarone, cimetidine, fluconazole, fluoxetine, fluvoxamine, isoniazid, metronidazole, or voriconazole. If carbamazepine, phenobarbital, phenytoin, primidone, or rifampin is used with leukotrienes, the effectiveness of the leukotrienes could be reduced.
- Zileuton and montelukast are metabolized by CYP3A4 and thus could increase the risk of toxicity if used with amiodarone, cimetidine, clarithromycin, cyclosporine, erythromycin, fluoxetine, fluvoxamine, grapefruit juice, itraconazole, ketoconazole, metronidazole, or voriconazole and could result in decreased effectiveness if used with carbamazepine, efavirenz, garlic supplements, modafinil, nevirapine, oxcarbazepine, phenobarbital, phenytoin, primidone, rifabutin, rifampin, or St. John's wort.

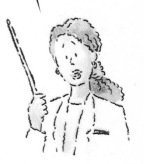

Leukotrienes can be very trying for asthma sufferers. Montelukast, zafirlukast, and zileuton help to inhibit their action.

• Zileuton is metabolized by CYP1A2 and thus could increase the risk of toxicity if used with cimetidine, clarithromycin, erythromycin, fluvoxamine, or isoniazid and could result in decreased effectiveness if used with carbamazepine, phenobarbital, phenytoin, primidone, rifampin, ritonavir, or St. John's wort or if used by a smoker. (See *Adverse reactions to leukotriene modifiers*.)

# Mast cell stabilizers

*Mast cell stabilizers* are used to prevent asthma attacks, especially in a child or a patient with mild disease. They're also used in an adult or child with mild to moderate persistent asthma. Drugs in this class include:
• cromolyn
• nedocromil.

## Pharmacokinetics

Mast cell stabilizers are minimally absorbed from the GI tract; they're available in inhaled forms that exert their effects locally.

## Pharmacodynamics

These drugs stabilize the mast cell membrane, possibly by inhibiting calcium channels, thus preventing the release of inflammatory mediators.

## Pharmacotherapeutics

Mast cell stabilizers are used for the prevention and long-term control of asthma symptoms. They do this by controlling the inflammatory process.

*Number 1 for children*

Mast cell stabilizers are often used for children and patients with exercise-induced asthma.

## Drug interactions

Interactions are uncommon when using inhaled forms. (See *Adverse reactions to mast cell stabilizers*.)

**Warning!**

## Adverse reactions to leukotriene modifiers

Adverse reactions that may occur with leukotriene modifiers include:
• headache
• dizziness
• nausea and vomiting
• myalgia.

**Warning!**

## Adverse reactions to mast cell stabilizers

Inhaled mast cell stabilizers may cause these adverse reactions:
• pharyngeal and tracheal irritation
• cough
• wheezing
• bronchospasm
• headache.

# Methylxanthines

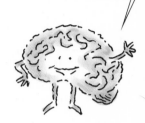

Xanthines stimulate my medulla!

*Methylxanthines*, also called *xanthines*, are used to treat respiratory disorders.

## Types of methylxanthines

Methylxanthines include *anhydrous theophylline* and its derivative salt aminophylline.

Theophylline is the most commonly prescribed oral methylxanthine. Aminophylline is preferred when an I.V. methylxanthine is required. Caffeine is also a xanthine derivative.

## Pharmacokinetics

The pharmacokinetics of methylxanthines vary according to which drug the patient is receiving, the dosage form, and the administration route.

### Absorption

When theophylline is given as an oral solution or a rapid-release tablet, it's absorbed rapidly and completely. High-fat meals can increase theophylline concentrations and the risk of toxicity.

## Gastric measures

Absorption of some of theophylline's slow-release forms depends on the gastric pH. Food can alter absorption. When converting the patient from I.V. aminophylline to oral theophylline, the dosage is decreased by 20%.

### Distribution

Theophylline is approximately 56% protein-bound in adults and 36% protein-bound in neonates. It readily crosses the placental barrier and is secreted in breast milk. Smokers and patients on dialysis may need higher doses.

### Metabolism and excretion

Theophylline is metabolized primarily in the liver by the CYP1A2 enzyme. In adults and children, about 10% of a dose is excreted unchanged in urine; therefore, no dosage adjustment is required in patients with renal insufficiency. Elderly patients and those with liver dysfunction may require a lower dose. Because an infant has an immature liver with reduced metabolic functioning, as much as one-half of a dose may be excreted unchanged in his urine.

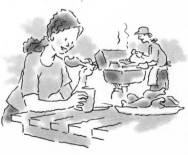

High-fat meals can increase the risk of theophylline toxicity.

## Blood levels matter

Theophylline levels must be measured to evaluate efficacy and avoid toxicity. The therapeutic serum concentration is 10 to 20 mcg/ml (SI, 44 to 111 µmol/L). Levels must be assessed when drug therapy is initiated, when the dosage is changed, and when drugs are added or removed from the patient's regimen.

### Pharmacodynamics

Methylxanthines act in many ways.

## Relax and breathe deeply

Methylxanthines decrease airway reactivity and relieve bronchospasm by relaxing bronchial smooth muscle. Theophylline is believed to inhibit phosphodiesterase, resulting in smooth-muscle relaxation, bronchodilation, and decreased inflammatory mediators (namely mast cells, T cells, and eosinophils). Much of theophylline's toxicity may be due to increased catecholamine release.

## A stimulating conversation

In nonreversible obstructive airway disease (chronic bronchitis, emphysema, and apnea), methylxanthines appear to increase the sensitivity of the brain's respiratory center to carbon dioxide and to stimulate the respiratory drive.

## Pumping you up

In chronic bronchitis and emphysema, these drugs reduce fatigue of the diaphragm, the respiratory muscle that separates the abdomen from the thoracic cavity. They also improve ventricular function and, therefore, the heart's pumping action.

### Pharmacotherapeutics

Theophylline and its salts are used as second- or third-line therapy for the long-term control and prevention of symptoms related to:
- asthma
- chronic bronchitis
- emphysema.

## Useful for neonates?

Theophylline has been used to treat neonatal apnea (periods of not breathing in the neonate) and has been effective in reducing severe bronchospasm in an infant with cystic fibrosis.

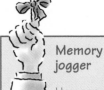

**Memory jogger**

How can you remember what theophylline and its salts are used to treat? Simple: Just remember that you really need to "ACE" this one! It's used for long-term control and prevention of symptoms related to:
A— asthma
C—chronic bronchitis
E—emphysema.

**Warning!**

# Adverse reactions to methylxanthines

Adverse reactions to methylxanthines may be transient or symptomatic of toxicity.

**Gut reactions**
Adverse GI system reactions include:
- nausea and vomiting
- abdominal cramping
- epigastric pain
- anorexia
- diarrhea.

**Nerve racking**
Adverse central nervous system reactions include:
- headache
- irritability
- restlessness
- anxiety
- insomnia
- dizziness.

**Heart of the matter**
Adverse cardiovascular reactions include:
- tachycardia
- palpitations
- arrhythmias.

## Drug interactions

Theophylline drug interactions occur with substances that inhibit or induce the CYP1A2 enzyme. (See *Adverse reactions to methylxanthines.*)

- Inhibitors of the CYP1A2 enzyme (including cimetidine, ciprofloxacin, clarithromycin, erythromycin, fluvoxamine, hormonal contraceptives, isoniazid, ketoconazole, ticlopidine, and zileuton) decrease theophylline metabolism, thus increasing its serum level as well as the risk of adverse reactions and toxicity. The dosage of theophylline may need to be reduced.
- Inducers of the CYP1A2 enzyme (including carbamazepine, phenobarbital, phenytoin, rifampin, St. John's wort, and charbroiled meats) increase theophylline metabolism, thus decreasing its serum level and possibly its effectiveness. The dosage of theophylline may need to be increased.
- Smoking cigarettes or marijuana increases theophylline elimination, thus decreasing its serum level and effectiveness.
- Taking adrenergic stimulants or drinking beverages that contain caffeine or caffeinelike substances may result in additive adverse reactions to theophylline or signs and symptoms of methylxanthine toxicity.
- Activated charcoal may decrease theophylline levels.
- The use of enflurane or isoflurane with theophylline or theophylline derivatives increases the risk of cardiac toxicity.
- Theophylline and its derivatives may reduce the effects of lithium by increasing its rate of excretion.
- Thyroid hormones may reduce theophylline levels; antithyroid drugs may increase theophylline levels.

Smoking increases the elimination of theophylline, which reduces its effectiveness.

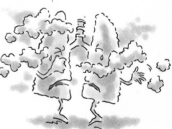

# Monoclonal antibodies

*Monoclonal antibodies*, particularly anti-immunoglobin (Ig) E monoclonal antibodies, are used in patients with moderate-to-severe asthma with a positive skin test and who are inadequately controlled with inhaled corticosteroids. Omalizumab is the only drug in this class.

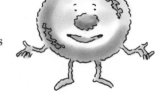

When inhaled corticosteroids aren't up to the task, monoclonal antibodies may be used to control a patient's moderate-to-severe asthma.

## Omalizumab

### Pharmacokinetics

Omalizumab is slowly absorbed after subcutaneous injection. It's metabolized by the liver, but the rate of metabolization depends on IgG clearance.

### Pharmacodynamics

Omalizumab inhibits the binding of IgE to its receptor on the mast cell and basophils. This in turns inhibits the release of allergic substances which potentiate asthma symptoms.

### Pharmacotherapeutics

Omalizumab is used in patients with moderate-to-severe asthma with a positive skin test and insufficient control on inhaled corti-costeroids. Dosing for the drug is based on pretreatment serum IgE levels.

---

**Warning!**

## Adverse reactions to monoclonal antibodies

Adverse reactions to monoclonal antibodies include:
• injection site reactions
• upper respiratory tract infections
• sinusitis
• headache
• pharyngitis

• allergic reaction.
    Allergic reactions may be severe enough to be life-threatening and typically occur within 2 hours of administration. However, in rare cases, delayed anaphylactic reactions (occurring more than 24 hours after administration) may occur.

### Drug interactions

No formal drug-interaction studies have been done. (See *Adverse reactions to monoclonal antibodies.*)

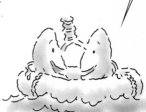

Expectorants thin mucus, helping me cough up clogging secretions more productively.

## Expectorants

*Expectorants* thin mucus so it's cleared more easily out of the airways. They also soothe mucous membranes in the respiratory tract. The result is a more productive cough.

## Guaifenesin

The most commonly used expectorant is *guaifenesin.*

### Pharmacokinetics

Guaifenesin is absorbed through the GI tract, metabolized by the liver, and excreted primarily by the kidneys.

### Pharmacodynamics

By increasing production of respiratory tract fluids, expectorants reduce the thickness, adhesiveness, and surface tension of mucus, making it easier to clear from the airways. Expectorants also provide a soothing effect on the mucous membranes of the respiratory tract.

### Pharmacotherapeutics

Guaifenesin is used to relieve symptoms due to ineffective, productive coughs from many disorders, such as:
- bronchial asthma
- bronchitis
- colds
- emphysema
- influenza
- minor bronchial irritation
- sinusitis.

### Drug interactions

Guaifenesin isn't known to have specific drug interactions; however, it does cause some adverse reactions. (See *Adverse reactions to guaifenesin.*)

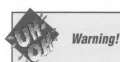

*Warning!*

### Adverse reactions to guaifenesin

Adverse reactions to guaifenesin include:
- nausea
- vomiting (if taken in large doses)
- diarrhea
- abdominal pain
- drowsiness
- headache
- hives
- rash.

# Antitussives

*Antitussive drugs* suppress or inhibit coughing.

## Types of antitussives

Antitussives are typically used to treat dry, nonproductive coughs. The major antitussives include:
• benzonatate
• codeine
• dextromethorphan
• hydrocodone bitartrate.

### Pharmacokinetics

Antitussives are absorbed well through the GI tract, metabolized in the liver, and excreted in urine.

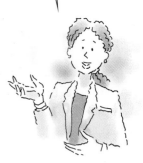

### Pharmacodynamics

Antitussives act in slightly different ways.

## Removing the sensation

Benzonatate acts by anesthetizing stretch receptors throughout the bronchi, alveoli, and pleurae.

## Taking direct action

Codeine, dextromethorphan, and hydrocodone suppress the cough reflex by direct action on the cough center in the medulla of the brain, thus lowering the cough threshold.

### Pharmacotherapeutics

The uses of these drugs vary slightly, but each treats a serious, nonproductive cough that interferes with a patient's ability to rest or carry out activities of daily living.

## Put it to the test

Benzonatate relieves cough caused by pneumonia, bronchitis, the common cold, and chronic pulmonary diseases such as emphysema. It can also be used during bronchial diagnostic tests, such as bronchoscopy, when the patient must avoid coughing.

## Top of the charts

Dextromethorphan is the most widely used cough suppressant in the United States and may provide better antitussive effects than codeine. Its popularity may stem from the fact that it isn't associ-

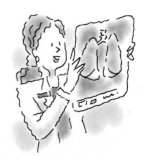

ated with sedation, respiratory depression, or addiction at usual doses.

## For really tough coughs

The opioid antitussives (typically codeine and hydrocodone) are reserved for treating an intractable cough.

### Drug interactions

Antitussives may interact with other drugs.
- Codeine and hydrocodone may cause excitation, an extremely elevated temperature, hypertension or hypotension, and coma when taken with monoamine oxidase inhibitors (MAOIs).
- Dextromethorphan use with MAOIs may produce excitation, an elevated body temperature, hypotension, and coma.
- Codeine taken with other central nervous system (CNS) depressants, including alcohol, barbiturates, phenothiazines, and sedative-hypnotics, may increase CNS depression, resulting in drowsiness, lethargy, stupor, respiratory depression, coma, and even death. (See *Adverse reactions to antitussives*.)

# Mucolytics

*Mucolytics* act directly on mucus, breaking down sticky, thick secretions so that they're more easily eliminated.

# Acetylcysteine

*Acetylcysteine* is the only mucolytic used clinically in the United States for the patient with abnormal or thick mucus.

## Pharmacokinetics

Inhaled acetylcysteine is absorbed from the pulmonary epithelium. When taken orally, the drug is absorbed from the GI tract.

### Metabolism and excretion

Acetylcysteine is metabolized in the liver; its excretion is unknown.

## Pharmacodynamics

Acetylcysteine decreases the thickness of respiratory tract secretions by altering the molecular composition of mucus. It also irritates the mucosa to stimulate clearance and restores glutathione, a substance that plays an important role in oxidation-reduction processes.

Liver cleaner

Glutathione's enzymatic action in the liver reduces acetaminophen toxicity from overdose.

## Pharmacotherapeutics

Mucolytics are used with other therapies to treat the patient with abnormal or thick mucus secretions, such as the patient with:
• atelectasis caused by mucus obstruction, as may occur in pneumonia, bronchiectasis, or chronic bronchitis
• bronchitis
• pulmonary complications related to cystic fibrosis.

Patient preparations

Mucolytics may also be used to prepare the patient for bronchography and other bronchial studies.

Overdose antidote

Acetylcysteine is the antidote for acetaminophen overdose. However, it doesn't fully protect against liver damage caused by acetaminophen toxicity.

## Drug interactions

Activated charcoal decreases acetylcysteine's effectiveness. When using acetylcysteine to treat an acetaminophen overdose, remove

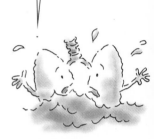

When thick secretions overwhelm me, mucolytics thin mucus quickly so I can breathe better.

activated charcoal from the stomach before administering. (See *Adverse reactions to acetylcysteine.*)

# Decongestants

*Decongestants* may be classified as systemic or topical, depending on how they're administered.

## Types of decongestants

As sympathomimetic drugs, systemic decongestants stimulate the sympathetic nervous system to reduce swelling of the respiratory tract's vascular network. Systemic decongestants include:
• ephedrine
• phenylephrine
• pseudoephedrine.

## Topical concerns

Topical decongestants are also powerful vasoconstrictors. When applied directly to swollen mucous membranes of the nose, they provide immediate relief from nasal congestion. These drugs include:
• ephedrine, epinephrine, and phenylephrine (sympathomimetic amines)
• naphazoline and tetrahydrozoline (imidazoline derivatives of sympathomimetic amines).

## Pharmacokinetics

The pharmacokinetic properties of decongestants vary.

### Absorbed quickly...

When taken orally, the systemic decongestants are absorbed readily from the GI tract and widely distributed throughout the body into various tissues and fluids, including cerebrospinal fluid, the placenta, and breast milk.

### ...metabolized slowly

Systemic decongestants are slowly and incompletely metabolized by the liver and excreted largely unchanged in urine within 24 hours of oral administration.·

### Direct action

Topical decongestants act locally on the alpha receptors of the vascular smooth muscle in the nose, causing the arterioles to constrict. As a result of this local action, absorption of the drug is negligible.

**Warning!**

## Adverse reactions to acetylcysteine

During administration, acetylcysteine has a "rotten egg" odor that may cause nausea. With prolonged or persistent use, acetylcysteine may produce:
• bronchospasm
• drowsiness
• nausea and vomiting
• severe runny nose
• stomatitis.
   Acetylcysteine isn't recommended for the patient with asthma because it may cause bronchospasm.

## Pharmacodynamics

The properties of systemic and topical decongestants vary slightly.

### System(ic) analysis

Systemic decongestants cause vasoconstriction by stimulating alpha-adrenergic receptors in the blood vessels of the body. This reduces the blood supply to the nose, which decreases swelling of the nasal mucosa. They also cause contraction of urinary and GI sphincters, dilated pupils, and decreased insulin secretion.

### Indirect hit

These drugs may also act indirectly, causing the release of norepinephrine from storage sites in the body, which results in peripheral vasoconstriction.

### On topic(al)

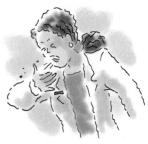

With sneezing usually comes congestion. Better get a decongestant!

Like systemic decongestants, topical decongestants stimulate alpha-adrenergic receptors in the smooth muscle of nasal blood vessels, resulting in vasoconstriction. The combination of reduced blood flow to the nasal mucous membranes and decreased capillary permeability reduces swelling. This action improves respiration by helping to drain sinuses, clear nasal passages, and open eustachian tubes.

## Pharmacotherapeutics

Systemic and topical decongestants are used to relieve the symptoms of swollen nasal membranes resulting from:
• acute coryza (profuse discharge from the nose)
• allergic rhinitis (hay fever)
• the common cold
• sinusitis
• vasomotor rhinitis.

### Team tactics

Systemic decongestants are commonly given with other drugs, such as antihistamines, antimuscarinics, antipyretic analgesics, and antitussives.

### Advantage, topical

Topical decongestants provide two major advantages over systemics: minimal adverse reactions and rapid symptom relief.

## Drug interactions

Because they produce vasoconstriction, which reduces drug absorption, topical decongestants seldom produce drug interactions.

**Warning!**

## Adverse reactions to decongestants

Most adverse reactions to decongestants result from central nervous system stimulation and include:
• nervousness
• restlessness
• insomnia
• nausea
• palpitations
• tachycardia
• difficulty urinating
• elevated blood pressure.

Systemic decongestants exacerbate hypertension, hyperthyroidism, diabetes, benign prostatic hypertrophy, glaucoma, and heart disease. They're also secreted in breast milk in a breast-feeding woman.

**Topical decongestants**
The most common adverse reaction associated with prolonged use (more than 5 days) of topical decongestants is rebound nasal congestion.

Other reactions include:
• burning and stinging of the nasal mucosa
• sneezing
• mucosal dryness or ulceration.

**Issue of sensitivity**
The patient who's hypersensitive to other sympathomimetic amines may also be hypersensitive to decongestants.

Systemic decongestants, however, may interact with other drugs. (See *Adverse reactions to decongestants*.)
• Increased CNS stimulation may occur when systemic decongestants are taken with other sympathomimetic drugs, including epinephrine, norepinephrine, dopamine, dobutamine, isoproterenol, metaproterenol, terbutaline, and phenylephrine, and tyramine-containing foods.
• Use of systemic decongestants with MAOIs may cause severe hypertension or a hypertensive crisis, which can be life-threatening. These drugs shouldn't be used together.
• Alkalinizing drugs may increase the effects of pseudoephedrine by reducing its urinary excretion.

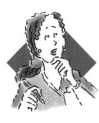

## Quick quiz

**1.** Which adverse reaction can occur if guaifenesin is taken in larger doses than necessary?
    A. Constipation
    B. Vomiting
    C. Insomnia
    D. Diarrhea

*Answer:* B. Vomiting can occur if guaifenesin is taken in abnormally large doses.

**2.** Which medication should the patient avoid when taking dextromethorphan?

    A.    Acetaminophen

    B.    Guaifenesin

    C.    Phenelzine

    D.    Famotidine

*Answer:* C. MAOIs, such as phenelzine, should be avoided by the patient taking dextromethorphan; concurrent use may cause life-threatening reactions.

**3.** Besides bronchitis, acetylcysteine may also be used to treat:

    A.    acetaminophen overdose.

    B.    severe rhinorrhea.

    C.    stomatitis.

    D.    diarrhea.

*Answer:* A. Acetylcysteine is an effective antidote for acetaminophen overdose.

**4.** Which adverse reaction most commonly occurs with a decongestant, such as tetrahydrozoline, especially if it's taken more often than recommended?

    A.    Nausea

    B.    Dizziness

    C.    Diarrhea

    D.    Rebound nasal congestion

*Answer:* D. Rebound nasal congestion commonly occurs when tetrahydrozoline is taken more frequently than recommended.

## Scoring

☆☆☆  If you answered all four items correctly, you're slicker than a mucolytic in action!

  ☆☆  If you answered three items correctly, you're as relaxed as bronchial smooth muscle on xanthines.

    ☆  If you answered fewer than three items correctly, you may need to clear your head with a decongestant. Review the chapter once more and try again!

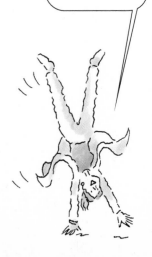

Great job on respiratory drugs! Now let's flip on over to GI drugs.

# Gastrointestinal drugs

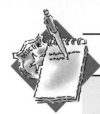

## Just the facts

In this chapter, you'll learn:

♦ classes of drugs used to improve GI function

♦ uses and varying actions of these drugs

♦ how these drugs are absorbed, distributed, metabolized, and excreted

♦ drug interactions and adverse reactions to these drugs.

## Drugs and the GI system

The GI tract is basically a hollow, muscular tube that begins at the mouth and ends at the anus; it encompasses the pharynx, esophagus, stomach, and the small and large intestines. Its primary functions are to digest food and absorb nutrients and fluids and excrete metabolic waste.

### Getting on tract

Classes of drugs used to improve GI function include:
• peptic ulcer drugs
• adsorbent, antiflatulent, and digestive drugs
• obesity drugs
• antidiarrheal and laxative drugs
• antiemetic and emetic drugs.

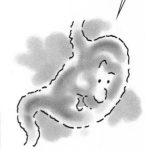

I'm very important to the GI tract. I help digest food and absorb nutrients!

## Antiulcer drugs

A *peptic ulcer* is a circumscribed lesion that develops in the mucous membranes of the lower esophagus, stomach, duodenum, or jejunum.

## Counting causes

The five major causes of peptic ulcers are:

 bacterial infection with *Helicobacter pylori*

the use of nonsteroidal anti-inflammatory drugs (NSAIDs)

hypersecretory states such as Zollinger-Ellison syndrome (a condition in which excessive secretion of gastric acid causes peptic ulcers)

cigarette smoking, which causes hypersecretion and impairs ulcer healing

a genetic predisposition, which accounts for 20% to 50% of peptic ulcers.

## Balancing act

*Peptic ulcer drugs* are aimed at either eradicating *H. pylori* or restoring the balance between acid and pepsin secretions and the GI mucosal defense. These drugs include:
- systemic antibiotics
- antacids
- Histamine-2 ($H_2$) receptor antagonists
- proton pump inhibitors
- other peptic ulcer drugs, such as misoprostol and sucralfate.

# Systemic antibiotics

*H. pylori* is a gram-negative bacterium that's thought to be a major causative factor in the formation of peptic ulcers and gastritis (inflammation of the stomach lining). Eradication of the bacteria helps to heal ulcers and decrease their recurrence.

## Teamwork is a must

Successful treatment involves the use of two or more antibiotics in combination with other drugs such as acid suppressants. *Systemic antibiotics* used to treat *H. pylori* include:
- amoxicillin
- clarithromycin
- metronidazole
- tetracycline.

### Pharmacokinetics (how drugs circulate)

Systemic antibiotics are variably absorbed from the GI tract.

## Dairy delay

Food, especially dairy products, decreases the absorption of tetracycline but doesn't significantly delay the absorption of the other antibiotics.

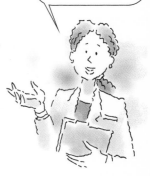

Food decreases the absorption of tetracycline.

### Distribution and excretion

All of these antibiotics are distributed widely and are excreted primarily in urine.

## Pharmacodynamics (how drugs act)

Antibiotics act by treating the *H. pylori* infection. They're usually combined with an H₂-receptor antagonist or a proton pump inhibitor to decrease stomach acid and further promote healing.

## Pharmacotherapeutics (how drugs are used)

They are indicated for *H. pylori* eradication to reduce the risk of a duodenal ulcer. For this reason they may be used in conjunction with other medications such as proton pump inhibitors.

## Successful strategy

Successful treatment plans use at least two antibiotics and a proton pump inhibitor for 14 days and then use a proton pump inhibitor for 6 more weeks to help reduce acid in patients with a peptic ulcer.

## Drug interactions

Tetracycline and metronidazole can interact with many other medications.
• Tetracycline increases digoxin levels.
• Metronidazole and tetracycline increase the risk of bleeding when taken with oral anticoagulants.
• Metronidazole can cause a severe reaction when combined with alcohol. (See *Adverse reactions to antibiotics*.)

# Antacids

*Antacids* are over-the-counter (OTC) medications that are used as adjunct therapy to treat peptic ulcers. They include:
• aluminum carbonate gel
• calcium carbonate
• magaldrate (aluminum-magnesium complex)
• magnesium hydroxide and aluminum hydroxide
• simethicone.

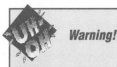

*Warning!*

## Adverse reactions to antibiotics

Antibiotics used to improve GI tract function may lead to adverse reactions.
• Metronidazole, clarithromycin, and tetracycline commonly cause mild GI disturbances.
• Clarithromycin and metronidazole may also produce abnormal tastes.
• Amoxicillin may cause diarrhea.

## Pharmacokinetics

Antacids work locally in the stomach by neutralizing gastric acid. They don't need to be absorbed to treat peptic ulcers.

### Distribution and excretion

Antacids are distributed throughout the GI tract and are eliminated primarily in stool.

## Pharmacodynamics

The acid-neutralizing action of antacids reduces the total amount of acid in the GI tract, allowing peptic ulcers to heal.

### The more it works, the sooner it rests

Pepsin, one of the stomach secretions, acts more effectively when the stomach is highly acidic; therefore, as acidity drops, pepsin action is also reduced. Contrary to popular belief, antacids don't work by coating peptic ulcers or the lining of the GI tract.

## Pharmacotherapeutics

Antacids are primarily prescribed to relieve pain and are used adjunctively in peptic ulcer disease.

### Settling the GI system

Antacids also relieve symptoms of acid indigestion, heartburn, dyspepsia (burning or indigestion), or gastroesophageal reflux disease (GERD), in which the contents of the stomach and duodenum flow back into the esophagus.

### Fighting phosphate

Antacids may be used to control hyperphosphatemia (elevated blood phosphate levels) in kidney failure. Because calcium binds with phosphate in the GI tract, calcium carbonate antacids prevent phosphate absorption.

## Drug interactions

All antacids can interfere with the absorption of oral drugs given at the same time. Absorption of digoxin, phenytoin, ketoconazole, iron salts, isoniazid, quinolones, and tetracyclines may be reduced if taken within 2 hours of antacids. (See *Adverse reactions to antacids.*)

*Warning!*

**Adverse reactions to antacids**

All adverse reactions to antacids are dose-related and include:
- diarrhea
- constipation
- electrolyte imbalances
- aluminum accumulation in serum.

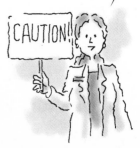

Antacids can interfere with the absorption of other orally administered drugs.

# H$_2$-receptor antagonists

*H$_2$-receptor antagonists* are commonly prescribed antiulcer drugs in the United States. They include:
• cimetidine
• famotidine
• nizatidine
• ranitidine.

## Pharmacokinetics

Cimetidine, nizatidine, and ranitidine are absorbed rapidly and completely from the GI tract. Famotidine isn't completely absorbed. Antacids may reduce the absorption of H$_2$-receptor antagonists.

### Distribution, metabolism, and excretion

H$_2$-receptor antagonists are distributed widely throughout the body, metabolized by the liver, and excreted primarily in urine.

## Pharmacodynamics

H$_2$-receptor antagonists block histamine from stimulating the acid-secreting parietal cells of the stomach.

*The acid test*

Acid secretion in the stomach depends on the binding of gastrin, acetylcholine, and histamine to receptors on the parietal cells. If the binding of one of these substances is blocked, acid secretion is reduced. The H$_2$-receptor antagonists, by binding with H$_2$ receptors, block the action of histamine in the stomach and reduce acid secretion. (See *How H$_2$-receptor antagonists work*, page 200.)

## Pharmacotherapeutics

H$_2$-receptor antagonists are used therapeutically to:
• promote healing of duodenal and gastric ulcers
• provide long-term treatment of pathologic GI hypersecretory conditions such as Zollinger-Ellison syndrome
• reduce gastric acid production and prevent stress ulcers in the severely ill patient and in the patient with reflux esophagitis or upper GI bleeding.

## Drug interactions

H$_2$-receptor antagonists may interact with antacids and other drugs.

*Now I get it!*

# How H$_2$-receptor antagonists work

These illustrations show how histamine-2 (H$_2$) receptor antagonists reduce the release of gastric acid.

To stimulate gastric acid secretion, certain endogenous substances—primarily histamine, but also acetylcholine and gastrin—attach to receptors on the surface of parietal cells. These substances activate the enzyme adenyl cyclase, which converts adenosine triphosphate (ATP) to the intracellular catalyst cyclic adenosine monophosphate (cAMP).

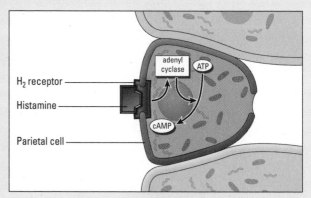

The cAMP ultimately stimulates proton-pump (H/K ATPase) activity. The pump catalyzes the exchange of extracellular potassium (K) ions for intracellular hydrogen (H) ions. When the H$^+$ ions combine with extracellular chloride (Cl) ions excreted by gastric cells at a different site, the result is hydrochloric (HCl), or gastric, acid.

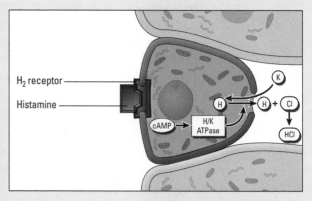

H$_2$-receptor antagonists competitively bind to H$_2$-receptor sites on the surface of parietal cells and inhibit the common pathway that histamine and the other substances must travel to stimulate proton-pump activity and promote gastric acid secretion.

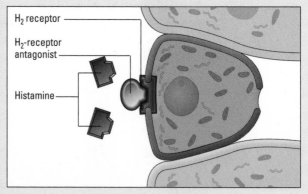

- Antacids reduce the absorption of cimetidine, famotidine, nizatidine, and ranitidine.
- Cimetidine may increase the blood levels of oral anticoagulants, propranolol (and possibly other beta-adrenergic blockers), benzodiazepines, tricyclic antidepressants, theophylline, procainamide, quinidine, lidocaine, phenytoin, calcium channel blockers, cyclosporine, carbamazepine, and opioid analgesics by reducing their metabolism in the liver and subsequent excretion.
- Cimetidine taken with carmustine increases the risk of bone marrow toxicity.
- Cimetidine inhibits metabolism of ethyl alcohol in the stomach, resulting in higher blood alcohol levels. (See *Adverse reactions to H₂-receptor antagonists.*)

# Proton pump inhibitors

*Proton pump inhibitors* disrupt chemical binding in stomach cells to reduce acid production, lessening irritation and allowing peptic ulcers to better heal. They include:
- esomeprazole
- lansoprazole
- omeprazole
- pantoprazole
- rabeprazole.

## Pharmacokinetics

Proton pump inhibitors are given orally in enteric-coated formulas to bypass the stomach because they're highly unstable in acid. When in the small intestine, they dissolve and are absorbed rapidly.

### Metabolism and excretion

These medications are highly protein-bound and are extensively metabolized by the liver to inactive compounds and then eliminated in urine.

## Pharmacodynamics

Proton pump inhibitors block the last step in the secretion of gastric acid by combining with hydrogen, potassium, and adenosine triphosphate in the parietal cells of the stomach.

## Pharmacotherapeutics

Proton pump inhibitors are indicated for:
- short-term treatment of active gastric ulcers

**Warning!**

## Adverse reactions to H₂-receptor antagonists

The use of H₂-receptor antagonists may lead to adverse reactions, especially in the elderly patient and the patient with altered hepatic or renal function.
- Cimetidine and ranitidine may produce headache, dizziness, malaise, muscle pain, nausea, diarrhea or constipation, rash, itching, loss of sexual desire, gynecomastia (cimetidine), and impotence.
- Famotidine and nizatidine produce few adverse reactions; headache is the most common, followed by constipation or diarrhea and rash.

- active duodenal ulcers
- erosive esophagitis
- symptomatic GERD unresponsive to other therapies
- active peptic ulcers associated with *H. pylori* infection, in combination with antibiotics
- long-term treatment of hypersecretory states such as Zollinger-Ellison syndrome.

## Drug interactions

Proton pump inhibitors may interfere with the metabolism of diazepam, phenytoin, and warfarin, causing increased half-life and elevated plasma levels of these drugs.

*Absorbing talk*

Proton pump inhibitors may also interfere with the absorption of drugs that depend on gastric pH for absorption, such as ketoconazole, digoxin, ampicillin, and iron salts. (See *Adverse reactions to proton pump inhibitors*.)

**Warning!**

## Adverse reactions to proton pump inhibitors

Adverse reactions to proton pump inhibitors include:
- abdominal pain
- diarrhea
- nausea and vomiting.

# Other antiulcer drugs

Research continues on the usefulness of other drugs in treating peptic ulcer disease. Two other drugs currently in use are:
- misoprostol (a synthetic form of prostaglandin $E_1$)
- sucralfate.

## Pharmacokinetics

Each drug has a slightly different pharmacokinetic property.

### Absorption, metabolism, and excretion

After an oral dose, misoprostol is absorbed extensively and rapidly. It's metabolized to misoprostol acid, which is clinically active, meaning that it can produce a pharmacologic effect. Misoprostol acid is highly protein-bound and is excreted primarily in urine.

Sucralfate is minimally absorbed from the GI tract and is excreted in stool.

## Pharmacodynamics

The actions of these drugs vary.

*Nay-saying NSAIDs*

Misoprostol protects against peptic ulcers caused by NSAIDs by reducing the secretion of gastric acid and boosting the production of gastric mucus, a natural defense against peptic ulcers.

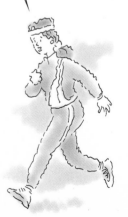

That misoprostol is one active drug!

### Safe and sound

## Dangers of misoprostol use during pregnancy

Use of misoprostol during pregnancy can lead to premature birth, birth defects, or fetal abortion. When used after the 8th week of pregnancy to induce labor or abortion, misoprostol can cause uterine rupture as well. Misoprostol-induced abortions may be incomplete. For these reasons, the drug is contraindicated for gastric ulcer prevention during pregnancy.

### Warning!

## Adverse reactions to other peptic ulcer drugs

**Misoprostol**
• Diarrhea (common and usually dose-related)
• Abdominal pain
• Gas
• Indigestion
• Nausea and vomiting

**Sucralfate**
• Constipation
• Nausea and vomiting
• Metallic taste

## Protective paste

Sucralfate works locally in the stomach, rapidly reacting with hydrochloric acid to form a thick, pastelike substance that adheres to the gastric mucosa and, especially, to ulcers. By binding to the ulcer site, sucralfate actually protects the ulcer from the damaging effects of acid and pepsin to promote healing. This binding usually lasts for 6 hours.

### Pharmacotherapeutics

Each of these drugs has its own therapeutic use.

## Making it less complicated

Misoprostol prevents gastric ulcers caused by NSAIDs in the patient at high risk for complications resulting from gastric ulcers. (See *Dangers of misoprostol use during pregnancy*.)

## In the short run

Sucralfate is used for the short-term treatment (up to 8 weeks) of duodenal or gastric ulcers and for the prevention of recurrent ulcers or stress ulcers.

### Drug interactions

Misoprostol and sucralfate may interact with other drugs.
• Antacids may bind with misoprostol or decrease its absorption. However, this effect doesn't appear to be clinically significant.
• Antacids may reduce the binding of sucralfate to the gastric and duodenal mucosa, reducing its effectiveness.
• Cimetidine, digoxin, norfloxacin, phenytoin, fluoroquinolones, ranitidine, tetracycline, and theophylline decrease the absorption of sucralfate. (See *Adverse reactions to other peptic ulcer drugs*.)

> Sucralfate reacts with hydrochloric acid to form a substance that adheres to ulcer sites.

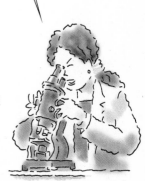

# Adsorbent, antiflatulent, and digestive drugs

Adsorbent, antiflatulent, and digestive drugs are used to fight undesirable toxins, acids, and gases in the GI tract, aiding healthy GI function.

## Adsorbent drugs

Natural and synthetic *adsorbents* are prescribed as antidotes for the ingestion of toxins, substances that can lead to poisoning or overdose.

*Charcoal sketch*

The most commonly used clinical adsorbent is activated charcoal, a black powder residue obtained from the distillation of various organic materials.

### Pharmacokinetics

Activated charcoal must be administered soon after toxic ingestion because it can bind only with drugs or poisons that haven't yet been absorbed from the GI tract.

*Vicious cycle*

After initial absorption, some poisons move back into the intestines, where they're reabsorbed. Activated charcoal may be administered repeatedly to break this cycle.

#### Absorption, metabolism, and excretion

Activated charcoal, which isn't absorbed or metabolized by the body, is excreted unchanged in stool.

### Pharmacodynamics

Because adsorbents attract and bind to toxins in the intestine, they inhibit toxins from being absorbed by the GI tract. However, this binding doesn't change toxic effects caused by earlier absorption of the poison.

### Pharmacotherapeutics

Activated charcoal is a general-purpose antidote used for many types of acute oral poisoning. It isn't indicated in acute poisoning from mineral acids, alkalines, cyanide, ethanol, methanol, iron,

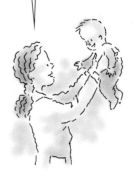

Don't worry. We know not to give you activated charcoal until you're at least 1 year old.

lithium, sodium chloride alkali, inorganic acids, or organic solvents. It also shouldn't be used in a child who's younger than age 1 year. In addition, it shouldn't be used in a patient who has a risk of GI obstruction, perforation, or hemorrhage or decreased or absent bowel sounds, or who has had recent GI surgery.

## Drug interactions

Activated charcoal can decrease absorption of oral medications; therefore, medications (other than those used to treat the ingested toxin) shouldn't be taken orally within 2 hours of taking the activated charcoal. The effectiveness of activated charcoal may be decreased by vomiting induced by ipecac syrup. If both drugs are used to treat oral poisoning, activated charcoal should be used after vomiting has ceased. (See *Adverse reactions to activated charcoal*.)

# Antiflatulent drugs

*Antiflatulents* disperse gas pockets in the GI tract. They're available alone or in combination with antacids. A major antiflatulent drug currently in use is simethicone.

## Pharmacokinetics

Antiflatulents aren't absorbed from the GI tract. They're distributed only in the intestinal lumen and are eliminated intact in stool.

## Pharmacodynamics

Antiflatulents provide defoaming action in the GI tract. By producing a film in the intestines, simethicone disperses mucus-enclosed gas pockets and helps prevent their formation.

## Pharmacotherapeutics

Antiflatulents are prescribed to treat conditions in which excess gas is a problem, such as:
• functional gastric bloating
• postoperative gaseous bloating
• diverticular disease
• spastic or irritable colon
• air swallowing.

## Drug interactions

Simethicone doesn't interact significantly with other drugs and doesn't cause known adverse reactions.

**Warning!**

## Adverse reactions to activated charcoal

Activated charcoal turns stools black and may cause constipation.

**Teaming up**
A laxative, such as sorbitol, usually is given with activated charcoal to prevent constipation and improve taste.

Antiflatulent drugs create a film in the intestines that collapses and disperses gas bubbles.

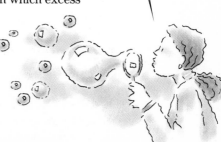

# Digestive drugs

*Digestive drugs* (digestants) aid digestion in the patient who's missing enzymes or other substances needed to digest food. Digestants that function in the GI tract, liver, and pancreas include:

- pancreatin
- pancrelipase
- lipase
- protease
- amylase (pancreatic enzymes).

## Pharmacokinetics

Digestants aren't absorbed; they act locally in the GI tract and are excreted in stool.

## Pharmacodynamics

The action of digestants resembles the action of the body substances they replace. Pancreatic enzymes replace normal pancreatic enzymes. They exert their effect in the duodenum and upper jejunum of the upper GI tract.

### Breaking it down

These drugs contain trypsin to digest proteins, amylase to digest carbohydrates, and lipase to digest fats.

## Pharmacotherapeutics

Because their action resembles the action of the body substances they replace, each digestant has its own indication.

### Mirror images

Pancreatic enzymes are administered to the patient with insufficient levels of pancreatic enzymes, such as the patient with pancreatitis or cystic fibrosis. They may also be used to treat steatorrhea (disorder of fat metabolism characterized by fatty, foul-smelling stool).

## Drug interactions

Antacids reduce the effects of pancreatic enzymes and shouldn't be given at the same time. Pancreatic enzymes may decrease the absorption of folic acid and iron. (See *Adverse reactions to digestive drugs.*)

**Warning!**

## Adverse reactions to digestive drugs

**Pancreatic enzymes**
- Abdominal cramping
- Diarrhea
- Nausea

# Obesity drugs

*Obesity drugs* are used for patients who are morbidly obese and have health problems that are likely to improve with weight loss. They're used in combination with a weight management program that includes diet, physical activity, and behavioral modification. Drug therapy should be used to improve health rather than promote cosmetic weight loss.

Drugs for obesity fall into two categories:
• appetite suppressants (phentermine and sibutramine)
• fat blockers (orlistat).

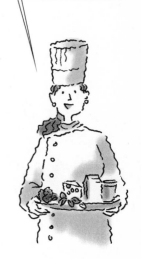

Obesity drugs should only be used for morbidly obese patients as part of a combined regimen that includes diet, physical activity, and behavioral modification.

## Pharmacokinetics

Sibutramine is rapidly absorbed from the intestines and rapidly distributed to most body tissues. It's metabolized in the liver and excreted in the urine and feces. Orlistat isn't absorbed systemically; its action occurs in the GI tract. Orlistat is excreted in the feces.

## Pharmacodynamics

Appetite suppressants increase the amount of norepinephrine and dopamine in the brain, thereby suppressing the appetite. The fat-blocking drug orlistat binds to gastric and pancreatic lipases in the GI tract, making them unavailable to break down fats. This blocks absorption of 30% of the fat ingested in a meal.

## Pharmacotherapeutics

Appetite suppressants and fat blockers are used primarily for weight loss when losing weight will improve the patient's health and prevent death.

## Drug interactions

Obesity drugs interact with other drugs.
• Appetite suppressants taken with cardiovascular stimulants may increase the risk of hypertension and arrhythmias.
• Appetite suppressants taken with central nervous system (CNS) stimulants can cause increased anxiety and insomnia.
• Appetite suppressants taken with serotonergic drugs (including fluoxetine, sumatriptan, dextromethorphan, and lithium) can cause agitation, confusion, hypomania, impaired coordination, loss of consciousness, nausea, or tachycardia.

> **Warning!**
>
> ## Adverse reactions to obesity drugs
>
> Adverse reactions to obesity drugs include the following:
> - Phentermine can cause nervousness, dry mouth, constipation, and hypertension.
> - Sibutramine can cause dry mouth, headache, insomnia, nervousness, constipation, hypertension, tachycardia, and palpitations.
> - Orlistat causes abdominal pain, oily spotting, fecal urgency, flatulence with discharge, fatty stools, fecal incontinence, and increased defecation. These effects usually subside after a few weeks.

- Orlistat blocks the absorption of fat-soluble vitamins if taken together. (See *Adverse reactions to obesity drugs.*)

# Antidiarrheal and laxative drugs

Diarrhea and constipation are the two major symptoms related to disturbances of the large intestine.

## Is it local?

*Antidiarrheals* act systemically or locally and include:
- opioid-related drugs
- kaolin and pectin
- 5-HT$_3$ receptor antagonists (alosetron).

## Loosen up!

*Laxatives* stimulate defecation and include:
- hyperosmolar drugs
- dietary fiber and related bulk-forming substances
- emollients
- stimulants
- lubricants.

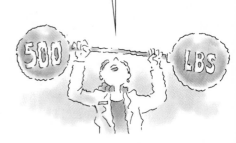

> Although many over-the-counter laxatives are available, diet and lifestyle changes are probably the best first line of defense against constipation.

# Opioid-related drugs

*Opioid-related drugs* decrease peristalsis (involuntary, progressive, wavelike intestinal movement that pushes fecal matter along) in the intestines and include:
- diphenoxylate with atropine

• loperamide.

## Pharmacokinetics

The combination drug diphenoxylate with atropine is readily absorbed from the GI tract. However, loperamide isn't absorbed well after oral administration.

### Distribution, metabolism, and excretion

Both drugs are distributed in serum, metabolized in the liver, and excreted primarily in stool. Diphenoxylate with atropine is metabolized to difenoxin, its biologically active major metabolite.

## Pharmacodynamics

Diphenoxylate with atropine and loperamide slow GI motility by depressing peristalsis in the large and small intestines. These drugs also decrease expulsive contractions throughout the colon.

## Pharmacotherapeutics

Diphenoxylate with atropine and loperamide are used to treat acute, nonspecific diarrhea. Loperamide is used to treat chronic diarrhea.

## Drug interactions

Diphenoxylate with atropine and loperamide may enhance the depressant effects of barbiturates, alcohol, opioids, tranquilizers, and sedatives. (See *Adverse reactions to opioid-related drugs*.)

**Warning!**

### Adverse reactions to opioid-related drugs

Adverse reactions to diphenoxylate with atropine and loperamide include:
• nausea and vomiting
• abdominal discomfort or distention
• drowsiness
• fatigue
• central nervous system depression
• tachycardia (fast heart rate)
• paralytic ileus (reduced or absent peristalsis in the intestines).

# Kaolin and pectin

*Kaolin* and *pectin* mixtures are locally acting OTC antidiarrheals. They work by adsorbing irritants and soothing the intestinal mucosa.

## Pharmacokinetics

Kaolin and pectin aren't absorbed and, therefore, aren't distributed throughout the body. They're excreted in stool.

## Pharmacodynamics

Kaolin and pectin act as adsorbents, binding with bacteria, toxins, and other irritants in the intestinal mucosa. Pectin decreases the pH in the intestinal lumen and provides a soothing effect on the irritated mucosa.

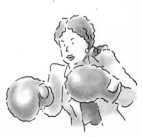

Kaolin and pectin give diarrhea the one-two punch.

## Pharmacotherapeutics

Kaolin and pectin are used to relieve mild to moderate acute diarrhea. They may also be used to temporarily relieve chronic diarrhea until the cause is determined and definitive treatment begun.

## Drug interactions

These antidiarrheals can interfere with the absorption of digoxin and other drugs by the intestinal mucosa if administered at the same time. (See *Adverse reactions to kaolin and pectin*.)

# 5-HT$_3$ receptor antagonists

*Alosetron* is a selective 5-HT$_3$ receptor antagonist used for short-term treatment of women with irritable bowel syndrome (IBS) with severe diarrhea as the main symptom. This drug is available only through a restricted marketing program because of reported serious GI adverse effects. Only prescribers enrolled in the prescribing program for alosetron may write a prescription for it.

## Pharmacokinetics

Alosetron is rapidly absorbed after oral administration and is metabolized by the cytochrome P450 pathway.

## Pharmacodynamics

Alosetron is thought to block serotonin in the GI system, thereby reducing the abdominal cramping and discomfort, urgency, and diarrhea commonly associated with IBS.

## Pharmacotherapeutics

Alosetron is used for the short-term treatment of a woman with IBS whose primary symptom is diarrhea. The drug shouldn't be taken if the patient is constipated and should be stopped if constipation develops.

## Drug interactions

Alosetron produces a 30% inhibition of *N*-acetyltransferase and CYP1A2. Although studies haven't been done, the inhibition of *N*-acetyltransferase may have clinical significance when alosetron is given with such drugs as isoniazid, procainamide, and hydralazine. Alosetron given with other drugs that decrease GI motility could cause constipation. (See *Adverse reactions to alosetron*.)

**Warning!**

## Adverse reactions to kaolin and pectin

Kaolin and pectin mixtures cause few adverse reactions. However, constipation may occur, especially in an elderly or a debilitated patient and with overdose or prolonged use.

**Warning!**

## Adverse reactions to alosetron

Alosetron can cause serious and sometimes fatal adverse reactions, such as ischemic colitis, and complications of constipation, including obstruction, perforation, and toxic megacolon.

**Elderly patients**
Older adults may have increased sensitivity to alosetron's effects, thus increasing their risk of developing serious constipation.

# Hyperosmolar laxatives

*Hyperosmolar laxatives* work by drawing water into the intestine, thereby promoting bowel distention and peristalsis. They include:
• glycerin
• lactulose
• saline compounds (magnesium salts, sodium biphosphate, sodium phosphate, polyethylene glycol [PEG], and electrolytes).

## Pharmacokinetics

The pharmacokinetic properties of hyperosmolar laxatives vary.

### Direct placement

Glycerin is placed directly into the colon by enema or suppository and isn't absorbed systemically.

### Minimal absorption

Lactulose enters the GI tract orally and is minimally absorbed. As a result, the drug is distributed only in the intestine. It's metabolized by bacteria in the colon and excreted in stool.

### Introducing ions

After saline compounds are introduced into the GI tract orally or as an enema, some of their ions are absorbed. Absorbed ions are excreted in urine, the unabsorbed drug in stool.

### Pegging PEG

PEG is a nonabsorbable solution that acts as an osmotic drug, but doesn't alter electrolyte balance.

## Pharmacodynamics

Hyperosmolar laxatives produce a bowel movement by drawing water into the intestine. Fluid accumulation distends the bowel and promotes peristalsis, resulting in a bowel movement.

## Pharmacotherapeutics

The uses of hyperosmolar laxatives vary.
• Glycerin is helpful in bowel retraining.
• Lactulose is used to treat constipation and to reduce ammonia production and absorption from the intestines in the patient with an elevated ammonia level, as occurs in cirrhosis and liver failure.
• Saline compounds are used when prompt and complete bowel evacuation is required.

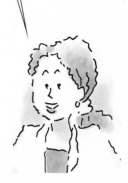

Hyperosmolar laxatives help the colon draw the water necessary for distention, peristalsis, and eventual bowel movement.

**Warning!**

## Adverse reactions to hyperosmolar laxatives

Adverse reactions to most hyperosmolar laxatives involve fluid and electrolyte imbalances.

**Glycerin**
- Weakness
- Fatigue

**Lactulose**
- Abdominal distention and cramps, gas
- Nausea and vomiting
- Diarrhea
- Hypokalemia

- Hypovolemia
- Increased blood glucose level

**Saline compounds**
- Weakness
- Lethargy
- Dehydration
- Hypernatremia
- Hypermagnesemia

- Hyperphosphatemia
- Hypocalcemia
- Cardiac arrhythmias
- Shock

**Polyethylene glycol**
- Nausea
- Explosive diarrhea
- Bloating

### Drug interactions

Hyperosmolar laxatives don't interact significantly with other drugs. However, oral drugs given 1 hour before administering PEG have significantly decreased absorption. (See *Adverse reactions to hyperosmolar laxatives.*)

# Dietary fiber and related bulk-forming laxatives

A high-fiber diet is the most natural way to prevent or treat constipation. *Dietary fiber* is the part of plants not digested in the small intestine.

Bulking up

*Bulk-forming laxatives*, which resemble dietary fiber, contain natural and semisynthetic polysaccharides and cellulose. These laxatives include:
- methylcellulose
- polycarbophil
- psyllium hydrophilic mucilloid.

### Pharmacokinetics

Dietary fiber and bulk-forming laxatives aren't absorbed systemically. The polysaccharides in these drugs are converted by intestinal bacterial flora into osmotically active metabolites that draw water into the intestine.

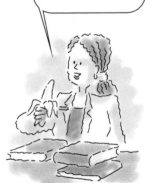

A diet high in fiber is the best way to prevent constipation.

### Excretion

Dietary fiber and bulk-forming laxatives are excreted in stool.

## Pharmacodynamics

Dietary fiber and bulk-forming laxatives increase stool mass and water content, promoting peristalsis.

## Pharmacotherapeutics

Bulk-forming laxatives are used to:
• treat simple cases of constipation, especially constipation resulting from a low-fiber or low-fluid diet
• aid patients recovering from acute myocardial infarction (MI) or cerebral aneurysms who need to avoid Valsalva's maneuver (forced expiration against a closed airway) and maintain soft stool
• manage patients with IBS and diverticulosis.

## Drug interactions

Decreased absorption of digoxin, warfarin, and salicylates occurs if these drugs are taken within 2 hours of taking fiber or bulk-forming laxatives. (See *Adverse reactions to dietary fiber and related bulk-forming laxatives.*)

# Emollient laxatives

*Emollients*—also known as *stool softeners*—include the calcium, potassium, and sodium salts of docusate.

## Pharmacokinetics

Administered orally, emollients are absorbed and excreted through bile in stool.

## Pharmacodynamics

Emollients soften stool and make bowel movements easier by emulsifying the fat and water components of stool in the small and large intestines. This detergent action allows water and fats to penetrate stool, making it softer and easier to eliminate.

*Stimulating talk*

Emollients also stimulate electrolyte and fluid secretion from intestinal mucosal cells.

**Warning!**

## Adverse reactions to dietary fiber and related bulk-forming laxatives

Adverse reactions to dietary fiber and related bulk-forming laxatives include:
• gas
• abdominal fullness
• intestinal obstruction
• fecal impaction (hard stool that can't be removed from the rectum)
• esophageal obstruction (if sufficient liquid hasn't been administered with the drug)
• severe diarrhea.

## Pharmacotherapeutics

Emollients are the drugs of choice for softening stools in patients who should avoid straining during a bowel movement, including those with:
- recent MI or surgery
- disease of the anus or rectum
- increased intracranial pressure (ICP)
- hernias.

## Drug interactions

Taking oral doses of mineral oil with oral emollients increases the systemic absorption of mineral oil and may result in tissue deposits of the oil.

### Proceed with caution

Because emollients may enhance the absorption of many oral drugs, drugs with low margins of safety (narrow therapeutic index) should be administered cautiously with emollients. (See *Adverse reactions to emollient laxatives*.)

> Emollients help soften the stool, easing the strain of defecation.

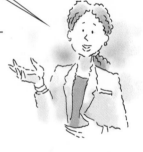

**Warning!**

## Adverse reactions to emollient laxatives

Although adverse reactions to emollients seldom occur, they may include:
- bitter taste
- diarrhea
- throat irritation
- mild, transient abdominal cramping.

# Stimulant laxatives

*Stimulant laxatives*, also known as *irritant cathartics*, include:
- bisacodyl
- castor oil
- senna.

## Pharmacokinetics

Stimulant laxatives are minimally absorbed and are metabolized in the liver. The metabolites are excreted in urine and stool.

## Pharmacodynamics

Stimulant laxatives promote peristalsis and produce a bowel movement by irritating the intestinal mucosa or stimulating nerve endings of the intestinal smooth muscle.

### No job is too small

Castor oil also increases peristalsis in the small intestine.

## Pharmacotherapeutics

Stimulant laxatives are the preferred drugs for emptying the bowel before general surgery, sigmoidoscopic or proctoscopic procedures, and radiologic procedures such as barium studies of the GI tract.

They're also used to treat constipation caused by prolonged bed rest, neurologic dysfunction of the colon, and constipating drugs such as opioids.

## Drug interactions

No significant drug interactions occur with the stimulant laxatives. However, because these laxatives produce increased intestinal motility, they reduce the absorption of other oral drugs administered at the same time, especially sustained-release forms. (See *Adverse reactions to stimulant laxatives.*)

# Lubricant laxatives

Mineral oil is the main *lubricant laxative* currently in clinical use.

## Pharmacokinetics

In its nonemulsified form, mineral oil is minimally absorbed; the emulsified form is about half absorbed. Absorbed mineral oil is distributed to the mesenteric lymph nodes, intestinal mucosa, liver, and spleen.

### Metabolism and excretion

Mineral oil is metabolized by the liver and excreted in stool.

## Pharmacodynamics

Mineral oil lubricates stool and the intestinal mucosa and prevents water reabsorption from the bowel lumen. The increased fluid content of stool increases peristalsis. Administration by enema also produces distention.

## Pharmacotherapeutics

Mineral oil is used to treat constipation and maintain soft stool when straining is contraindicated, such as after a recent MI (to avoid Valsalva's maneuver), eye surgery (to prevent increased pressure in the eye), or cerebral aneurysm repair (to avoid increased ICP).

*Warning!*

## Adverse reactions to stimulant laxatives

Adverse reactions to stimulant laxatives include:
• weakness
• nausea
• abdominal cramps
• mild inflammation of the rectum and anus
• urine discoloration (with senna).

**Warning!**

## Adverse reactions to mineral oil

Adverse reactions to mineral oil include:
• nausea and vomiting
• diarrhea
• abdominal cramping.

### Impacting impaction

Administered orally or by enema, this lubricant laxative is also used to treat the patient with fecal impaction.

#### Drug interactions

Mineral oil can interact with other drugs.
• Mineral oil may impair the absorption of many oral drugs, including fat-soluble vitamins, hormonal contraceptives, and anticoagulants.
• Mineral oil may interfere with the antibacterial activity of nonabsorbable sulfonamides. To minimize drug interactions, administer mineral oil at least 2 hours before these medications. (See *Adverse reactions to mineral oil.*)

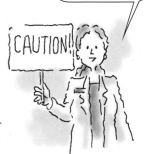

Mineral oil can impair the absorption of some oral drugs.

# Antiemetic and emetic drugs

*Antiemetics* and *emetics* are two groups of drugs with opposing actions. Antiemetic drugs decrease nausea, reducing the urge to vomit. Emetic drugs, which are derived from plants, produce vomiting.

## Antiemetics

The major antiemetics are:
• antihistamines, including buclizine, cyclizine, dimenhydrinate, diphenhydramine, hydroxyzine hydrochloride, hydroxyzine pamoate, meclizine, and trimethobenzamide
• phenothiazines, including chlorpromazine, perphenazine, prochlorperazine maleate, promethazine, and thiethylperazine maleate

- serotonin 5-HT$_3$ receptor antagonists, including dolasetron, granisetron, and ondansetron.

## Top of the charts

Ondansetron is currently the antiemetic of choice in the United States.

## Pharmacokinetics

The pharmacokinetic properties of antiemetics may vary slightly.

### Absorption, metabolism, and excretion

Oral antihistamine antiemetics are absorbed well from the GI tract and are metabolized primarily by the liver. Their inactive metabolites are excreted in urine.

Phenothiazine antiemetics and serotonin 5-HT$_3$ receptor antagonists are absorbed well, extensively metabolized by the liver, and excreted in urine and stool.

## Pharmacodynamics

The action of antiemetics may vary.

## What's going on here?

The mechanism of action that produces the antiemetic effect of antihistamines is unclear.

## Don't pull the trigger!

Phenothiazines produce their antiemetic effect by blocking the dopaminergic receptors in the chemoreceptor trigger zone in the brain. (This area of the brain, near the medulla, stimulates the vomiting center in the medulla, causing vomiting.) These drugs may also directly depress the vomiting center.

## Stopping serotonin stimulation

The serotonin 5-HT$_3$ receptor antagonists block serotonin stimulation centrally in the chemoreceptor trigger zone and peripherally in the vagal nerve terminals, both of which stimulate vomiting.

## Pharmacotherapeutics

The uses of antiemetics may vary.

## Lend me your ear

Antihistamines are specifically used for nausea and vomiting caused by inner ear stimulation. As a consequence, these drugs prevent or treat motion sickness. They usually prove most effec-

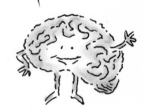

Some antiemetics block the vomiting center in my medulla or nearby areas that stimulate vomiting.

## Other antiemetics

Here are other antiemetics currently in use.

### Scopolamine

Scopolamine prevents motion sickness, but its use is limited because of its sedative and anticholinergic effects. One transdermal preparation, Transderm-Scōp, is highly effective without producing the usual adverse effects.

### Metoclopramide

Metoclopramide is used primarily to treat GI motility disorders including gastroparesis in diabetic patients. It's also used to prevent chemotherapy-induced nausea and vomiting.

### Diphenidol

Diphenidol is used to prevent vertigo (whirling sensation) and to prevent or treat generalized nausea and vomiting. However, its use is limited because of the auditory and visual hallucinations, confusion, and disorientation that may occur.

### Dronabinol

Dronabinol, a purified derivative of cannabis, is a Schedule II drug (meaning it has a high potential for abuse) used to treat chemotherapy-induced nausea and vomiting in the patient who doesn't respond adequately to conventional antiemetics. It has also been used to stimulate appetite in the patient with acquired immunodeficiency syndrome. However, dronabinol can accumulate in the body, and the patient can develop tolerance or physical and psychological dependence.

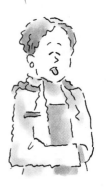

When you're not feeling so hot, it might be time for an antiemetic.

tive when given before activities that produce motion sickness and are much less effective when nausea or vomiting has already begun.

*Severe cases*

Phenothiazine antiemetics and serotonin 5-HT$_3$ receptor antagonists control severe nausea and vomiting from various causes. They're used when vomiting becomes severe and potentially hazardous, such as postsurgical or viral nausea and vomiting. Both types of drugs are also prescribed to control the nausea and vomiting resulting from chemotherapy and radiotherapy. (See *Other antiemetics*.)

## Drug interactions

Antiemetics may have many significant interactions.
• Antihistamines and phenothiazines can produce additive CNS depression and sedation when taken with CNS depressants, such as barbiturates, tranquilizers, antidepressants, alcohol, and opioids.
• Antihistamines can cause additive anticholinergic effects, such as constipation, dry mouth, vision problems, and urine retention, when taken with anticholinergic drugs, including tricyclic antidepressants, phenothiazines, and antiparkinsonian drugs.

*Warning!*

## Adverse reactions to antiemetics

Use of these antiemetic drugs may lead to adverse reactions:
• Antihistamine and phenothiazine antiemetics produce drowsiness and sometimes paradoxical central nervous system (CNS) stimulation.
• CNS effects associated with phenothiazine and serotonin 5-HT$_3$ receptor antagonist antiemetics include confusion, anxiety, euphoria, agitation, depression, headache, insomnia, restlessness, and weakness.

• The anticholinergic effect of antiemetics may cause constipation, dry mouth and throat, painful or difficult urination, urine retention, impotence, and visual and auditory disturbances.
• Phenothiazine antiemetics commonly cause hypotension and orthostatic hypotension with an increased heart rate, fainting, and dizziness.

• Phenothiazine antiemetics taken with anticholinergic drugs increase the anticholinergic effect and decrease the antiemetic effects.
• Droperidol used with phenothiazine antiemetics increases the risk of extrapyramidal (abnormal involuntary movements) effects. (See *Adverse reactions to antiemetics*.)

# Emetics

*Emetics* are used to induce vomiting in a person who has ingested toxic substances. *Ipecac syrup* is used to induce vomiting in early management of oral poinsoning or drug overdose.

*Controversy?*

The use of ipecac syrup has become controversial, however, because it delays the use of activated charcoal. There's a risk of potential abuse by individuals with eating disorders. The American Academy of Pediatrics no longer recommends the routine use of ipecac syrup. The first action parents or caregivers should take if a child has ingested a poisonous substance is to call the poison control center and emergency medical services.

## Pharmacokinetics

Little information exists concerning the absorption, distribution, and excretion of ipecac syrup. After administration of ipecac syrup, vomiting occurs within 10 to 30 minutes.

## Measuring success

The success of treatment is directly linked to fluid intake with ipecac administration.

### Pharmacodynamics

Ipecac syrup induces vomiting by stimulating the vomiting center located in the brain's medulla.

### Pharmacotherapeutics

Ipecac syrup is used to induce vomiting in the early management of oral poisoning and drug overdose in individuals who are fully conscious. It shouldn't be used after ingestion of petroleum products, volatile oils, or caustic substances, such as lye, because of the risk of additional esophageal injury or aspiration.

### Drug interactions

Because ipecac syrup is used only in acute situations, drug interactions rarely occur. If poisoning results from ingestion of a phenothiazine, the phenothiazine's antiemetic effect may decrease the emetic effect of ipecac syrup. Ipecac syrup shouldn't be administered concurrently with activated charcoal, which will absorb and inactivate it. (See *Adverse reactions to ipecac syrup*.)

**Warning!**

## Adverse reactions to ipecac syrup

Ipecac syrup rarely produces adverse reactions when used in the recommended dosages. However, prolonged vomiting (for more than 1 hour) or repeated vomiting (more than six episodes in 1 hour), lethargy, and diarrhea may occur with regular dosage as well. Some people are very sensitive to ipecac syrup.

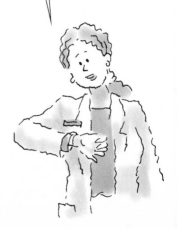

After administration of ipecac syrup, vomiting occurs within 10 to 30 minutes.

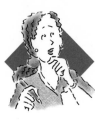

# Quick quiz

**1.** A patient is asked why he's taking antibiotics for an ulcer. The practitioner explains that antibiotics will:

    A.    destroy the bacteria causing the ulcer.

    B.    destroy the virus causing the ulcer.

    C.    prevent infection from entering through open areas in the gastric mucosa.

    D.    prevent infection from occurring.

*Answer:* A. Antibiotics destroy bacteria responsible for ulcer formation.

**2.** What's a common adverse reaction to misoprostol?

    A.    Indigestion

    B.    Constipation

    C.    Headache

    D.    Diarrhea

*Answer:* D. Diarrhea is a common adverse reaction to misoprostol.

**3.** How does simethicone relieve gas in the GI tract?

    A.    It disperses and prevents gas pocket formation.

    B.    It facilitates expulsion of gas pockets.

    C.    It neutralizes gastric contents and reduces gas.

    D.    It coats and protects the lining of the stomach.

*Answer:* A. Simethicone relieves gas in the GI tract by producing a film in the intestines that disperses mucus-enclosed gas pockets and helps prevent their formation.

**4.** The antiemetic drug that would probably be best for a patient who experiences motion sickness on an airplane is:

    A.    chlorpromazine.

    B.    dronabinol.

    C.    dimenhydrinate.

    D.    dolasetron.

*Answer:* C. An antihistamine, such as dimenhydrinate, is the most effective antiemetic for a patient who experiences motion sickness during air travel.

**5.** To prevent a postsurgical patient from straining during a bowel movement, the practitioner is most likely to prescribe:

    A.    docusate.

    B.    magnesium citrate.

    C.    bisacodyl.

    D.    castor oil.

*Answer:*   A. Docusate is commonly prescribed to prevent straining during a bowel movement after surgery.

## Scoring

☆☆☆  If you answered all five items correctly, well done! You digested this GI information admirably!

☆☆  If you answered four items correctly, keep up the good work (preferably without emetics).

☆  If you answered fewer than four items correctly, you may need extra stimulation. Reread this chapter and see what you can do!

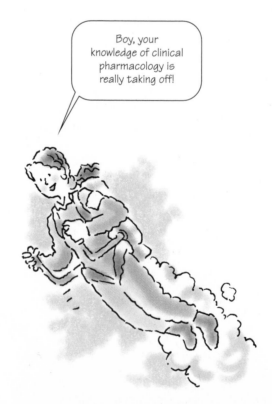

Boy, your knowledge of clinical pharmacology is really taking off!

# 9

# Genitourinary drugs

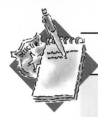

## Just the facts

In this chapter, you'll learn:

♦ classes of drugs used to treat genitourinary (GU) disorders

♦ uses and varying actions of these drugs

♦ absorption, distribution, metabolization, and excretion of these drugs

♦ drug interactions and adverse reactions to these drugs.

## Drugs and the genitourinary system

The GU system consists of the reproductive system (the sex organs) and the urinary system, which includes the kidneys, ureters, bladder, and urethra. The kidneys perform most of the work of the urinary system.

### Multitalented

The kidneys perform several vital tasks, including:
• disposing of wastes and excess ions in the form of urine
• filtering blood, which regulates its volume and chemical make-up
• helping to maintain fluid, electrolyte, and acid-base balances
• producing several hormones and enzymes
• converting vitamin D to a more active form
• helping to regulate blood pressure and volume by secreting renin.

### Helping hands

Types of drugs used to treat GU disorders include:
• diuretics
• urinary tract antispasmodics
• erectile dysfunction therapy drugs
• hormonal contraceptives.

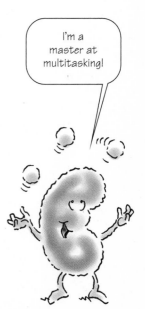

I'm a master at multitasking!

# Diuretics

Diuretics trigger the excretion of water and electrolytes from the kidneys, making these drugs a primary choice in the treatment of renal disease, edema, hypertension, and heart failure.

## Thiazide and thiazide-like diuretics

Derived from sulfonamides, thiazide and thiazide-like diuretics are used to treat edema and to prevent the development and recurrence of renal calculi. They're also used for such cardiovascular diseases as hypertension and heart failure.

Thiazide diuretics include:
- bendroflumethiazide
- chlorothiazide
- hydrochlorothiazide
- hydroflumethiazide
- methyclothiazide
- polythiazide.

Thiazide-like diuretics include:
- chlorthalidone
- indapamide
- metolazone.

### Pharmacokinetics (how drugs circulate)

Thiazide diuretics are absorbed rapidly but incompletely from the GI tract after oral administration. They cross the placenta and are secreted in breast milk. These drugs differ in how well they're metabolized, but all are excreted primarily in urine.

Thiazide-like diuretics are absorbed from the GI tract. Chlorthalidone is 90% bound to erythrocytes; little is known about its metabolism. Indapamide is distributed widely into body tissues and metabolized in the liver. Little is also known about the metabolism of metolazone. All of these drugs are primarily excreted in urine.

### Pharmacodynamics (how drugs act)

Thiazide and thiazide-like diuretics promote the excretion of water by preventing the reabsorption of sodium in the kidneys. As the kidneys excrete the excess sodium, they excrete water along with it. These drugs also increase the excretion of chloride, potassium, and bicarbonate, which can result in electrolyte imbalances. With long-term use, thiazide diuretics also lower blood pressure by causing arteriolar vasodilation.

## Turning down the volume

Initially, diuretic drugs decrease circulating blood volume, leading to reduced cardiac output. However, if therapy is maintained, cardiac output stabilizes but plasma fluid volume decreases.

### Pharmacotherapeutics (how drugs are used)

Thiazides are used for the long-term treatment of hypertension; they're also used to treat edema caused by kidney or liver disease, mild or moderate heart failure, and corticosteroid and estrogen therapy. Because these drugs decrease the level of calcium in urine, they may be used alone or with other drugs to prevent the development and recurrence of renal calculi.

## Pointing out a paradox

In patients with diabetes insipidus (a disorder characterized by excessive urine production and excessive thirst resulting from reduced secretion of antidiuretic hormone), thiazides paradoxically decrease urine volume, possibly through sodium depletion and plasma volume reduction.

### Drug interactions

Drug interactions related to thiazide and thiazide-like diuretics result in altered fluid volume, blood pressure, and serum electrolyte levels:
• These drugs may decrease excretion of lithium, causing lithium toxicity.
• Nonsteroidal anti-inflammatory drugs, including cyclooxygenase-2 (COX-2) inhibitors, may reduce the antihypertensive effect of these diuretics.
• Use of these drugs with other potassium-depleting drugs and digoxin may cause an additive effect, increasing the risk of digoxin toxicity.
• These diuretics may increase the response to skeletal muscle relaxants.
• Use of these drugs may increase blood glucose levels, requiring higher doses of insulin or oral antidiabetic drugs.
• These drugs may produce additive hypotension when used with antihypertensives. (See *Adverse reactions to thiazide and thiazide-like diuretics*.)

**Warning!**

## Adverse reactions to thiazide and thiazide-like diuretics

The most common adverse reactions to thiazide and thiazide-like diuretics include:
• reduced blood volume
• orthostatic hypotension
• hypokalemia
• hyperglycemia
• hyponatremia.

> Administering thiazide diuretics along with antihypertensives can result in additive hypotension. I don't like the way this is adding up!

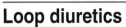

# Loop diuretics

Loop (high ceiling) diuretics are highly potent drugs. They include bumetanide, ethacrynic acid, and furosemide.

## Pharmacokinetics

Loop diuretics are absorbed well in the GI tract and are rapidly distributed. These diuretics are highly protein bound. They undergo partial or complete metabolism in the liver, except for furosemide, which is excreted primarily unchanged. Loop diuretics are excreted primarily by the kidneys.

## Pharmacodynamics

Loop diuretics are the most potent diuretics available, producing the greatest volume of diuresis (urine production). Bumetanide—which is 40 times more potent than furosemide—is the shortest-acting diuretic. Loop diuretics also have a high potential for causing severe adverse reactions. (See *Loop diuretics warning.*)

### The scoop on the loop

Loop diuretics received their name because they act primarily on the thick, ascending loop of Henle (the part of the nephron responsible for concentrating urine) to increase the secretion of sodium, chloride, and water. These drugs also inhibit sodium, chloride, and water reabsorption in the proximal tubule.

## Pharmacotherapeutics

Loop diuretics are used to treat edema associated with renal disease, hepatic cirrhosis, and heart failure, as well as to treat hypertension (usually with a potassium-sparing diuretic or potassium supplement to prevent hypokalemia).

Ethacrynic acid may also be used for the short-term management of ascites due to malignancy, idiopathic edema, or lymphedema. Furosemide may be used with mannitol to treat cerebral edema.

## Drug interactions

Loop diuretics produce a variety of drug interactions:
• The risk of ototoxicity (damage to the organs of hearing) increases when aminoglycosides and cisplatin are taken with loop diuretics (especially with high doses of furosemide). (See *Adverse reactions to loop diuretics.*)
• Loop diuretics reduce the hypoglycemic effects of oral antidiabetic drugs, possibly resulting in hyperglycemia.
• These drugs may increase the risk of lithium toxicity.
• The risk of electrolyte imbalances that can trigger arrhythmias increases when cardiac glycosides and loop diuretics are taken together.

*Safe and sound*

## Loop diuretics warning

Loop diuretics, with the exception of ethacrynic acid, contain sulfa. A patient who has an allergy to sulfa may experience an allergic reaction to loop diuretics. Use with caution, and alert the patient to this possibility.

• Use with digoxin may cause additive toxicity, increasing the risk of digoxin toxicity and arrhythmias.

# Potassium-sparing diuretics

Potassium-sparing diuretics have weaker diuretic and antihypertensive effects than other diuretics but provide the advantage of conserving potassium. These drugs include amiloride, spironolactone, and triamterene.

## Pharmacokinetics

Potassium-sparing diuretics are only available orally and are absorbed in the GI tract. They're metabolized by the liver (except for amiloride, which isn't metabolized) and excreted primarily in urine.

## Pharmacodynamics

The direct action of potassium-sparing diuretics on the distal tubule of the kidneys results in urinary excretion of sodium, water, bicarbonate, and calcium. The drug also decreases the excretion of potassium and hydrogen ions. These effects lead to reduced blood pressure and increased serum potassium levels.

### Compare and contrast

Structurally similar to aldosterone, spironolactone acts as an aldosterone antagonist. Aldosterone promotes the retention of sodium and water and the loss of potassium, whereas spironolactone counteracts these effects by competing with aldosterone for receptor sites. As a result, sodium, chloride, and water are excreted and potassium is retained.

## Pharmacotherapeutics

Potassium-sparing diuretics are used to treat:
• edema
• diuretic-induced hypokalemia in patients with heart failure
• cirrhosis
• nephrotic syndrome (abnormal condition of the kidneys)
• heart failure
• hypertension.

### A hairy situation

Spironolactone also is used to treat hyperaldosteronism (excessive secretion of aldosterone) and hirsutism (excessive hair growth), including hirsutism associated with Stein-Leventhal

**Warning!**

## Adverse reactions to loop diuretics

The most common adverse reactions to loop diuretics include:
• fluid and electrolyte imbalances (including metabolic alkalosis, hypovolemia, hypochloremia, hypochloremic alkalosis, hyperglycemia, hyperuricemia, dehydration, hyponatremia, hypokalemia, and hypomagnesemia)
• transient deafness
• tinnitus
• diarrhea
• nausea
• vomiting
• abdominal pain
• impaired glucose tolerance
• dermatitis
• paresthesia
• hepatic dysfunction
• photosensitivity
• orthostatic hypotension.

(polycystic ovary) syndrome. Potassium-sparing diuretics are commonly used with other diuretics to potentiate their action or counteract their potassium-wasting effects.

## Drug interactions

Giving potassium-sparing diuretics with potassium supplements or angiotensin-converting enzyme inhibitors increases the risk of hyperkalemia. Concurrent use of spironolactone and digoxin increases the risk of digoxin toxicity. (See *Adverse reactions to potassium-sparing diuretics.*)

# Osmotic diuretics

Osmotic diuretics cause diuresis through osmosis, moving fluid into the extracellular spaces. They include mannitol and urea.

## Pharmacokinetics

Administered I.V. for rapid distribution, osmotic diuretics are freely filtered by the glomeruli of the kidney—except for mannitol, which is only slightly metabolized. Osmotic diuretics are excreted primarily in urine.

## Pharmacodynamics

Osmotic diuretics receive their name because they increase the osmotic pressure of the glomerular filtrate, which inhibits the reabsorption of sodium and water. They create an osmotic gradient in the glomerular filtrate and the blood. In the glomerular filtrate, the gradient prevents sodium and water reabsorption. In the blood, the gradient allows fluid to be drawn from the intracellular into the intravascular spaces.

## Pharmacotherapeutics

Osmotic diuretics are used to treat acute renal failure and cerebral edema and to reduce intracranial and intraocular pressure. Mannitol is used to promote diuresis in acute renal failure and to promote urinary excretion of toxic substances.

## Drug interactions

Taking osmotic diuretics with lithium may increase renal excretion of lithium, which in turn decreases the effectiveness of lithium. Patients taking both drugs require lithium level monitoring. (See *Adverse reactions to osmotic diuretics.*)

*Warning!*

### Adverse reactions to potassium-sparing diuretics

Few adverse drug reactions occur with potassium-sparing diuretics. However, their potassium-sparing effects can lead to hyperkalemia, especially if given with a potassium supplement or high-potassium diet.

*Warning!*

### Adverse reactions to osmotic diuretics

Adverse reactions to osmotic diuretics include:
• hyponatremia
• dehydration
• circulatory overload (from osmotic effects)
• thrombophlebitis or local irritation at the infusion site.

# Carbonic anhydrase inhibitors

Carbonic anhydrase inhibitors are diuretics that block the action of carbonic anhydrase. They include acetazolamide and methazolamide.

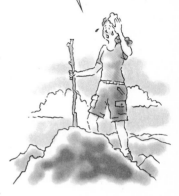

Acetazolamide... (huff)... may be used... (puff)... to treat acute mountain sickness...

## Pharmacokinetics

Carbonic anhydrase inhibitors are absorbed through the GI tract. Some systemic absorption also occurs after ophthalmic administration. They're distributed in tissues with high carbonic anhydrase content, such as erythrocytes, plasma, kidneys, eyes, liver, and muscle. Carbonic anhydrase inhibitors are excreted by the kidneys in urine.

## Pharmacodynamics

In the kidneys, carbonic anhydrase inhibitors decrease the availability of hydrogen ions, which blocks the sodium-hydrogen exchange mechanisms. As a result, urinary excretion of sodium, potassium, bicarbonate, and water increases.

### Don't lose your sense of humor

In the eyes, carbonic anhydrase inhibition reduces aqueous humor production, which reduces intraocular pressure.

## Pharmacotherapeutics

Carbonic anhydrase inhibitors are used for diuresis and to treat glaucoma. Acetazolamide may also be used to treat epilepsy and acute mountain sickness.

## Drug interactions

Carbonic anhydrase inhibitors produce a variety of drug interactions:
• Salicylates may cause carbonic anhydrase inhibitor toxicity, including central nervous system depression and metabolic acidosis.
• Diflunisal may increase intraocular pressure when given with a carbonic anhydrase inhibitor.
• Acetazolamide used concurrently with cyclosporine may increase cyclosporine levels and the risk of neurotoxicity.
• Acetazolamide used concurrently with primidone may decrease serum and urine levels of primidone. (See *Adverse reactions to carbonic anhydrase inhibitors.*)

*Warning!*

## Adverse reactions to carbonic anhydrase inhibitors

Adverse reactions to carbonic anhydrase inhibitors include:
• hypokalemia
• metabolic acidosis
• electrolyte imbalances.

# Urinary tract antispasmodics

Urinary tract antispasmodics help decrease urinary tract muscle spasms. They include darifenacin, flavoxate, oxybutynin, solifenacin, tolterodine, and trospium.

## Pharmacokinetics

Flavoxate, oxybutynin, tolterodine, darifenacin, and solifenacin are most often administered orally and are rapidly absorbed. Trospium is administered orally but is poorly absorbed. Oxybutynin is also available as a dermal patch. These drugs are all widely distributed, metabolized in the liver, and excreted in urine. Urinary tract antispasmodics also cross the placenta and are excreted in breast milk.

## Pharmacodynamics

Urinary tract antispasmodics relieve smooth muscle spasms by inhibiting parasympathetic activity, which causes the detrusor and urinary muscles to relax. Flavoxate and oxybutynin also exhibit many anticholinergic effects.

## Pharmacotherapeutics

Urinary tract antispasmodics are used for patients with overactive bladders who have symptoms of urinary frequency, urgency, or incontinence.

### Urgent symptoms

Trospium is also indicated for patients with overactive bladders who have symptoms of urge urinary incontinence, and oxybutynin acts as an antispasmodic for uninhibited or reflex neurogenic bladder. (See *How oxybutynin works*.)

## Drug interactions

Urinary tract antispasmodics have few drug interactions:
• Use with anticholinergic agents may increase dry mouth, constipation, and other anticholinergic effects. (See *Adverse reactions to urinary tract antispasmodics*.)
• Urinary tract antispasmodics may decrease the effectiveness of phenothiazines and haloperidol.
• Trospium may interfere with the elimination of certain drugs excreted through the kidneys (such as digoxin, metformin, and vancomycin), resulting in increased blood levels of these drugs.

*Now I get it!*

## How oxybutynin works

When acetylcholine is released within the bladder, it attaches to receptors on the surface of smooth muscle in the bladder, stimulating bladder contractions. Oxybutynin suppresses these involuntary contractions by blocking the release of acetylcholine. This anticholinergic effect is what makes oxybutynin useful in the treatment of overactive bladder.

**Warning!**

## Adverse reactions to urinary tract antispasmodics

Possible adverse reactions to urinary tract antispasmodics include:

- blurred vision
- headache
- somnolence
- urinary retention
- dry mouth
- dyspepsia
- constipation
- nausea
- vomiting
- weight gain
- pain
- acute and secondary angle-closure glaucoma.

# Erectile dysfunction therapy drugs

Erectile dysfunction therapy drugs treat penile erectile dysfunction that results from a lack of blood flowing through the corpus cavernosum. This type of erectile dysfunction usually stems from vascular and neurologic conditions. Drugs used for erectile dysfunction include alprostadil, sildenafil, tadalafil, and vardenafil.

## Pharmacokinetics

Erectile dysfunction drugs are well absorbed in the GI tract. Distribution of these drugs isn't known. The majority of these drugs—including sildenafil, tadalafil, and vardenafil—are given orally, metabolized in the liver, and excreted in feces.

### An exceptional drug

Alprostadil is the exception: it's administered directly into the corpus cavernosum, metabolized in the lungs, and excreted in urine.

## Pharmacodynamics

Sildenafil, tadalafil, and vardenafil selectively inhibit the phosphodiesterase type 5 receptors, which causes an increase in blood levels of nitric oxide. This increase in nitric oxide levels activates the cGMP enzyme, which relaxes smooth muscles and allows blood to flow into the corpus cavernosum, causing an erection.

Alprostadil acts locally, promoting smooth muscle relaxation, which causes an increase in blood flow to the corpus cavernosum and produces an erection.

**Warning!**

## Adverse reactions to erectile dysfunction drugs

Adverse reactions to erectile dysfunction drugs include:
• decreased supine blood pressure and cardiac output
• increased risk of cardiovascular events, including myocardial infarction, sudden cardiac death, ventricular arrhythmias, cerebrovascular hemorrhage, transient ischemic attack, and hypertension

• headache
• dizziness
• flushing
• dyspepsia
• vision changes
• prolonged erections (more than 4 hours), which can result in irreversible damage to erectile tissue
• penile pain (with alprostadil).

## Pharmacotherapeutics

Alprostadil, sildenafil, tadalafil, and vardenafil are all used in the treatment of erectile dysfunction. Sildenafil is also indicated for the treatment of pulmonary arterial hypertension.

## Drug interactions

Erectile dysfunction drugs may interact with other drugs in the following ways:
• Nitrates and alpha-adrenergic blockers used in combination with erectile dysfunction drugs may cause severe hypotension and potentially serious cardiac events. (See *Adverse reactions to erectile dysfunction drugs.*)
• Ketoconazole, itraconazole, and erythromycin may result in increased levels of vardenafil or tadalafil.
• Protease inhibitors, such as indinavir or ritonavir, may cause increased tadalafil or vardenafil levels.

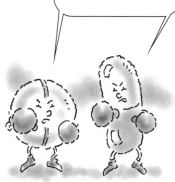

Sometimes we just can't get along: Nitrates and alpha-adrenergic blockers used with erectile dysfunction drugs can cause severe hypotension and potentially serious cardiac events.

# Hormonal contraceptives

Hormonal contraceptives inhibit ovulation. Contraceptives typically contain a combination of hormones. For example, ethinyl estradiol may be combined with desogestrel, drospirenone, levonorgestrel, norethindrone, norgestimate, or norgestrel. Also, mestranol may be combined with norethindrone. Ethinyl estradiol or ethynodiol diacetate may also be used alone as a contraceptive.

## Pharmacokinetics

Hormonal contraceptives are absorbed from the GI tract and are widely distributed. They're metabolized in the kidneys and excreted in urine and feces.

*Patch power*

Some forms of hormonal contraceptives are available in a transdermal patch form. These contraceptives are absorbed through the skin but have the same distribution, metabolism, and excretion as orally administered contraceptives.

## Pharmacodynamics

The primary mechanism of action of combination hormonal contraceptives (estrogen and progestin) is the suppression of gonadotropins, which inhibits ovulation. Estrogen suppresses secretion of follicle-stimulating hormone, which blocks follicular development and ovulation. Progestin suppresses the secretion of luteinizing hormone, which prevents ovulation, even if the follicle develops. Progestin also thickens the cervical mucus; this interferes with sperm migration and causes endometrial changes that prevent implantation of a fertilized ovum.

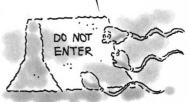

It looks like we're not welcome here, guys!

## Pharmacotherapeutics

The primary purpose for taking hormonal contraceptives is the prevention of pregnancy in women. The combination of ethinyl estradiol and norgestimate is also used to treat moderate acne in females younger than age 15.

## Drug interactions

Hormonal contraceptives can interact with other medications in various ways:

• Antibiotics, oxcarbazepine, phenobarbital, phenytoin, topiramate, and modafinil may decrease the effectiveness of oral contraceptives. A patient taking these drugs with a hormonal contraceptive needs to use a barrier contraceptive.

• Atorvastatin may increase serum estrogen levels.

• Cyclosporin and theophylline have an increased risk of toxicity when taken with hormonal contraceptives.

• Prednisone increases the therapeutic and possibly toxic effects of hormonal contraceptives. (See *Adverse reactions to hormonal contraceptives*.)

• Several herbal medications can affect serum levels of hormonal contraceptives.

*Warning!*

## Adverse reactions to hormonal contraceptives

Potentially serious adverse reactions to hormonal contraceptives include arterial thrombosis, thrombophlebitis, pulmonary embolism, myocardial infarction, cerebral hemorrhage or thrombosis, hypertension, gallbladder disease, and hepatic adenomas.

Other adverse reactions include:
• acne
• bleeding or spotting between menstrual periods
• bloating
• breast tenderness or enlargement
• changes in libido
• diarrhea
• difficulty wearing contact lenses
• unusual hair growth
• weight fluctuations
• upset stomach
• vomiting.

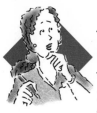

# Quick quiz

**1.** When caring for a patient taking a hydrochlorothiazide, you should monitor the patient for:

    A.   hypertension.
    B.   hypernatremia.
    C.   hypokalemia.
    D.   hypoglycemia.

*Answer:*   C. Watch for signs of hypokalemia in a patient receiving hydrochlorothiazide.

**2.** When teaching a patient about diuretics, you should tell him to:

    A.   take the drug in the evening.
    B.   call his practitioner if he loses more that 2 lb (0.9 kg) per day.
    C.   eat a high-sodium diet.
    D.   avoid sun exposure for several hours after taking the medication to prevent a photosensitivity reaction.

*Answer:*   B. A weight loss of more that 2 lb per day indicates excessive diuresis.

**3.** Urinary tract antispasmodics are used to treat:

    A.   overactive bladder.
    B.   erectile dysfunction.
    C.   hypertension.
    D.   seizures.

*Answer:*   A. Urinary tract antispasmodics are used to treat an overactive bladder.

**4.** Which drug necessitates use of an additional form of contraception for a patient taking hormonal contraceptives?

    A.   Atorvastatin
    B.   Theophylline
    C.   Cyclosporine
    D.   Antibiotics

*Answer:*   D. Advise the patient taking hormonal contraceptives and an antibiotic to use additional form of birth control if she's also taking certain antibiotics because antibiotics may decrease the effectiveness of hormonal contraceptives.

## Scoring

☆☆☆ If you answered all four questions correctly, terrific! Everything's flowing smoothly for you when it comes to GU drugs.

☆☆ If you answered three questions correctly, super! Your stream of knowledge about GU drugs is impressive.

☆ If you answered fewer than three questions correctly, don't spaz out! Relax, review the chapter, and try again.

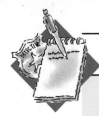

# 10

# Anti-infective drugs

## Just the facts

In this chapter, you'll learn:

♦ classes of drugs that act as anti-infectives

♦ the uses and varying actions of these drugs

♦ how these drugs are absorbed, distributed, metabolized, and excreted

♦ drug interactions and adverse reactions to these drugs.

# Selecting an antimicrobial drug

Selecting an appropriate antimicrobial drug to treat a specific infection involves several important factors:
• First, the microorganism must be isolated and identified—generally through growing a culture.
• Then its susceptibility to various drugs must be determined. Because culture and sensitivity results take 48 hours, treatment usually starts at assessment and then is reevaluated when test results are obtained.
• The location of the infection must be considered. For therapy to be effective, an adequate concentration of the antimicrobial must be delivered to the infection site.
• Lastly, the cost of the drug must be considered as well as its potential adverse effects and the possibility of patient allergies.

## Preventing pathogen resistance

The usefulness of antimicrobial drugs is limited by pathogens that may develop resistance to a drug's action.

Resistance is the ability of a microorganism to live and grow in the presence of an antimicrobial drug that's either bacteriostatic (inhibits the growth or multiplication of bacteria) or bactericidal

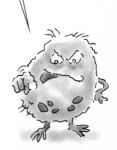

Because I'm a sensitive guy, I'm responsive only to certain drugs.

(kills bacteria). Resistance usually results from genetic mutation of the microorganism. (See *The rise of the resistance movement.*)

# Antibacterial drugs

*Antibacterial drugs*, also known as *antibiotics* (drugs that inhibit the growth of bacteria), are used mainly to treat systemic (involving the whole body rather than a localized area) bacterial infections. The antibacterials include:
- aminoglycosides
- penicillins
- cephalosporins
- tetracyclines
- lincomycin derivatives
- macrolides
- vancomycin
- carbapenems
- monobactams
- fluoroquinolones
- sulfonamides
- nitrofurantoin (nitrofuran).

## Aminoglycosides

*Aminoglycosides* provide effective bactericidal activity against:
- gram-negative bacilli
- some aerobic gram-positive bacteria
- mycobacteria
- some protozoa.

### Common aminoglycosides

Aminoglycosides currently in use include:
- amikacin sulfate
- gentamicin sulfate
- kanamycin sulfate
- neomycin sulfate
- paromomycin sulfate
- streptomycin sulfate
- tobramycin sulfate.

### Pharmacokinetics (how drugs circulate)

Because aminoglycosides are absorbed poorly from the GI tract, they're usually given parenterally. After I.V. or I.M. administration, aminoglycoside absorption is rapid and complete.

*Yea or nay?*

## The rise of the resistance movement

Indiscriminate use of antimicrobial drugs has serious consequences. Unnecessary exposure of organisms to these drugs encourages the emergence of resistant strains, which are likely to do far more damage than their predecessors.

**Make reservations**
The use of antimicrobial drugs should be reserved for patients with infections caused by susceptible organisms and should be used in high enough doses and for an appropriate period. New antimicrobial drugs should be reserved for severely ill patients with serious infections that don't respond to conventional drugs.

### Distribution

Aminoglycosides are distributed widely in extracellular fluid. They readily cross the placental barrier, but don't cross the blood-brain barrier.

### Metabolism and excretion

Aminoglycosides aren't metabolized. They're excreted primarily unchanged by the kidneys.

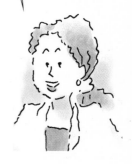

Aminoglycosides are usually given parenterally because they're poorly absorbed from the GI tract.

## Pharmacodynamics (how drugs act)

Aminoglycosides act as bactericidal drugs (remember, this means they kill bacteria) against susceptible organisms by binding to the bacterium's 30S subunit, a specific ribosome in the microorganism, thereby interrupting protein synthesis and causing the bacterium to die.

### Rising resistance

Bacterial resistance to aminoglycosides may be related to:
• failure of the drug to cross the cell membrane
• altered binding to ribosomes
• destruction of the drug by bacterial enzymes.

### One-two punch

Some gram-positive enterococci resist aminoglycoside transport across the cell membrane. When penicillin is used with aminoglycoside therapy, the cell wall is altered, allowing the aminoglycoside to penetrate the bacterial cell.

## Pharmacotherapeutics (how drugs are used)

Aminoglycosides are most useful in treating:
• infections caused by gram-negative bacilli
• serious nosocomial (hospital-acquired) infections, such as gram-negative bacteremia (abnormal presence of microorganisms in the bloodstream), peritonitis (inflammation of the peritoneum, the membrane that lines the abdominal cavity), and pneumonia, in critically ill patients
• urinary tract infections (UTIs) caused by enteric bacilli that are resistant to less toxic antibiotics, such as penicillins and cephalosporins
• infections of the central nervous system (CNS) and the eye (treated with local instillation).

### Works well with others

Aminoglycosides are used in combination with penicillins to treat gram-positive organisms, such as staphylococcal or enterococcal infections. Combination therapy increases the drugs' effectiveness.

### Inactive duty

Aminoglycosides are inactive against anaerobic bacteria.

### Role call

Individual aminoglycosides may have their own particular usefulness:
• Streptomycin is active against many strains of mycobacteria, including *Mycobacterium tuberculosis*, and against the gram-positive bacteria *Nocardia* and *Erysipelothrix*.
• Amikacin, gentamicin, and tobramycin are active against *Acinetobacter*, *Citrobacter*, *Enterobacter*, *Klebsiella*, *Proteus* (indole-positive and indole-negative), *Providencia*, *Serratia*, *Escherichia coli*, and *Pseudomonas aeruginosa*.

## Drug interactions

Carbenicillin and ticarcillin reduce the effects of amikacin, gentamicin, kanamycin, neomycin, streptomycin, and tobramycin. This is especially true if the penicillin and aminoglycoside are mixed in the same container or I.V. line.

### Putting up a blockade

Amikacin, gentamicin, kanamycin, neomycin, streptomycin, and tobramycin administered with neuromuscular blockers increase neuromuscular blockade, resulting in increased muscle relaxation and respiratory distress.

### Kidney punch

Toxicity to the kidneys may result in renal failure; toxicity to the neurologic system results in peripheral neuropathy with numbness and tingling of the extremities. The risk of renal toxicity also increases when amikacin, gentamicin, kanamycin, or tobramycin is taken with cyclosporine, amphotericin B, or acyclovir.

### What? Say that again...

The symptoms of ototoxicity (damage to the ear) caused by aminoglycosides may be masked by antiemetic drugs. Loop diuretics taken with aminoglycosides increase the risk of ototoxicity. Hearing loss may occur in varying degrees and may be irreversible. (See *Adverse reactions to aminoglycosides*.)

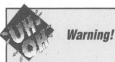

**Warning!**

## Adverse reactions to aminoglycosides

Serious adverse reactions limit the use of aminoglycosides. They include:
• neuromuscular reactions, ranging from peripheral nerve toxicity to neuromuscular blockade
• ototoxicity
• renal toxicity.

**Oral history**
Adverse reactions to oral aminoglycosides include:
• nausea and vomiting
• diarrhea.

# Penicillins

*Penicillins* remain one of the most important and useful antibacterials, despite the availability of numerous others. The penicillins
can be divided into four groups:
• natural penicillins (penicillin G benzathine, penicillin G potassium, penicillin G procaine, penicillin G sodium, penicillin V potassium)
• penicillinase-resistant penicillins (dicloxacillin, nafcillin,
oxacillin)
• aminopenicillins (amoxicillin, ampicillin)
• extended-spectrum penicillins (carbenicillin, ticarcillin).

## Pharmacokinetics

After oral administration, penicillins are absorbed mainly in the
duodenum and the upper jejunum of the small intestine.

### Absorb these factors

Absorption of oral penicillin varies and depends on such factors
as the:
• particular penicillin used
• pH of the patient's stomach and intestine
• presence of food in the GI tract.
    Most penicillins should be given on an empty stomach (1 hour
before or 2 hours after a meal) to enhance absorption. Penicillins
that can be given without regard to meals include amoxicillin,
penicillin V, and amoxicillin/clavulanate potassium.

### Distribution

Penicillins are distributed widely to most areas of the body, including the lungs, liver, kidneys, muscle, bone, and placenta. High
concentrations also appear in urine, making penicillins useful in
treating UTIs.

### Metabolism and excretion

Penicillins are metabolized to a limited extent in the liver to inactive metabolites and are excreted 60% unchanged by the kidneys.
Nafcillin and oxacillin are excreted in bile.

## Pharmacodynamics

Penicillins are usually bactericidal in action. They bind reversibly
to several enzymes outside the bacterial cytoplasmic membrane.

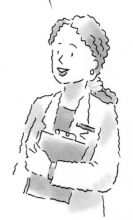

Despite the
wide variety of
antibacterials in
use, penicillins are
still among the
most useful.

## Playing with PBPs

These enzymes, known as *penicillin-binding proteins* (PBPs), are involved in cell-wall synthesis and cell division. Interference with these processes inhibits cell-wall synthesis, causing rapid destruction of the cell.

## Pharmacotherapeutics

No other class of antibacterial drugs provides as wide a spectrum of antimicrobial activity as the penicillins. As a class, they cover gram-positive, gram-negative, and anaerobic organisms, although specific penicillins are more effective against specific organisms.

### Oral vs. I.M. route

Penicillin is given by I.M. injection when oral administration is inconvenient or a patient's compliance is questionable. Because long-acting preparations of penicillin G (penicillin G benzathine and penicillin G procaine) are relatively insoluble, they must be administered by the I.M. route.

## Drug interactions

Penicillins may interact with various drugs.
• Probenecid increases the plasma concentration of penicillins.
• Penicillins reduce tubular secretion of methotrexate in the kidney, increasing the risk of methotrexate toxicity.
• Tetracyclines and chloramphenicol reduce the bactericidal action of penicillins.
• Neomycin decreases the absorption of penicillin V.
• The effectiveness of hormonal contraceptives is reduced when they're taken with penicillin V or ampicillin. Be sure to advise the patient to use a reliable, alternative method of contraception in addition to hormonal contraceptives during penicillin therapy.
• Large doses of I.V. penicillins can increase the bleeding risk of anticoagulants by prolonging bleeding time. Nafcillin and dicloxacillin have been implicated in warfarin resistance.

### Acting against aminoglycosides

High dosages of penicillin G and extended-spectrum penicillins (carbenicillin and ticarcillin) inactivate aminoglycosides. Moreover, penicillins shouldn't be mixed in the same I.V. solutions with aminoglycosides. (See *Adverse reactions to penicillins*.)

Let's move in. We'll be just fine unless they bring on the penicillins!

### Warning!

## Adverse reactions to penicillins

Hypersensitivity reactions are the major adverse reactions to penicillins. They may include:
• anaphylactic reactions
• serum sickness (a hypersensitivity reaction occurring 1 to 2 weeks after injection of a foreign serum)
• drug fever
• various rashes.

**Oral penicillins**
Adverse GI reactions associated with oral penicillins include:

• tongue inflammation
• nausea and vomiting
• diarrhea.

**Aminopenicillins and extended-spectrum penicillins**
The aminopenicillins and extended-spectrum penicillins can produce pseudomembranous colitis (diarrhea caused by a change in the flora of the colon or an overgrowth of a toxinproducing strain of *Clostridium difficile*).

**Oxacillin**
Oxacillin therapy may cause liver toxicity.

# Cephalosporins

Many antibacterial drugs introduced for clinical use in recent years have been *cephalosporins*.

## Through the generations

Cephalosporins are grouped into generations according to their effectiveness against different organisms, their characteristics, and their development.
• First-generation cephalosporins include cefadroxil, cefazolin sodium, and cephalexin monohydrate.
• Second-generation cephalosporins include cefaclor, cefprozil, cefoxitin, cefuroxime axetil, and cefuroxime sodium.
• Third-generation cephalosporins include cefdinir, cefixime, cefotaxime sodium, cefpodoxime proxetil, ceftazidime, ceftibuten, and ceftriaxone sodium.
• Fourth-generation cephalosporins include cefepime hydrochloride.

## A sensitive issue

Because penicillins and cephalosporins are chemically similar (they have what's called a *beta-lactam molecular structure*), cross-sensitivity occurs in 10% to 15% of patients. This means that someone who has had a reaction to penicillin is also at risk for a reaction to cephalosporins.

## Pharmacokinetics

Many cephalosporins are administered parenterally because they aren't absorbed from the GI tract. Some cephalosporins are absorbed from the GI tract and can be administered orally, but food usually decreases the absorption rate of these oral cephalosporins, though not the amount absorbed. Two cephalosporins (oral cefuroxime and cefpodoxime) actually have increased absorption when given with food.

### Distribution

After absorption, cephalosporins are distributed widely and readily cross the placenta.

### Generational divide

Cefuroxime (second-generation) and the third-generation drugs cefotaxime, ceftriaxone, and ceftazidime cross the blood-brain barrier after I.V. or I.M. administration. Cefepime (fourth-generation) also crosses the blood-brain barrier, but to what extent isn't known.

### Metabolism

Many cephalosporins aren't metabolized at all. Cefotaxime sodium is metabolized to the nonacetyl forms, which provide less antibacterial activity than the parent compounds. To a small extent, ceftriaxone is metabolized in the intestines to inactive metabolites, which are excreted via the biliary system.

### Excretion

All cephalosporins are excreted primarily unchanged by the kidneys with the exception of ceftriaxone, which is excreted in stool via bile.

## Pharmacodynamics

Like penicillins, cephalosporins inhibit cell-wall synthesis by binding to the bacterial enzymes known as PBPs, located on the cell membrane. After the drug damages the cell wall by binding with the PBPs, the body's natural defense mechanisms destroy the bacteria. (See *How cephalosporins attack bacteria.*)

## Pharmacotherapeutics

The four generations of cephalosporins have particular therapeutic uses.
• First-generation cephalosporins, which act primarily against gram-positive organisms, may be used as alternative therapy in

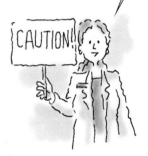
Be careful! A person who has had a reaction to penicillin may also have a reaction to cephalosporins.

*Now I get it!*

# How cephalosporins attack bacteria

The antibacterial action of cephalosporins depends on their ability to penetrate the bacterial wall and bind with proteins on the cytoplasmic membrane, as shown below.

**Mature bacterial cell**

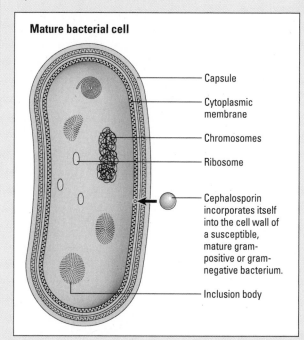

- Capsule
- Cytoplasmic membrane
- Chromosomes
- Ribosome
- Cephalosporin incorporates itself into the cell wall of a susceptible, mature gram-positive or gram-negative bacterium.
- Inclusion body

**Daughter cells after division**

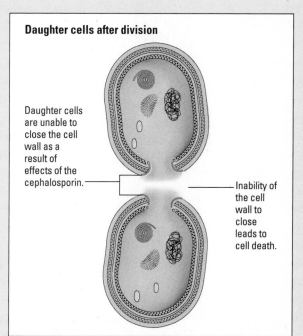

Daughter cells are unable to close the cell wall as a result of effects of the cephalosporin.

Inability of the cell wall to close leads to cell death.

the patient who's allergic to penicillin, depending on how sensitive to penicillin he is. They're also used to treat staphylococcal and streptococcal infections, including pneumonia, cellulitis (skin infection), and osteomyelitis (bone infection).

- Second-generation cephalosporins act against gram-negative bacteria. Cefoxitin is the only cephalosporin effective against anaerobes (organisms that live without oxygen).
- Third-generation cephalosporins, which act primarily against gram-negative organisms, are the drugs of choice for infections caused by *Enterobacter*, *P. aeruginosa*, and anaerobic organisms.
- Fourth-generation cephalosporins are active against many gram-positive and gram-negative bacteria.

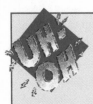

## Adverse reactions to cephalosporins

Adverse reactions to cephalosporins include:
- confusion
- seizures
- bleeding
- nausea
- vomiting
- diarrhea.

Ceftriaxone may be associated with a decrease in prothrombin activity (prothrombin time and partial thromboplastin time), leading to an increased risk of bleeding. Patients at risk include those with renal impairment, liver disease, or impaired vitamin K synthesis or storage.

**An issue of sensitivity**

Hypersensitivity reactions are the most common systemic adverse reactions to cephalosporins. They include:
- hives
- itching
- measles-type rash
- serum sickness (reaction after injection of a foreign serum characterized by edema, fever, hives, and inflammation of the blood vessels and joints)
- anaphylaxis (in rare cases).

## Drug interactions

The patient receiving cephalosporins who drinks alcoholic beverages with or up to 72 hours after taking a dose may experience acute alcohol intolerance, with such signs and symptoms as headache, flushing, dizziness, nausea, vomiting, or abdominal cramps within 30 minutes of alcohol ingestion. This reaction can occur up to 3 days after discontinuing the antibiotic. (See *Adverse reactions to cephalosporins.*)

### In use with uricosurics

Uricosurics (drugs to relieve gout), such as probenecid and sulfinpyrazone, can reduce kidney excretion of some cephalosporins. Probenecid is used therapeutically to increase and prolong plasma cephalosporin concentrations.

Cephalosporins may also decrease estrogen absorption, leading to decreased efficacy of oral contraceptives containing estrogen and progesterone.

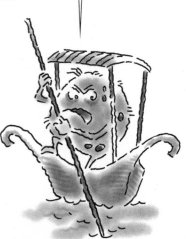

Cephalosporins penetrate and bind. That's how they wipe me out.

# Tetracyclines

*Tetracyclines* are broad-spectrum antibiotics. They may be classified as:
- intermediate-acting compounds such as demeclocycline hydrochloride
- long-acting compounds, such as doxycycline hyclate and minocycline hydrochloride.

## Pharmacokinetics

Tetracyclines are absorbed from the stomach and small intestine when taken orally.

### Distribution and excretion

Tetracyclines are distributed widely into body tissues and fluids, concentrated in bile, and excreted primarily by the kidneys. Doxycycline is also excreted in stool. Minocycline undergoes enterohepatic recirculation.

## Pharmacodynamics

All tetracyclines are primarily bacteriostatic, meaning they inhibit the growth or multiplication of bacteria. They penetrate the bacterial cell by an energy-dependent process. Within the cell, they bind primarily to a subunit of the ribosome, inhibiting the protein synthesis needed to maintain the bacterial cell.

## Pharmacotherapeutics

Tetracyclines provide a broad spectrum of activity against:
- gram-positive and gram-negative aerobic and anaerobic bacteria
- spirochetes
- mycoplasma
- rickettsiae
- chlamydiae
- some protozoa.

### Longer equals broader

The long-acting compounds doxycycline and minocycline provide more action against various organisms than other tetracyclines.

### Taking aim

Tetracyclines are used to treat Rocky Mountain spotted fever, Q fever, and Lyme disease. They're the drugs of choice for treating nongonococcal urethritis caused by *Chlamydia* and *Ureaplasma*.

Combination therapy with a tetracycline and streptomycin is the most effective treatment for brucellosis.

## Zit zapper

Tetracyclines in low dosages effectively treat acne because they can decrease the fatty acid content of sebum.

## Drug interactions

Tetracyclines can reduce the effectiveness of hormonal contraceptives, which may result in breakthrough bleeding or ineffective contraception. The patient taking hormonal contraceptives should use a reliable, secondary method of contraception. Tetracyclines may also decrease the bactericidal action of penicillin.

Other interactions commonly affect the ability of tetracyclines to move through the body.
• Aluminum, calcium, and magnesium antacids reduce the absorption of oral tetracyclines.
• Iron salts, bismuth subsalicylate, and zinc sulfate reduce the absorption of tetracyclines. Reduced absorption can be prevented by separating doses of tetracyclines and these agents by 2 to 3 hours.
• Barbiturates, carbamazepine, and phenytoin increase the metabolism and reduce the antibiotic effect of doxycycline.

## Be wary of dairy

These drugs, with the exception of doxycycline and minocycline, may also interact with milk and milk products, which bind with the drugs and prevent their absorption. To prevent decreased absorption, administer the tetracycline 1 hour before or 2 hours after meals. (See *Adverse reactions to tetracyclines.*)

# Lincomycin derivatives

Because of its high potential for causing serious adverse effects, *clindamycin* is another antibacterial prescribed only when there's no therapeutic alternative. It's used for many gram-positive and anaerobic organisms.

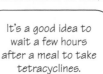

It's a good idea to wait a few hours after a meal to take tetracyclines.

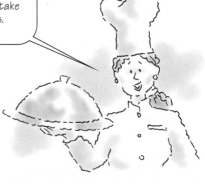

## Less from lincomycin

*Lincomycin* is less effective than clindamycin and is rarely used. Lincomycin shouldn't be used in the treatment of minor infections but would be used to treat serious respiratory or skin infections in the patient who's allergic to other antibiotics indicated for the infection.

## Pharmacokinetics

When taken orally, clindamycin is absorbed well and distributed widely throughout the body. It's metabolized by the liver and excreted by the kidneys and biliary pathways. About 20% to 30% of lincomycin, when taken orally, is absorbed from the GI tract; food delays its absorption. Lincomycin is partially metabolized in the liver and is excreted in the urine, stool, and bile.

## Pharmacodynamics

Clindamycin and lincomycin inhibit bacterial protein synthesis by inhibiting the binding of bacterial ribosomes. At therapeutic concentrations, clindamycin is primarily bacteriostatic against most organisms.

## Pharmacotherapeutics

Because of their potential for causing serious toxicity and pseudomembranous colitis (characterized by severe diarrhea, abdominal pain, fever, and mucus and blood in stool), these drugs are limited to a few clinical situations in which safer alternative antibacterials aren't available.

• Clindamycin is potent against most aerobic gram-positive organisms, including staphylococci, streptococci (except *Enterococcus faecalis*), and pneumococci.

• Clindamycin is effective against most clinically important anaerobes and is used primarily to treat anaerobic intraabdominal, pleural, or pulmonary infections caused by *Bacteroides fragilis*. It's also used as an alternative to penicillin in treating *Clostridium perfringens* infections.

• Clindamycin and lincomycin may be used as alternatives to penicillin in treating staphylococcal infections in a patient who's allergic to penicillin.

## Drug interactions

Clindamycin and lincomycin have neuromuscular blocking properties and may enhance the neuromuscular blocking action of neuromuscular blockers. This can lead to profound respiratory depression. (See *Adverse reactions to clindamycin*.)

# Macrolides

*Macrolides* are used to treat a number of common infections. They include erythromycin and its derivatives, such as:
• erythromycin estolate
• erythromycin ethylsuccinate

### Warning!

## Adverse reactions to clindamycin

Pseudomembranous colitis may occur with clindamycin. This syndrome can be fatal and requires prompt discontinuation of the drug as well as aggressive fluid and electrolyte management.

Although this is the most serious reaction to clindamycin and limits its use, other reactions may also occur, such as:
• diarrhea
• stomatitis (mouth inflammation)
• nausea and vomiting
• hypersensitivity reactions.

- erythromycin lactobionate
- erythromycin stearate.

## These aren't derivatives

Other macrolides include:
- azithromycin
- clarithromycin.

## Pharmacokinetics

Because erythromycin is acid-sensitive, it must be buffered or have an enteric coating to prevent destruction by gastric acid. Erythromycin is absorbed in the duodenum. It's distributed to most tissues and body fluids except, in most cases, for cerebrospinal fluid (CSF). However, as a class, macrolides can enter the CSF when meninges are inflamed.

### Metabolism and excretion

Erythromycin is metabolized by the liver and excreted in bile in high concentrations; small amounts are excreted in urine. It also crosses the placental barrier and is secreted in breast milk.

## Pharmacodynamics

Macrolides inhibit ribonucleic acid (RNA)–dependent protein synthesis by acting on a small portion of the ribosome, much like clindamycin.

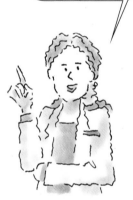

Erythromycin needs to be buffered or coated to prevent destruction by gastric acid.

## Pharmacotherapeutics

Erythromycin has a range of therapeutic uses.
- It provides a broad spectrum of antimicrobial activity against gram-positive and gram-negative bacteria, including *Mycobacterium*, *Treponema*, *Mycoplasma*, and *Chlamydia*.
- It's also effective against pneumococci and group A streptococci. *Staphylococcus aureus* is sensitive to erythromycin; however, resistant strains may appear during therapy.
- Erythromycin is the drug of choice for treating *Mycoplasma pneumoniae* infections as well as pneumonia caused by *Legionella pneumophila*.

## An alternative to penicillin

In the patient who's allergic to penicillin, erythromycin is effective for infections produced by group A beta-hemolytic streptococci or *Streptococcus pneumoniae*. It may also be used to treat gonorrhea and syphilis in the patient who can't tolerate penicillin G or the tetracyclines. Erythromycin may also be used to treat minor staphylococcal infections of the skin.

## Ranging far and wide...

Azithromycin provides a broad spectrum of antimicrobial activity against gram-positive and gram-negative bacteria, including *Mycobacterium*, *S. aureus*, *Haemophilus influenzae*, *Moraxella catarrhalis*, and *Chlamydia*. It's also effective against pneumococci and groups C, F, and G streptococci.

Clarithromycin is a broad-spectrum antibacterial that's active against gram-positive aerobes, such as *S. aureus*, *S. pneumoniae*, and *Streptococcus pyogenes*; gram-negative aerobes, such as *H. influenzae* and *M. catarrhalis*; and other aerobes such as *M. pneumoniae*.

Clarithromycin has also been used in combination with antacids, histamine-2 blockers, and proton pump inhibitors to treat *Helicobacter pylori*–induced duodenal ulcer disease.

### Drug interactions

Macrolides may interact with these drugs.
• Erythromycin, azithromycin, and clarithromycin can increase theophylline levels in the patient receiving high dosages of theophylline, increasing the risk of theophylline toxicity.
• Clarithromycin may increase the concentration of carbamazepine when used together. (See *Adverse reactions to macrolides*.)

# Vancomycin

*Vancomycin hydrochloride* is used increasingly to treat methicillin-resistant *S. aureus*, which has become a major concern in the United States and other parts of the world. Because of the emergence of vancomycin-resistant enterococci, vancomycin must be used judiciously. As a rule of thumb, it should be used only when culture and sensitivity test results confirm the need for it.

## Pharmacokinetics

Because vancomycin is absorbed poorly from the GI tract, it must be given I.V. to treat systemic infections. However, an oral form of vancomycin is used to treat pseudomembranous colitis. Vancomycin diffuses well into pleural (around the lungs), pericardial (around the heart), synovial (joint), and ascitic (in the peritoneal cavity) fluids.

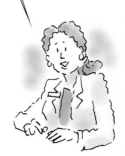

Macrolides are broad-spectrum antibiotics used to treat a number of common infections.

*Warning!*

## Adverse reactions to macrolides

Erythromycin produces few adverse effects, which may include:
• epigastric distress
• nausea and vomiting
• diarrhea (especially with large doses)
• rash
• fever
• eosinophilia (an increase in the number of eosinophils, a type of white blood cell)
• anaphylaxis.

## No switching!

Remember that I.V. vancomycin can't be used in place of oral vancomycin and vice versa. The two forms aren't interchangeable.

### Metabolism and excretion

The metabolism of vancomycin is unknown. About 85% of the dose is excreted unchanged in urine within 24 hours. A small amount may be eliminated through the liver and biliary tract.

## Pharmacodynamics

Vancomycin inhibits bacterial cell-wall synthesis, damaging the bacterial plasma membrane. When the bacterial cell wall is damaged, the body's natural defenses can attack the organism.

## Pharmacotherapeutics

Vancomycin is active against gram-positive organisms, such as *S. aureus*, *S. epidermidis*, *S. pyogenes*, *Enterococcus*, and *S. pneumoniae*.

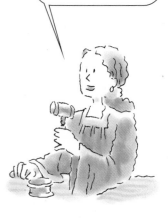

Vancomycin must be used judiciously because of the emergence of vancomycin-resistant enterococci.

## In the I.V. league

I.V. vancomycin is the therapy of choice for the patient with a serious resistant staphylococcal infection who's hypersensitive to penicillins.

## Oral history

Oral vancomycin is used for the patient with antibiotic-associated *Clostridium difficile* colitis who can't take or has responded poorly to metronidazole.

## The 1 in the 1-2 punch

Vancomycin, when used with an aminoglycoside, is also the treatment of choice for *E. faecalis* endocarditis in the patient who's allergic to penicillin.

## Drug interactions

Vancomycin may increase the risk of toxicity when administered with other drugs toxic to the kidneys and organs of hearing, such as aminoglycosides, amphotericin B, bacitracin, cisplatin, colistin, and polymyxin B. (See *Adverse reactions to vancomycin.*)

**Warning!**

## Adverse reactions to vancomycin

Adverse reactions to vancomycin, although rare, include:
- hypersensitivity and anaphylactic reactions
- drug fever
- eosinophilia (an increased number of eosinophils, a type of white blood cell [WBC])
- neutropenia (a decreased number of neutrophils, another type of WBC)
- hearing loss (transient or permanent), especially with excessive doses (as when it's given with other ototoxic drugs).

**Rash behavior**

Severe hypotension may occur with rapid I.V. administration of vancomycin and may be accompanied by a red rash with flat and raised lesions on the face, neck, chest, and arms (red man's syndrome).

Dosages of 1 g or less should be given over 1 hour, and dosages of more than 1 g should be given over 1½ to 2 hours.

# Carbapenems

*Carbapenems* are a class of beta-lactam antibacterials that includes:
- ertapenem
- imipenem-cilastatin sodium (a combination drug)
- meropenem.

## The Broadway of antibacterials

The antibacterial spectrum of activity for imipenem-cilastatin is broader than that of any other antibacterial studied to date. Because of this broad spectrum of activity, it's used for serious or life-threatening infection, especially gram-positive and gram-negative health-care acquired infections. Broad-spectrum antibacterials cover many organisms; narrow-spectrum antibacterials are effective against a select few organisms.

## Pharmacokinetics

The pharmacokinetic properties of carbapenems vary slightly.

### Distribution, metabolism, and excretion

Imipenem must be given with cilastatin because imipenem alone is rapidly metabolized in the tubules of the kidneys, rendering it ineffective. After parenteral administration, imipenem-cilastatin is distributed widely. It's metabolized by several mechanisms and excreted primarily in urine.

Ertapenem is completely absorbed after I.V. administration and is more highly protein-bound than the other two carbapenems. It's metabolized by hydrolysis and excreted mainly in urine.

## Mostly unchanged

After parenteral administration, meropenem is distributed widely, including to the CNS. Metabolism is insignificant; 70% of the drug is excreted unchanged in urine.

## Pharmacodynamics

Imipenem-cilastatin, ertapenem, and meropenem are bactericidal. They exert antibacterial activity by inhibiting bacterial cell-wall synthesis.

## Pharmacotherapeutics

Imipenem has the broadest spectrum of activity of currently available beta-lactam antibiotics.
• It's effective against aerobic gram-positive species, such as *Streptococcus*, *S. aureus*, and *S. epidermidis*.
• It inhibits most *Enterobacter* species.
• It also inhibits *P. aeruginosa* (including strains resistant to piperacillin and ceftazidime) and most anaerobic species, including *B. fragilis*.

## Lone ranger

Imipenem may also be used alone to treat serious health-care acquired infections and infections in immunocompromised patients caused by mixed aerobic and anaerobic organisms.

## Don't forget the other carbapenems

Meropenem is indicated for the treatment of intra-abdominal infections as well as for the management of bacterial meningitis caused by susceptible organisms.

Ertapenem's spectrum of activity includes intra-abdominal, skin, urinary tract, and gynecologic infections as well as community-acquired pneumonias caused by a variety of gram-positive, gram-negative, and anaerobic organisms.

## Drug interactions

Carbapenems may interact with these drugs.
• Taking probenecid with imipenem-cilastatin increases the serum level of cilastatin, but only slightly increases the serum level of imipenem.
• Probenecid may cause meropenem and ertapenem to accumulate to toxic levels.

• The combination of imipenem-cilastatin and an aminoglycoside acts synergistically against *E. faecalis*, *Staphylococcus aureus* and *Listeria monocytogenes*. (See *Adverse reactions to carbapenems*.)

# Monobactams

*Aztreonam* is the first member in the class of monobactam antibiotics and the only one currently available. It's a synthetic monobactam with a narrow spectrum of activity that includes many gram-negative aerobic bacteria.

## Pharmacokinetics

After parenteral administration, aztreonam is rapidly and completely absorbed and widely distributed throughout the body. It's metabolized partially and excreted primarily in urine as unchanged drug.

## Pharmacodynamics

Aztreonam's bactericidal activity results from inhibition of bacterial cell-wall synthesis. It binds to the PBP-3 of susceptible gram-negative bacterial cells, inhibiting cell-wall division and resulting in lysis.

## Pharmacotherapeutics

Aztreonam is indicated in a range of therapeutic situations.
• It's effective against a wide variety of gram-negative aerobic organisms, including *P. aeruginosa*.
• It's effective against most strains of the following organisms: *E. coli*, *Enterobacter*, *Klebsiella pneumoniae*, *K. oxytoca*, *Proteus mirabilis*, *Serratia marcescens*, *H. influenzae*, and *Citrobacter*.
• It's also used to treat complicated and uncomplicated UTIs, septicemia, and lower respiratory tract, skin and skin-structure, intra-abdominal, and gynecologic infections caused by susceptible gram-negative aerobic bacteria.
• It's usually active against gram-negative aerobic organisms that are resistant to antibiotics hydrolyzed by beta-lactamases. (Beta-lactamase is an enzyme that makes an antibiotic ineffective.)

*It can need help*

Aztreonam shouldn't be used alone as empiric therapy (treatment based on clinical experience rather than on medical data) in a se-

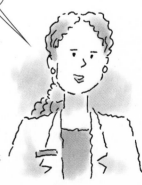

> Aztreonam inhibits bacterial cell-wall synthesis.

riously ill patient who may have a gram-positive bacterial infection or a mixed aerobic-anaerobic bacterial infection.

## Drug interactions

Aztreonam may interact with several other drugs.
• Synergistic or additive effects occur when aztreonam is used with aminoglycosides or other antibiotics, such as cefoperazone, cefotaxime, clindamycin, and piperacillin.
• Potent inducers of beta-lactamase production (cefoxitin, imipenem) may inactivate aztreonam. Concomitant use isn't recommended.
• Taking aztreonam with clavulanic acid–containing antibiotics may produce synergistic or antagonistic effects, depending on the organism involved. (See *Adverse reactions to aztreonam*.)

# Fluoroquinolones

*Fluoroquinolones* are structurally similar synthetic antibiotics. They are primarily administered to treat UTIs, upper respiratory tract infections, pneumonia, and gonorrhea and include:
• ciprofloxacin
• levofloxacin
• moxifloxacin
• norfloxacin
• ofloxacin.

## Pharmacokinetics

After oral administration, fluoroquinolones are absorbed well.

### Metabolism and excretion

Fluoroquinolones aren't highly protein-bound, are minimally metabolized in the liver, and are excreted primarily in urine.

## Pharmacodynamics

Fluoroquinolones interrupt deoxyribonucleic acid (DNA) synthesis during bacterial replication by inhibiting DNA gyrase, an essential enzyme of replicating DNA. As a result, the bacteria can't reproduce.

## Pharmacotherapeutics

Fluoroquinolones can be used to treat many UTIs. Each drug in this class also has specific indications.

**Warning!**

## Adverse reactions to aztreonam

Aztreonam can cause some adverse reactions, including:
• diarrhea
• hypersensitivity and skin reactions
• hypotension
• nausea and vomiting
• transient electrocardiogram changes (including ventricular arrhythmias)
• transient increases in serum liver enzyme levels.

- Ciprofloxacin is used to treat lower respiratory tract infections, infectious diarrhea, and skin, bone, and joint infections.
- Levofloxacin is indicated for the treatment of lower respiratory tract infections, skin infections, and UTIs.
- Moxifloxacin is used to treat acute bacterial sinusitis and mild to moderate community-acquired pneumonia.
- Norfloxacin is used to treat UTIs and prostatitis.
- Ofloxacin is used to treat selected sexually transmitted diseases, lower respiratory tract infections, skin and skin-structure infections, and prostatitis (inflammation of the prostate gland).

## Drug interactions

Several drug interactions may occur with the fluoroquinolones.
- Administration with antacids that contain magnesium or aluminum hydroxide results in decreased absorption of the fluoroquinolone.
- Some fluoroquinolones, such as ciprofloxacin, norfloxacin, and ofloxacin, interact with xanthine derivatives, such as aminophylline and theophylline, increasing the plasma theophylline level and the risk of theophylline toxicity.
- Giving ciprofloxacin or norfloxacin with probenecid results in decreased kidney elimination of these fluoroquinolones, increasing their serum levels and half-life.
- Drugs that prolong the QT interval, such as antiarrhythmics, should be used cautiously during moxifloxacin therapy. (See *Adverse reactions to fluoroquinolones*.)

# Sulfonamides

*Sulfonamides* were the first effective systemic antibacterial drugs. They include:
- co-trimoxazole (sulfamethoxazole and trimethoprim)
- sulfadiazine.

## Pharmacokinetics

Most sulfonamides are well absorbed and widely distributed in the body. They're metabolized in the liver to inactive metabolites and excreted by the kidneys.

### Lots and lots and lots of liquid

Because crystalluria and subsequent kidney stone formation may occur during the metabolic excretory phase, adequate fluid intake is highly recommended during sulfonamide therapy. The patient taking oral sulfonamides should take the medication with 8 oz of

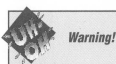

**Warning!**

## Adverse reactions to fluoroquinolones

Fluoroquinolones are well tolerated by most patients, but some serious adverse effects may occur, including:
- dizziness
- nausea and vomiting
- diarrhea
- abdominal pain.

**Serious reactions**
Moderate to severe phototoxic reactions have occurred with direct and indirect sunlight and with artificial ultraviolet lights, with and without sunscreen. Light should be avoided for several days after stopping fluoroquinolone therapy.

water and should drink plenty of fluids throughout therapy (2 to 3 L daily).

## Pharmacodynamics

Sulfonamides are bacteriostatic drugs that prevent the growth of microorganisms by inhibiting folic acid production. The decreased folic acid synthesis decreases the number of bacterial nucleotides and inhibits bacterial growth.

## Pharmacotherapeutics

Sulfonamides are commonly used to treat acute UTIs. With recurrent or chronic UTIs, the infecting organism may not be susceptible to sulfonamides. Therefore, the choice of therapy should be based on bacteria susceptibility tests.

*Infectious behavior*

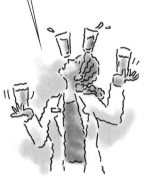

If you're taking sulfonamides, you'd better be drinking lots of fluids!

Sulfonamides also are used to treat infections caused by *Nocardia asteroides* and *Toxoplasma gondii*. Co-trimoxazole (a combination of a sulfa drug and a folate antagonist) is used for a variety of other infections, such as *Pneumocystis carinii* (*Pneumocystis jiroveci*) pneumonia, acute otitis media (due to *H. influenzae* and *S. pneumoniae*), and acute exacerbations of chronic bronchitis (due to *H. influenzae* and *S. pneumoniae*). Sulfonamides exhibit a wide spectrum of activity against gram-positive and gram-negative bacteria.

## Drug interactions

Sulfonamides have few significant interactions.
• They increase the hypoglycemic effects of the sulfonylureas (oral antidiabetic drugs), which may decrease blood glucose levels.
• When taken with methenamine, they may lead to the development of crystals in urine.
• Co-trimoxazole may increase the anticoagulant effect of coumarin anticoagulants.
• Co-timoxazole and methotrexate may cause increased methotrexate levels and increase the risk of toxicity.
• Co-trimoxazole plus cyclosporine increases the risk of kidney toxicity. (See *Adverse reactions to sulfonamides*.)

**Warning!**

## Adverse reactions to sulfonamides

Excessively high doses of less water-soluble sulfonamides can produce crystals in urine and deposits of sulfonamide crystals in the renal tubules. This complication isn't a problem with the newer water-soluble sulfonamides. Hypersensitivity reactions may occur and appear to increase as the dosage increases.

**Is it serum sickness?**
A reaction that resembles serum sickness may occur, producing fever, joint pain, hives, bronchospasm, and leukopenia (reduced white blood cell count).

**Photo finish**
Sulfonamides can also produce photosensitivity reactions.

# Nitrofurantoin

*Nitrofurantoin* is used to treat acute and chronic UTIs. It isn't useful in treating pyelonephritis or perinephric (around the kidney) diseases.

## Pharmacokinetics

After oral administration, nitrofurantoin is absorbed rapidly and well from the GI tract. Taking the drug with food enhances its bioavailability. It's available in a microcrystalline form and a macrocrystalline form. The microcrystalline form is absorbed more slowly because of slower dissolution and thus causes less GI distress.

### Distribution

The drug is 20% to 60% protein-bound. Nitrofurantoin crosses the placental barrier and is secreted in breast milk. It's also distributed in bile.

### Metabolism and excretion

Nitrofurantoin is partially metabolized by the liver, and 30% to 50% is excreted unchanged in urine.

## Pharmacodynamics

Usually bacteriostatic, nitrofurantoin may become bactericidal, depending on its urinary concentration and the susceptibility of the infecting organism.

## Reduces power?

Although its exact mechanism of action is unknown, nitrofurantoin appears to inhibit formation of acetyl coenzyme A from pyruvic acid, thereby inhibiting the energy production of the infecting organism. Nitrofurantoin may also disrupt bacterial cell-wall formation.

### Pharmacotherapeutics

Because the absorbed drug concentrates in urine, nitrofurantoin is used to treat UTIs. It has a higher antibacterial activity in acid urine. Nitrofurantoin isn't effective against systemic bacterial infections.

### Drug interactions

Nitrofurantoin has few significant interactions.
• Probenecid and sulfinpyrazone inhibit the excretion of nitrofurantoin by the kidneys, reducing its efficacy and increasing its toxic potential.
• Magnesium salts and magnesium-containing antacids can decrease the extent and rate of nitrofurantoin absorption.
• Nitrofurantoin may decrease the antibacterial activity of norfloxacin and nalidixic acid. (See *Adverse reactions to nitrofurantoin.*)

**Warning!**

### Adverse reactions to nitrofurantoin

Adverse reactions to nitrofurantoin include:
• GI irritation
• anorexia
• nausea and vomiting
• diarrhea
• dark yellow or brown urine
• abdominal pain
• chills
• fever
• joint pain
• anaphylaxis
• headache
• hypersensitivity reactions involving the skin, lungs, blood, and liver.

# Antiviral drugs

*Antiviral drugs* are used to prevent or treat viral infections ranging from influenza to human immunodeficiency virus (HIV). The major antiviral drug classes used to treat systemic infections include:
• synthetic nucleosides
• pyrophosphate analogues
• influenza A and syncytial virus drugs
• nucleoside analogue reverse transcriptase inhibitors (NRTIs)
• non-nucleoside reverse transcriptase inhibitors (NNRTIs)
• nucleotide analogue reverse transcriptase inhibitors
• protease inhibitors.

## Synthetic nucleosides

*Synthetic nucleosides* are a group of drugs used to treat many viral syndromes that can occur in an immunocompromised patient,

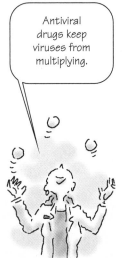

Antiviral drugs keep viruses from multiplying.

including herpes simplex virus (HSV) and cytomegalovirus (CMV). Drugs in this class include:

- acyclovir
- famciclovir
- ganciclovir
- valacyclovir
- valganciclovir.

Acyclovir sodium, used to treat HSV, is an effective antiviral drug that causes minimal toxicity to cells. A derivative of acyclovir, ganciclovir has potent antiviral activity against HSV and CMV.

## A prodrug drug

Famciclovir is used to treat acute herpes zoster, genital herpes, and recurrent HSV infections in the HIV-infected patient. Valacyclovir is used to treat herpes zoster, genital herpes, and herpes labialis. Valganciclovir is used to treat CMV retinitis in the patient with acquired immunodeficiency syndrome (AIDS).

## Pharmacokinetics

Each of these antiviral drugs travels its own route through the body.

## Slow by mouth

When given orally, acyclovir absorption is slow and only 10% to 30% complete. It's distributed throughout the body and metabolized primarily inside the infected cells; the majority of the drug is excreted in urine.

## Bound? Not much

Famciclovir is less than 20% bound to plasma proteins. It's extensively metabolized in the liver and excreted in urine.

## I.V. only

Ganciclovir is administered I.V. because it's absorbed poorly from the GI tract. More than 90% of ganciclovir isn't metabolized and is excreted unchanged by the kidneys.

## Metabolic changes

Valacyclovir is converted to acyclovir during its metabolism and has pharmacokinetic properties similar to those of acyclovir. Valganciclovir is metabolized in the intestinal wall and liver to ganciclovir; however, interchanging the two drugs isn't effective.

## Pharmacodynamics

To be effective, acyclovir, famciclovir, and ganciclovir must be metabolized to their active form in cells infected by HSV.

### Presto change-o

Acyclovir enters virus-infected cells, where it's changed through a series of steps to acyclovir triphosphate. Acyclovir triphosphate inhibits virus-specific DNA polymerase, an enzyme necessary for viral growth, thus disrupting viral replication.

On entry into CMV-infected cells, ganciclovir is converted to ganciclovir triphosphate, which is thought to produce its antiviral activity by inhibiting viral DNA synthesis.

Famciclovir enters viral cells (herpes simplex 1 and 2, varicella zoster), where it inhibits DNA polymerase, viral DNA synthesis and, thus, viral replication.

Valacyclovir rapidly converts to acyclovir; acyclovir then becomes incorporated into viral DNA and inhibits viral DNA polymerase, thus inhibiting viral multiplication.

Valganciclovir is converted to ganciclovir, which inhibits replication of viral DNA synthesis of CMV.

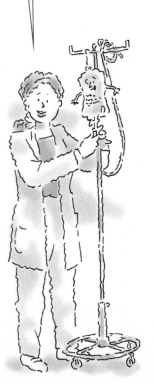

I.V. acyclovir treats shingles in an immunocompromised patient.

## Pharmacotherapeutics

Acyclovir is used to treat infection caused by herpes viruses, including HSV types 1 and 2 and the varicella-zoster virus. Oral acyclovir is used primarily to treat initial and recurrent HSV type 2 infections.

I.V. acyclovir is used to treat:
• severe initial HSV type 2 infections in a patient with a normal immune system
• initial and recurrent skin and mucous membrane HSV type 1 and 2 infections in an immunocompromised patient
• herpes zoster infections (shingles) caused by the varicella-zoster virus in an immunocompromised patient
• disseminated varicella-zoster virus in an immunocompromised patient
• varicella infections (chickenpox) caused by the varicella-zoster virus in an immunocompromised patient.

### RSVP for CMV

Ganciclovir is used to treat CMV retinitis in an immunocompromised patient, including a patient with AIDS or other CMV infections such as encephalitis.

### If it keeps coming back

Famciclovir is used to treat acute herpes zoster, genital herpes, and recurrent HSV infections in a patient with HIV.

## The valiant vals

Valganciclovir is used to treat CMV retinitis, and valacyclovir is effective against herpes zoster, genital herpes, and herpes labialis.

## Drug interactions

Synthetic nucleosides may interact with these drugs.
• Probenecid reduces kidney excretion and increases blood levels of ganciclovir, valganciclovir, valacyclovir, famciclovir, and acyclovir, increasing the risk of toxicity.
• Taking ganciclovir with drugs that are damaging to tissue cells, such as dapsone, pentamidine isethionate, flucytosine, vincristine, vinblastine, doxorubicin, amphotericin B, and co-trimoxazole, inhibits replication of rapidly dividing cells in the bone marrow, GI tract, skin, and sperm-producing cells.
• Imipenem-cilastatin increases the risk of seizures when taken with ganciclovir or valganciclovir.
• Zidovudine increases the risk of granulocytopenia (reduced number of granulocytes, a type of white blood cell) when taken with ganciclovir. (See *Adverse reactions to synthetic nucleosides.*)

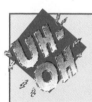

*Warning!*

## Adverse reactions to synthetic nucleosides

Treatment with these drugs may lead to particular adverse reactions.

### Acyclovir
Reversible kidney impairment may occur with rapid I.V. injection (less than 10 minutes) or infusion of acyclovir.

### Oral history
Common reactions to oral acyclovir include headache, nausea, vomiting, and diarrhea.

### Issues of sensitivity
Hypersensitivity reactions may occur with acyclovir.

### Ganciclovir
The most common adverse reactions to ganciclovir are granulocytopenia and thrombocytopenia.

### Famciclovir and valacyclovir
Common adverse reactions to famciclovir and valacyclovir include headache, nausea, and vomiting.

### Valganciclovir
Common adverse reactions to valganciclovir include headache, insomnia, seizures, retinal detachment, diarrhea, nausea, vomiting, abdominal pain, neutropenia, anemia, thrombocytopenia, pancytopenia, bone marrow depression, aplastic anemia, sepsis, and hypersensitivity reactions.

# Pyrophosphate analogues

The antiviral drug *foscarnet* is used to treat CMV retinitis in the patient with AIDS. It's also used to treat acyclovir-resistant HSV infections in the immunocompromised patient.

## Pharmacokinetics

Foscarnet is poorly bound to plasma proteins. In patients with normal kidney function, the majority of foscarnet is excreted unchanged in urine.

## Pharmacodynamics

Foscarnet prevents viral replication by selectively inhibiting DNA polymerase.

## Pharmacotherapeutics

Foscarnet's primary therapeutic use is treating CMV retinitis in the patient with AIDS. It's also used in combination therapy with ganciclovir for the patient who has relapsed with either drug.

## Drug interactions

Foscarnet has few drug interactions.
• Foscarnet and pentamidine together increase the risk of hypocalcemia (low blood calcium levels) and toxicity to the kidneys.
• The use of foscarnet and other drugs that alter serum calcium levels may result in hypocalcemia.
• Foscarnet given with amiodarone increases the risk of cardiotoxicity and QT prolongation.
• The risk of kidney impairment increases when drugs toxic to the kidneys, such as amphotericin B and aminoglycosides, are taken with foscarnet. Because of the risk of kidney toxicity, the patient should be aggressively hydrated during treatment. (See *Adverse reactions to foscarnet.*)

**Warning!**

### Adverse reactions to foscarnet

Adverse reactions to foscarnet may include:
• fatigue, depression, fever, confusion, headache, numbness and tingling, dizziness, and seizures
• nausea and vomiting, diarrhea, and abdominal pain
• granulocytopenia, leukopenia, and anemia
• involuntary muscle contractions and neuropathy
• breathing difficulties and coughing
• rash
• altered kidney function
• electrolyte disturbances.

# Influenza A and syncytial virus drugs

*Amantadine* and its derivative, *rimantadine hydrochloride*, are used to prevent or treat influenza A infections. *Ribavirin* is used to treat respiratory syncytial virus (RSV) infections in children.

## Breathe in

To treat RSV, ribavirin is administered by aerosol inhalation, using a small-particle aerosol generator.

## Pharmacokinetics

After oral administration, amantadine and rimantadine are well absorbed in the GI tract and widely distributed throughout the body. Ribavirin is administered by nasal or oral inhalation and is well absorbed. It has a limited, specific distribution, with the highest concentration found in the respiratory tract and in red blood cells (RBCs). Ribavirin capsules are rapidly absorbed after administration and are distributed in plasma.

### Metabolism and excretion

Amantadine is eliminated primarily in urine; rimantadine is extensively metabolized and then excreted in urine.

Ribavirin is metabolized in the liver and by RBCs. It's excreted primarily by the kidneys, with some excreted in stool.

## Pharmacodynamics

Although its exact mechanism of action is unknown, amantadine appears to inhibit an early stage of viral replication. Rimantadine inhibits viral RNA and protein synthesis.

The mechanism of action of ribavirin isn't known completely, but the drug's metabolites inhibit viral DNA and RNA synthesis, subsequently halting viral-replication.

## Pharmacotherapeutics

Amantadine and rimantadine are used to prevent and treat respiratory tract infections caused by strains of the influenza A virus. They can reduce the severity and duration of fever and other symptoms in patients already infected with influenza A.

Ribavirin, used to treat severe RSV infection in children, is also used in adults in combination with interferon alfa-2B for treatment of chronic hepatitic C.

## In the meantime

These drugs also protect the patient who has received the influenza vaccine during the 2 weeks needed for immunity to develop as well as the patient who can't take the influenza vaccine because of hypersensitivity.

**Warning!**

## Adverse reactions to amantadine and rimantadine

**Amantadine**
Adverse reactions include:
• anorexia
• anxiety
• confusion
• depression
• dizziness
• fatigue
• forgetfulness
• hallucinations
• hypersensitivity reactions
• insomnia
• irritability
• nausea
• nervousness
• psychosis.

**Rimantadine**
Adverse reactions to rimantadine are similar to those for amantadine. However, they tend to be less severe.

### Calming the shakes

Amantadine is also used to treat parkinsonism and drug-induced extrapyramidal reactions (abnormal involuntary movements).

## Drug interactions

Amantadine may interact with some drugs. (See *Adverse reactions to amantadine and rimantadine*, page 265.)
• Taking anticholinergics with amantadine increases adverse anticholinergic effects.
• Amantadine given with the combination drug hydrochlorothiazide and triamterene results in decreased urine excretion of amantadine, causing increased amantadine levels.
• Amantadine and co-trimoxazole levels are increased when used together.

### All quiet on the rimantadine front

No clinically significant drug interactions have been documented with rimantadine.
Ribavirin has few interactions with other drugs.
• Ribavirin reduces the antiviral activity of zidovudine, and concomitant use of these drugs may cause blood toxicity.
• Taking ribavirin and digoxin can cause digoxin toxicity, producing such effects as GI distress, CNS abnormalities, and cardiac arrhythmias. (See *Adverse reactions to ribavirin*.)

**Warning!**

## Adverse reactions to ribavirin

Adverse reactions to ribavirin include:
• apnea (lack of breathing)
• cardiac arrest
• hypotension
• nausea
• pneumothorax (air in the pleural space, causing the lung to collapse)
• worsening of respiratory function.

# Nucleoside analogue reverse transcriptase inhibitors

NRTIs are used to treat the patient with advanced HIV infection. Drugs in this class include:
• abacavir
• didanosine
• emtricitabine
• lamivudine
• stavudine
• zidovudine.

### First in the fight against AIDS

Zidovudine was the first drug to receive Food and Drug Administration (FDA) approval for treating AIDS and AIDS-related complex.

## Pharmacokinetics

Each of the NRTIs has its own pharmacokinetic properties.

## Into space

Abacavir is rapidly and extensively absorbed after oral administration. It's distributed in the extravascular space, and about 50% binds with plasma proteins. Abacavir is metabolized by the cytosolic enzymes and excreted primarily in urine with the remainder excreted in stool.

Lamivudine and stavudine are rapidly absorbed after administration and are excreted by the kidneys.

Emtricitabine is rapidly and extensively absorbed after oral administration and is excreted by the kidneys.

## Buffer needed

Because didanosine is degraded rapidly in gastric acid, didanosine tablets and powder contain a buffering drug to increase pH. The exact route of metabolism isn't fully understood. About one-half of an absorbed dose is excreted in urine.

## Well absorbed, widely distributed

Zidovudine is well absorbed from the GI tract, widely distributed throughout the body, metabolized by the liver, and excreted by the kidneys. The dosage may need to be adjusted in the patient with kidney or liver disease, as is the case with most of the NRTIs.

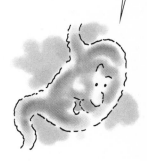

Gastric acid rapidly degrades didanosine.

## Pharmacodynamics

NRTIs must undergo conversion to their active metabolites to produce their action.
• Abacavir is converted to an active metabolite that inhibits the activity of HIV-1 transcriptase by competing with a natural component and incorporating into viral DNA.
• Didanosine undergoes cellular enzyme conversion to its active antiviral metabolite to block HIV replication.
• Emtricitabine inhibits the enzyme, reverse transcriptase, and thus inhibits viral DNA replication.
• Lamivudine and stavudine are converted in the cells to their active metabolites, which inhibit viral DNA replication.
• Zidovudine is converted by cellular enzymes to an active form, zidovudine triphosphate, which prevents viral DNA from replicating. (See *How zidovudine works*, page 268.)

## Pharmacotherapeutics

NRTIs are used to treat HIV and AIDS.

*Now I get it!*

# How zidovudine works

Zidovudine can inhibit replication of the human immunodeficiency virus (HIV). The first two illustrations show how HIV invades cells and then replicates itself. The bottom illustration shows how zidovudine blocks viral transformation.

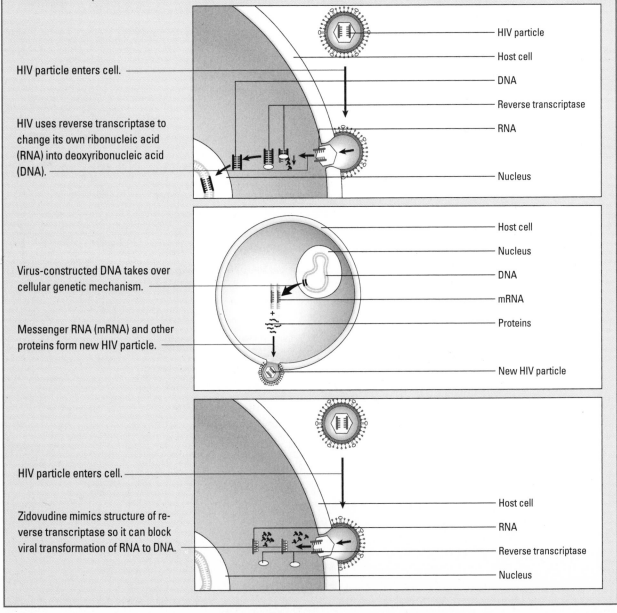

## When you're hospitalized

I.V. zidovudine is used for the hospitalized patient who can't take oral medication. It's also used to prevent transmission of HIV from the mother to her fetus and to treat AIDS-related dementia.

Like all drugs for HIV infection, oral zidovudine is used as part of a multidrug regimen.

## Getting a jump on HIV

Didanosine, in combination with other antiretrovirals (antivirals used to treat HIV infection), is an alternative initial treatment for HIV infection.

## Part of the combo...

Lamivudine, stavudine, and abacavir are used in combination with other antiretrovirals to treat HIV infection. *Combivir* is combination therapy that includes lamivudine and zidovudine. *Trizivir* is combination therapy that includes abacavir, lamivudine, and zidovudine; it was approved by the FDA in November 2000 to simplify dosing in the treatment of HIV.

Emtricitabine is used in combination with other antiretrovirals to treat HIV infection.

## ...but be careful here

Because of inhibition of phosphorylation (the process needed to form the active DNA-inhibiting metabolite), stavudine shouldn't be given in combination with zidovudine.

## Drug interactions

NRTIs may be responsible for many drug interactions.
• Potentially fatal lactic acidosis and severe hepatomegaly with steatosis have occurred in patients taking NRTIs alone or with other antiretrovirals such as tenofovir. The majority of patients were women, and obesity and prolonged NRTI exposure may be risk factors.
• An increased risk of cellular and kidney toxicity occurs when zidovudine is taken with such drugs as dapsone, pentamidine isethionate, flucytosine, vincristine, vinblastine, doxorubicin, interferon, and ganciclovir.
• Taking zidovudine with probenecid, aspirin, acetaminophen, indomethacin, cimetidine, or lorazepam increases the risk of toxicity of either drug.
• Zidovudine plus acyclovir may produce profound lethargy and drowsiness.
• Didanosine may reduce the absorption of tetracyclines, delavirdine, and fluoroquinolones.

## Adverse reactions to NRTIs

Each of the nucleoside reverse transcriptase inhibitors (NRTIs) can cause adverse reactions.

**Zidovudine**
- Blood-related reactions
- Headache and dizziness
- Muscle pain, fever, and rash
- Nausea, vomiting, abdominal pain, diarrhea

**Didanosine**
- Diarrhea, nausea, vomiting, abdominal pain, constipation, stomatitis, unusual taste or loss of taste, dry mouth, pancreatitis

- Headache, peripheral neuropathy, dizziness
- Muscle weakness, rash, itching, muscle pain, hair loss

**Abacavir**
- Potentially fatal hypersensitivity reactions

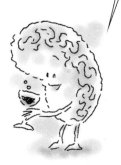

Abacavir levels increase with alcohol consumption.

- Abacavir levels increase with alcohol consumption.
- Emtricitabine has been studied in combination with indinavir, stavudine, famciclovir, and tenofovir; there were no clinically significant drug interactions. (See *Adverse reactions to NRTIs*.)

# Non-nucleoside reverse transcriptase inhibitors

NNRTIs are used in combination with other antiretrovirals to treat HIV infection. The three agents in this class include:
- delavirdine
- efavirenz
- nevirapine. (See *Combining antiretroviral drugs*.)

## Pharmacokinetics

Efavirenz and delavirdine are highly protein-bound after absorption and distribution, and nevirapine is widely distributed throughout the body. All three drugs are metabolized by the cytochrome P-450 liver enzyme system and excreted in urine and stool.

## Pharmacodynamics

Nevirapine and delavirdine bind to the reverse transcriptase enzyme, preventing it from exerting its effect, and thus preventing HIV replication. Efavirenz competes for the enzyme through noncompetitive inhibition.

## Combining antiretroviral drugs

Monotherapy (using a single drug) isn't recommended for human immunodeficiency virus infection. For the best results, a combination of antiretroviral agents is used.

## Pharmacotherapeutics

NNRTIs are used in combination with other antiretrovirals in HIV treatment; nevirapine is specifically indicated for the patient whose clinical condition and immune status have deteriorated.

## Drug interactions

NNRTIs may be responsible for many drug interactions.
• Nevirapine may decrease the activity of protease inhibitors and hormonal contraceptives; these drugs shouldn't be used together.
• Delavirdine may increase levels of benzodiazepines, clarithromycin, rifabutin, saquinavir, and warfarin; it may also significantly increase concentrations of indinavir, requiring a decrease in the indinavir dosage.
• The indinavir dosage will need to be increased when given with efavirenz.
• Nevirapine has been associated with a severe rash that may be life-threatening. If a rash occurs, discontinue the drug. (See *Adverse reactions to NNRTIs*.)

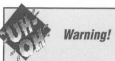

**Warning!**

## Adverse reactions to NNRTIs

Adverse reactions to nonnucleoside reverse transcriptase inhibitors (NNRTIs) include:
• headache
• dizziness
• asthenia
• nausea and vomiting
• diarrhea
• rash.

# Nucleotide analogue reverse transcriptase inhibitors

Nucleotide analogue reverse transcriptase inhibitors are used in combination with other antiretrovirals in the treatment of HIV. The only drug in this class to date is *tenofovir*, and it works much like the NRTIs.

## Pharmacokinetics

Tenofovir is absorbed much better after a high-fat meal. It's then distributed in small amounts into plasma and serum proteins. Metabolism isn't thought to be mediated by cytochrome P-450 liver enzymes, and the drug is excreted by the kidneys.

## Pharmacodynamics

Tenofovir competes with substrates and is subsequently incorporated into the DNA chain, thus halting HIV replication.

## Pharmacotherapeutics

Tenofovir is used in combination with other drugs to treat HIV infection.

## Drug interactions

Tenofovir may be responsible for some drug interactions.

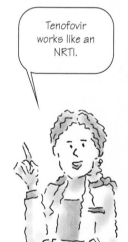

Tenofovir works like an NRTI.

• Drugs that are eliminated through the kidneys or that decrease kidney function may increase levels of tenofovir when given concurrently.

• Didanosine levels increase when it's given with tenofovir; watch for didanosine-based adverse effects.

• Potentially fatal lactic acidosis and severe hepatomegaly with steatosis have occurred in patients taking tenofovir alone or with other antiretrovirals. The majority of patients were women, and obesity and previous NRTI exposure may be risk factors. Patients with preexisting liver disease should take this drug with caution. Suspend treatment if hepatotoxicity is suspected. (See *Adverse reactions to tenofovir*.)

# Protease inhibitors

*Protease inhibitors* are drugs that act against the enzyme HIV protease, preventing it from dividing a larger viral precursor protein into the active smaller enzymes that the HIV virus needs to fully mature. The result is an immature, noninfectious cell. Drugs in this group include:

• amprenavir
• atazanavir
• darunavir
• fosamprenavir
• indinavir sulfate
• lopinavir and ritonavir
• nelfinavir mesylate
• ritonavir
• saquinavir mesylate
• tipranavir.

## Pharmacokinetics

Protease inhibitors may have different pharmacokinetic properties.

### Active and inactive

Amprenavir is metabolized in the liver to active and inactive metabolites and is minimally excreted in urine and stool.

Atazanavir is rapidly absorbed and is metabolized in the liver by the CYP3A. The drug is excreted mainly through stool and urine.

Darunavir is well absorbed when taken with food and highly protein-bound. It's metabolized in the liver and excreted in stool.

Fosamprenavir is well absorbed and highly protein-bound. It's rapidly metabolized by CYP3A4 and it is unknown how it is excreted.

*Warning!*

## Adverse reactions to tenofovir

Adverse reactions to the nucleotide analogue reverse transcriptase inhibitor tenofovir include:

• nausea and vomiting
• diarrhea
• anorexia
• abdominal pain
• severe hepatomegaly (enlargement of the liver)
• lactic acidosis (increased lactic acid production in the blood).

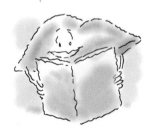

Says here I do a lot of absorbing and metabolizing. Hmmm. No wonder I'm tired by the end of the day!

## P-450 at it again

Lopinavir is extensively metabolized by the liver's cytochrome P-450 system; ritonavir acts as an inhibitor of lopinavir. This combination drug's antiviral activity is due to lopinavir.

## Availability unknown

Nelfinavir's bioavailability (the degree to which it becomes available to target tissue after administration) isn't determined. Food increases its absorption. It's highly protein-bound, metabolized in the liver, and excreted primarily in stool.

## Broken into five...

Ritonavir is well absorbed, metabolized by the liver, and broken down into at least five metabolites. It's mainly excreted in stool, with some elimination through the kidneys.

## ...and seven

Indinavir sulfate is rapidly absorbed and moderately bound to plasma proteins. It's metabolized by the liver into seven metabolites. The drug is excreted mainly in stool.

## Highly bound

Saquinavir mesylate is poorly absorbed from the GI tract. It's widely distributed, highly bound to plasma proteins, metabolized by the liver, and excreted mainly by the kidneys.

Tipranavir has limited absorption, but its bioavailability increases when it's taken with a high-fat meal. It's metabolized by the chromosome P-450 and excreted mostly unchanged in stool.

## Pharmacodynamics

All of these drugs inhibit the activity of HIV protease and prevent the cleavage of viral polyproteins.

## Pharmacotherapeutics

Protease inhibitors are used in combination with other antiretroviral agents for the treatment of HIV infection.

## Drug interactions

Protease inhibitors may interact with many drugs. Here are some common interactions.
• The action of saquinavir may be reduced by phenobarbital, phenytoin, dexamethasone, and carbamazepine.

## Blockers beware!

• Ritonavir may increase the effects of alpha-adrenergic blockers, antiarrhythmics, antidepressants, antiemetics, antifungals, antilipemics, antimalarials, antineoplastics, beta-adrenergic blockers, calcium channel blockers, cimetidine, corticosteroids, erythromycin, immunosuppressants, methylphenidate, pentoxifylline, phenothiazines, and warfarin.
• Indinavir sulfate inhibits the metabolism of midazolam and triazolam, increasing the risk of potentially fatal events such as cardiac arrhythmias.
• Didanosine decreases gastric absorption of indinavir sulfate; these drugs should be administered at least 1 hour apart.
• Rifampin markedly reduces plasma levels of most protease inhibitors, including atazanavir.
• Nelfinavir may greatly increase plasma levels of amiodarone, ergot derivatives, midazolam, rifabutin, quinidine, and triazolam.
• Lopinavir and ritonavir are used in combination because of their positive effects on HIV RNA levels and CD4 counts. When given together, ritonavir inhibits the metabolism of lopinavir, leading to increased plasma lopinavir levels.
• Carbamazepine, phenobarbital, and phenytoin may reduce the effectiveness of nelfinavir.
• Protease inhibitors may increase sildenafil levels, resulting in sildenafil-associated adverse reactions, including hypotension, vision changes, and priapism.
• Atazanavir shouldn't be given with drugs also metabolized by the CYPA3A pathway, such as HMG-CoA reductase inhibitors (including lovastatin, simvastatin, and atorvastatin). Concurrent use may increase the risk of myopathy and rhabdomyolysis.

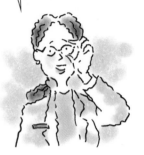

Adverse reactions to protease inhibitors include vision changes.

## Interval issues

• Drugs that prolong the PR interval, such as calcium channel blockers (including diltiazem) and beta-adrenergic blockers (including atenolol), should be used cautiously with atazanavir because atazanavir may also prolong the PR interval.
• Atazanavir shouldn't be given with benzodiazepines, such as midazolam and triazolam, because of the potential for increased sedation or respiratory depression.
• Atazanavir shouldn't be given with ergot derivatives, such as ergotamine and dihydroergotamine, because of the potential for life-threatening ergot toxicity resulting in peripheral vasospasm and ischemia of the extremities.
• St. John's wort may reduce plasma levels of atazanavir and darunavir.
• Tipranavir and sulfonyureas administered together may result in hypoglycemia.

**Warning!**

## Adverse reactions to protease inhibitors

These common adverse reactions occur with protease inhibitors:

- abdominal discomfort
- abdominal pain
- acid regurgitation
- anorexia
- back pain
- deep vein thrombosis
- depression
- diarrhea
- dizziness
- dry mouth
- encephalopathy
- fatigue
- flank pain
- headache

- hemorrhagic colitis
- hypercholesterolemia
- hyperglycemia
- hypertriglyceridemia
- insomnia
- leukopenia
- muscle weakness
- nausea and vomiting
- neutropenia
- pancreatitis
- paresthesis
- rash
- Stevens-Johnson syndrome
- taste perversion

- Indinavir and ritonavir may increase plasma nelfinavir levels. (See *Adverse reactions to protease inhibitors.*)

# Antitubercular drugs

*Antitubercular drugs* are used to treat tuberculosis (TB), which is caused by *Mycobacterium tuberculosis.* Not always curative, these drugs can halt the progression of a mycobacterial infection.

## Myco-versatility

These drugs also are effective against less common mycobacterial infections caused by *M. kansasii, M. avium-intracellulare, M. fortuitum,* and related organisms.

## Time consuming

Unlike most antibiotics, antitubercular drugs may need to be administered over many months. This creates problems, such as patient noncompliance, the development of bacterial resistance, and drug toxicity. (See *Directly observable therapy for TB*, page 276.)

*Yea or nay?*

## Directly observable therapy for TB

Among infectious diseases, tuberculosis (TB) remains a frequent killer worldwide. What makes treatment difficult is that it requires long-term medical therapy—typically for as long as 6 to 9 months. The long treatment period commonly creates problems with patient compliance (an inability or unwillingness to follow a treatment plan), and poor compliance contributes to reactivation of the disease and the development of drug-resistant TB.

**DOT on the spot**
Directly observable therapy (DOT) was developed to combat these treatment issues. DOT requires that a health care worker observe a patient take every dose of medication for the duration of therapy. A controversy exists over whether every individual with TB should be observed (universal DOT) or whether only the patient at risk for poor compliance should be observed (selective DOT).

**Who fails to comply?**
The patient at risk for poor compliance includes one with a history of poor compliance or drug or alcohol abuse, mental illness, homelessness, incarceration, or residence in a homeless shelter. Some areas, such as Mississippi and New York City, practice universal DOT; other areas, including Massachusetts, first evaluate a patient's ability and willingness to comply.

# Drug regimens for treating TB

Traditionally, isoniazid, rifampin, and ethambutol were the mainstays of multidrug TB therapy and successfully prevented the emergence of drug resistance.

## A new regimen to combat resistance

Because of the current incidence of drug-resistant TB strains, a four-drug regimen is now recommended for initial treatment:

 isoniazid

 rifampin

 pyrazinamide

 streptomycin or ethambutol.

## One regimen may succeed another

The antitubercular regimen should be modified if local testing shows resistance to one or more of these drugs. If local outbreaks of TB resistant to isoniazid and rifampin are occurring in facilities (for example, health care or correctional facilities), then five- or

## Other antitubercular drugs

Several other drugs are used as antitubercular drugs in combination with first-line drugs. Because these drugs have a greater incidence of toxicity, they're used primarily for the patient who's resistant or allergic to less toxic drugs.

### Fluoroquinolones

Fluoroquinolones, such as ciprofloxacin and ofloxacin, are effective against *Mycobacterium tuberculosis*. Of these two drugs, ofloxacin is more potent and may be an initial choice in retreatment. These drugs are administered orally and are generally well tolerated. GI adverse reactions are most commonly reported. However, resistance to fluoroquinolones develops rapidly when these drugs are used alone or in insufficient doses.

### Streptomycin

Streptomycin was the first drug recognized as effective in treating tuberculosis. Streptomycin is administered I.M. only. It appears to enhance the activity of oral antitubercular drugs and is of greatest value in the early weeks to months of therapy. However, I.M. administration limits its usefulness in long-term therapy. Rapidly absorbed from the I.M. injection site, streptomycin is excreted primarily by the kidneys as unchanged drug. Most patients tolerate streptomycin well, but those receiving large doses may exhibit eighth cranial nerve toxicity (ototoxicity).

six-drug regimens are recommended as initial therapy. (See *Other antitubercular drugs.*)

## Pharmacokinetics

Most antitubercular drugs are administered orally. When administered orally, these drugs are well absorbed from the GI tract and widely distributed throughout the body. They're metabolized primarily in the liver and excreted by the kidneys.

## Pharmacodynamics

Antitubercular drugs are specific for mycobacteria. At usual doses, ethambutol and isoniazid are tuberculostatic, meaning that they inhibit the growth of *M. tuberculosis.* In contrast, rifampin is tuberculocidal, meaning that it destroys the mycobacteria. Because bacterial resistance to isoniazid and rifampin can develop rapidly, they should always be used with other antitubercular drugs.

### Antireplication station

The exact mechanism of action of ethambutol remains unclear, but it may be related to inhibition of cell metabolism, arrest of multiplication, and cell death. Ethambutol acts only against replicating bacteria.

## Breaking down walls

Although isoniazid's exact mechanism of action isn't known, the drug is believed to inhibit the synthesis of mycolic acids, important components of the mycobacterium cell wall. This inhibition disrupts the cell wall. Only replicating, not resting, bacteria appear to be inhibited.

## Synthesis stopper

Rifampin inhibits RNA synthesis in susceptible organisms. The drug is effective primarily in replicating bacteria, but may have some effect on resting bacteria as well.

## Acid based

The exact mechanism of action of pyrazinamide isn't known, but the antimycobacterial activity appears to be linked to the drug's conversion to the active metabolite pyrazinoic acid. Pyrazinoic acid, in turn, creates an acidic environment where mycobacteria can't replicate.

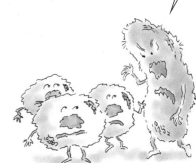

Bring it on! It can take as many as five or six drugs to wipe me out, so you cells are no problem!

# Pharmacotherapeutics

Isoniazid usually is used with ethambutol, rifampin, or pyrazinamide. This is because combination therapy for TB and other mycobacterial infections can prevent or delay the development of resistance.

## In uncomplicated cases

Ethambutol is used with isoniazid and rifampin to treat the patient with uncomplicated pulmonary TB. It's also used to treat infections resulting from *M. bovis* and most strains of *M. kansasii.*

## Isolating isoniazid

Although isoniazid is the most important drug for treating TB, bacterial resistance develops rapidly if it's used alone. However, resistance doesn't pose a problem when isoniazid is used alone to prevent TB in the patient who has been exposed to the disease, and no evidence exists of cross-resistance between isoniazid and other antitubercular drugs. Isoniazid is typically given orally, but may be given intravenously, if necessary.

## Pulmonary power

Rifampin is a first-line drug for treating pulmonary TB with other antitubercular drugs. It combats many gram-positive and some gram-negative bacteria, but is seldom used for nonmycobacterial infections because bacterial resistance develops rapidly. It's used to treat asymptomatic carriers of *Neisseria meningitidis* when the risk of meningitis is high, but it isn't used to treat *N. meningi-*

**Warning!**

# Adverse reactions to antitubercular drugs

Here are common adverse reactions to antitubercular drugs.

**Ethambutol**
Itching, joint pain, GI distress, malaise, leukopenia, headache, dizziness, numbness and tingling of the extremities, optic neuritis, and confusion may occur.

Although rare, hypersensitivity reactions to ethambutol may produce rash and fever. Anaphylaxis may also occur.

**Isoniazid**
Peripheral neuropathy is the most common adverse reaction. Severe and occasionally fatal hepatitis associated with isoniazid may occur even many months after treatment has

stopped. The patient must be monitored carefully.

**Rifampin**
The most common adverse reactions include epigastric pain, nausea, vomiting, abdominal cramps, flatulence, anorexia, and diarrhea.

**Pyrazinamide**
Liver toxicity is the major limiting adverse reaction. GI disturbances include nausea, vomiting, hyperuricemia, arthralgia, and anorexia.

*tidis* infections because of the potential for bacterial resistance.

## On the TB front

Pyrazinamide is currently recommended as a first-line TB drug in combination with ethambutol, rifampin, *and* isoniazid. Pyrazinamide is a highly specific drug that's active only against *M. tuberculosis.* Resistance to pyrazinamide may develop rapidly when it's used alone.

## Drug interactions

Antitubercular drugs may interact with many other drugs. (See *Adverse reactions to antitubercular drugs.*)
• Cycloserine and ethionamide may produce additive CNS effects, such as drowsiness, dizziness, headache, lethargy, depression, tremor, anxiety, confusion, and tinnitus (ringing in the ears), when administered with isoniazid.
• Isoniazid may increase levels of phenytoin, carbamazepine, diazepam, ethosuximide, primidone, theophylline, and warfarin.
• When corticosteroids and isoniazid are taken together, the effectiveness of isoniazid is reduced while the effects of corticosteroids are increased.

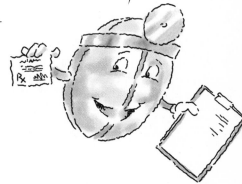

Rifampin is your first-line defense against pulmonary TB.

• Isoniazid may reduce the plasma levels of ketoconazole, itraconazole, and oral antidiabetic agents.
• Oral contraceptives and rifampin taken together may decrease the effectiveness of the oral contraceptive.
• When given together, rifampin, isoniazid, ethionamide, and pyrazinamide increase the risk of hepatotoxicity.
• Pyrazinamide combined with phenytoin may increase phenytoin levels.

# Antimycotic drugs

*Antimycotic*, or *antifungal*, *drugs* are used to treat fungal infections. The major antifungal drug groups include:
• polyenes
• fluorinated pyrimidine
• imidazole
• synthetic triazoles
• glucan synthesis inhibitors
• synthetic allylamine derivatives. (See *Other antimycotic drugs.*)

# Polyenes

The polyenes include *amphotericin B* and *nystatin*. Amphotericin B's potency has made it the most widely used antimycotic drug for severe systemic fungal infections. It's available in several forms, including lipid-based preparations that may decrease renal or systemic toxicity. Nystatin is used only topically or orally to treat local fungal infections because it's extremely toxic when administered parenterally.

## Pharmacokinetics

After I.V. administration, amphotericin B is distributed throughout the body and excreted by the kidneys. Its metabolism isn't well defined.

Oral nystatin undergoes little or no absorption, distribution, or metabolism. It's excreted unchanged in stool. Topical nystatin isn't absorbed through the skin or mucous membranes.

## Pharmacodynamics

Amphotericin B works by binding to sterol (a lipid) in the fungal cell membrane, altering cell permeability (ability to allow a sub-

## Other antimycotic drugs

Several other antimycotic drugs offer alternative forms of treatment for topical fungal infections.

### Clotrimazole

An imidazole derivative, clotrimazole is used:
• topically to treat dermatophyte and *Candida albicans* infections
• orally to treat oral candidiasis
• vaginally to treat vaginal candidiasis.

### Griseofulvin

Griseofulvin is used to treat fungal infections of the:
• skin (tinea corporis)
• feet (tinea pedis)
• groin (tinea cruris)
• beard area of the face and neck (tinea barbae)
• nails (tinea unguium)
• scalp (tinea capitis).

#### *Long-term treatment*

To prevent a relapse, griseofulvin therapy must continue until the fungus is eradicated and the infected skin or nails are replaced.

### Miconazole

Available as miconazole or miconazole nitrate, this imidazole derivative is used to treat local fungal infections, such as vaginal and vulvar candidiasis, and topical fungal infections such as chronic candidiasis of the skin and mucous membranes.

#### *Delivery options*

Miconazole may be administered:
• I.V. or intrathecally (into the subarachnoid space) to treat fungal meningitis
• I.V. or by bladder irrigation to treat fungal bladder infections
• locally to treat vaginal infections
• topically to treat topical infections.

### Other topical antimycotic drugs

Ciclopirox olamine, econazole nitrate, haloprogin, butoconazole nitrate, naftifine, tioconazole, terconazole, tolnaftate, butenafine, terbinafine, sulconazole, oxiconazole, clioquinol, triacetin, and undecylenic acid are available only as topical drugs.

stance to pass through) and allowing intracellular components to leak out.

## A license to kill

Amphotericin B usually acts as a fungistatic drug (inhibiting fungal growth and multiplication), but can become fungicidal (destroying fungi) if it reaches high concentrations in the fungi.

Nystatin binds to sterols in fungal cell membranes and alters the permeability of the membranes, leading to loss of cell components. Nystatin can act as a fungicidal or fungistatic drug, depending on the organism present.

## Pharmacotherapeutics

Amphotericin B usually is administered to treat severe systemic fungal infections and meningitis caused by fungi sensitive to the drug. It's never used for noninvasive forms of fungal disease because it's highly toxic. It's usually the drug of choice for severe infections caused by *Candida, Paracoccidioides brasiliensis, Blastomyces dermatitidis, Coccidioides immitis, Cryptococcus neo-*

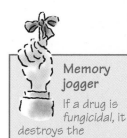

**Memory jogger**

If a drug is fungicidal, it destroys the fungus—*cidus* is a Latin term for "killing." If it's fungistatic, it prevents fungal growth and multiplication—*stasis* is a Greek term for "halting."

*formans*, and *Sporothrix schenckii*. It's also effective against *Aspergillus fumigatus*, *Microsporum audouinii*, *Rhizopus*, *Candida glabrata*, *Trichophyton*, and *Rhodotorula*.

## Last-ditch effort

Because amphotericin B is highly toxic, its use is limited to the patient who has a definitive diagnosis of life-threatening infection and is under close medical supervision.

## Topical concerns

Nystatin is used primarily to treat candidal skin infections. Different forms of nystatin are available for treating different types of candidal infections. Topical nystatin is used to treat candidal skin or mucous membrane infections, such as oral thrush, diaper rash, vaginal and vulvar candidiasis, and candidiasis between skin folds.

## Oral history

Oral nystatin is used to treat GI infections.

## Drug interactions

Nystatin doesn't interact significantly with other drugs, but amphotericin B may have significant interactions with many drugs.
• Because of the synergistic effects between flucytosine and amphotericin B, these two drugs commonly are combined in therapy for candidal or cryptococcal infections, especially for cryptococcal meningitis.
• The risk of kidney toxicity increases when amphotericin B is taken with aminoglycosides, cyclosporine, or acyclovir.
• Corticosteroids, extended-spectrum penicillins, and digoxin may worsen the hypokalemia (low blood potassium levels) produced by amphotericin B, possibly leading to heart problems. Moreover, the risk of digoxin toxicity is increased.
• Amphotericin B plus nondepolarizing skeletal muscle relaxants (such as pancuronium bromide) increase muscle relaxation.
• Electrolyte solutions may inactivate amphotericin B when diluted in the same solution. Amphotericin B preparations must be mixed with dextrose 5% in water; they can't be mixed with saline solution.
• Magnesium and potassium levels and kidney function must be monitored frequently in patients receiving amphotericin. (See *Adverse reactions to amphotericin B* and *Adverse reactions to nystatin*.)

**Warning!**

## Adverse reactions to nystatin

Reactions to nystatin seldom occur, but high dosages may produce:
• diarrhea
• nausea and vomiting
• abdominal pain
• a bitter taste.

**It can get under your skin**
Topical nystatin may also cause skin irritation, and a hypersensitivity reaction may occur with oral or topical administration.

### Warning!

## Adverse reactions to amphotericin B

Almost all patients receiving I.V. amphotericin B, particularly at the beginning of low-dose therapy, experience:
- chills
- fever
- nausea and vomiting
- anorexia
- muscle and joint pain
- indigestion.

**Anemia**

Most patients also develop normochromic (adequate hemoglobin in each red blood cell [RBC]) or normocytic anemia (too few RBCs) that significantly decreases the hematocrit. Hypomagnesemia and hypokalemia may occur, causing electrocardiographic changes and requiring replacement electrolyte therapy.

**Kidney concerns**

Up to 80% of patients may develop some degree of kidney toxicity, causing the kidneys to lose their ability to concentrate urine.

# Flucytosine

*Flucytosine* is the only antimetabolite (a substance that closely resembles one required for normal physiologic functioning and that exerts its effect by interfering with metabolism) that acts as an antimycotic. It's a purine and pyrimidine inhibitor that's used primarily with another antimycotic drug, such as amphotericin B, to treat systemic fungal infections.

## Pharmacokinetics

After oral administration, flucytosine is well absorbed from the GI tract and widely distributed. It undergoes little metabolism and is excreted primarily by the kidneys.

## Pharmacodynamics

Flucytosine penetrates fungal cells, where it's converted to its active metabolite fluorouracil. Fluorouracil then is incorporated into the RNA of the fungal cells, altering their protein synthesis and causing cell death.

## Pharmacotherapeutics

Although amphotericin B is effective in treating candidal and cryptococcal meningitis alone, flucytosine is given with it to reduce the dosage and the risk of toxicity. This combination therapy is the treatment of choice for cryptococcal meningitis.

## Standing alone

Flucytosine can be used alone to treat candidal infections of the lower urinary tract because it reaches a high urinary concentration. It's also effective in treating infections caused by *T. glabrata*, *Phialophora*, *Aspergillus*, and *Cladosporium*.

### Drug interactions

Cytarabine may antagonize the antifungal activity of flucytosine, possibly by competitive inhibition. Hematologic, kidney, and liver function must be closely monitored during flucytosine therapy because of the drug's serious risk of toxicity. (See *Adverse reactions to flucytosine*.)

# Imidazole

*Ketoconazole*, the most commonly used imidazole, is an effective oral antimycotic drug with a broad spectrum of activity.

## Pharmacokinetics

When given orally, ketoconazole is absorbed variably and distributed widely. It undergoes extensive liver metabolism and is excreted through bile and stool.

## Pharmacodynamics

Within the fungal cells, ketoconazole interferes with sterol synthesis, damaging the cell membrane and increasing its permeability. This leads to a loss of essential intracellular elements and inhibition of cell growth.

## Can inhibit or kill

Ketoconazole usually produces fungistatic effects, but can also produce fungicidal effects under certain conditions.

## Pharmacotherapeutics

Ketoconazole is used to treat topical and systemic infections caused by susceptible fungi, which include dermatophytes and most other fungi.

## Drug interactions

Ketoconazole may have significant interactions with other drugs.

**Warning!**

## Adverse reactions to flucytosine

Flucytosine may produce unpredictable adverse reactions, including:
• confusion
• headache
• drowsiness
• vertigo
• hallucinations
• difficulty breathing
• respiratory arrest
• rash
• nausea and vomiting
• abdominal distention
• diarrhea
• anorexia.

• Ketoconazole used with drugs that decrease gastric acidity, such as cimetidine, ranitidine, famotidine, nizatidine, antacids, and anticholinergic drugs, may decrease absorption of ketoconazole and reduce its antimycotic effects. If the patient must take these drugs, delay administration of ketoconazole by at least 2 hours.

• Taking ketoconazole with phenytoin may alter metabolism and increase blood levels of both drugs.

• When taken with theophylline, ketoconazole may decrease the serum theophylline level.

• Using ketoconazole with other liver-toxic drugs may increase the risk of liver disease.

• Combined with cyclosporine therapy, ketoconazole may increase cyclosporine and serum creatinine levels.

• Ketoconazole increases the effect of oral anticoagulants and can cause hemorrhage.

• Ketoconazole can inhibit the metabolism (and possibly increase levels) of quinidine, sulfonylureas, carbamazepine, and protease inhibitors.

• Ketoconazole shouldn't be given with rifampin because serum ketoconazole levels may decrease. (See *Adverse reactions to ketoconazole.*)

# Synthetic triazoles

The synthetic triazoles include:
• fluconazole
• itraconazole
• voriconazole.

*Fluconazole* belongs to a class of synthetic, broad-spectrum triazoles and is also referred to as a *bistriazole antimycotic drug.*

*Itraconazole* and *voriconazole* also belong to the synthetic triazole class of drugs. They inhibit the synthesis of ergosterol, a vital component of fungal cell membranes.

## Pharmacokinetics

After oral administration, fluconazole is about 90% absorbed. It's distributed into all body fluids, and more than 80% of the drug is excreted unchanged in urine.

Oral bioavailability is greatest when itraconazole is taken with food; voriconazole is more effective if taken 1 hour before or after a meal.

**Warning!**

## Adverse reactions to ketoconazole

The most common adverse reactions to ketoconazole are nausea and vomiting. Less frequent reactions include:
• anaphylaxis
• joint pain
• chills
• fever
• ringing in the ears
• impotence
• photophobia.

**Toxic topics**
Liver toxicity is rare and reversible when the drug is stopped.

## Bound and determined

Itraconazole and voriconazole are bound to plasma proteins and extensively metabolized in the liver into a large number of metabolites. They're minimally excreted in stool.

### Pharmacodynamics

Fluconazole inhibits fungal cytochrome P-450, an enzyme responsible for fungal sterol synthesis, causing fungal cell walls to weaken.

Itraconazole and voriconazole interfere with fungal cell-wall synthesis by inhibiting the formation of ergosterol and increasing cell-wall permeability, making the fungus susceptible to osmotic instability.

### Pharmacotherapeutics

Fluconazole is used to treat mouth, throat, and esophageal candidiasis and serious systemic candidal infections, including UTIs, peritonitis, and pneumonia. It's also used to treat cryptococcal meningitis.

## Osis, smosis

Itraconazole is used to treat blastomycosis, nonmeningeal histoplasmosis, candidiasis, aspergillosis, and fungal nail disease. Voriconazole is used to treat invasive aspergillosis and serious fungal infections caused by *Scedosporium apiospermum* and *Fusarium* species.

### Drug interactions

Fluconazole may have interactions with other drugs:
• Using fluconazole with warfarin may increase the risk of bleeding.
• It may increase levels of phenytoin and cyclosporine.
• It may increase the plasma levels of oral antidiabetic drugs, such as glyburide, tolbutamide, and glipizide, increasing the risk of hypoglycemia.
• Rifampin and cimetidine enhance the metabolism of fluconazole, reducing its plasma level.
• Fluconazole may increase the activity of zidovudine. (See *Adverse reactions to synthetic triazoles.*)

Itraconazole and voriconazole may have these interactions:
• Both may increase the risk of bleeding when combined with oral anticoagulants.
• Antacids, $H_2$-receptor antagonists, phenytoin, and rifampin lower plasma itraconazole levels.

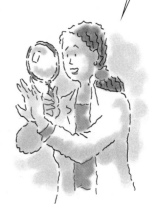

Itraconazole treats fungal nail disease. Hmm...might be time for a manicure.

**Warning!**

## Adverse reactions to synthetic triazoles

Adverse reactions to fluconazole include:
- abdominal pain
- diarrhea
- dizziness
- headache
- elevated liver enzyme levels
- nausea and vomiting
- rash.

Adverse reactions to itraconazole include:
- dizziness
- headache
- hypertension
- impaired liver function
- nausea.

Adverse reactions to voriconazole include:
- vision disturbances
- fever
- chills
- headache
- tachycardia
- nausea and vomiting
- rash
- elevated liver enzyme.

- Voriconazole may inhibit the metabolism of phenytoin, benzodiazepines, calcium channel blockers, sulfonylureas, and tacrolimus.
- Voriconazole is contraindicated with sirolimus and ergot alkaloids because voriconazole may increase plasma levels of sirolimus and ergots.
- Voriconazole is contraindicated with quinidine and pimozide because of the risk of prolonged QT interval and, rarely, torsades de pointes.

# Glucan synthesis inhibitors

*Caspofungin* is a drug in a new class of agents known as *glucan synthesis inhibitors* (also called *echinocandins*). Its major use is in the patient who hasn't responded to other antifungal therapies, such as amphotericin B or itraconazole.

## Pharmacokinetics

After being given intravenously, caspofungin is highly protein-bound, with little distribution into RBCs. The drug is slowly metabolized and is excreted in urine and stool.

## Pharmacodynamics

Caspofungin inhibits the synthesis of beta (1,3) *D*-glucan, an integral component of the fungal cell wall.

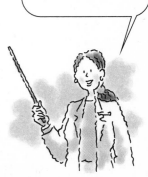

Caspofungin is used to treat invasive aspergillosis in the patient who hasn't responded to, or can't tolerate, other antifungals.

## Pharmacotherapeutics

Caspofungin is used to treat invasive aspergillosis in the patient who hasn't responded to, or can't tolerate, other antifungals. It hasn't been studied as an initial treatment for invasive aspergillosis.

## Drug interactions

• Patients taking caspofungin and tacrolimus may need higher doses of tacrolimus because caspofungin decreases the blood tacrolimus level.
• Inducers of drug clearance, such as phenytoin, carbamazepine, efavirenz, nevirapine, and nelfinavir, may lower caspofungin clearance.
• Concurrent use of caspofungin and cyclosporine may result in elevated liver enzyme levels and decreased caspofungin clearance, so use together isn't recommended. (See *Adverse reactions to caspofungin.*)

**Warning!**

## Adverse reactions to caspofungin

Adverse reactions to caspofungin include:
• paresthesia (burning or prickling sensation)
• tachycardia (excessively rapid heart beat)
• tachypnea (excessively rapid breathing)
• nausea and vomiting
• diarrhea
• rash
• facial swelling.

# Synthetic allylamine derivatives

*Terbinafine*, the most commonly used synthetic allylamine derivative, is an allylamine antifungal, which inhibits fungal cell growth by inhibiting an enzyme responsible for the manufacture of ergosterol.

## Pharmacokinetics

Terbinafine is well absorbed and distributed throughout the body, especially if taken with food. It's extensively metabolized; more than two-thirds of the drug is excreted in urine.

## Risk to liver

Rare cases of liver failure have occurred with terbinafine use, even in the patient with no known history of liver disease. Avoid using this drug if liver disease is suspected, and obtain baseline liver enzyme test results before use.

## Pharmacodynamics

Terbinafine is thought to inhibit squalene epoxidase, which blocks the biosynthesis of ergosterol, an essential component of fungal cell membranes.

### Pharmacotherapeutics

This drug is used to treat tinea unguium (fungal infections of the fingernail or toenail).

### Drug interactions

• Terbinafine clearance is decreased when it's taken with cimetidine and increased when it's taken with rifampin.
• Terbinafine increases plasma levels of caffeine and dextromethorphan and decreases levels of cyclosporine. (See *Adverse reactions to terbinafine.*)

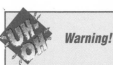

# Recombinant human activated protein C

Recombinant human activated protein C (rhAPC) is a relatively new class of drug possessing antithrombotic, anti-inflammatory, and fibrinolytic properties. Although its mechanism of action isn't well known, rhACP is used to treat patients with severe sepsis when the risk of death from acute organ dysfunction is extremely high.

## Drotrecogin alfa

*Drotrecogin alfa*, the first FDA-approved rhACP drug, is used to treat severe sepsis in adult patients with acute organ dysfunction when they are at risk for death.

### Pharmacokinetics

After I.V. infusion, drotrecogin alfa achieves a median steady state level in 2 hours. Information about its distribution, metabolism, and excretion isn't available.

### Pharmacodynamics

Although drotrecogin alfa's anti-infective action isn't known, it may work by producing dose-dependent reductions in D-dimer and interleukin-6. Activated protein C exerts an antithrombotic effect by inhibiting factors Va and VIIIa.

*Safe and sound*

## Contraindications for drotrecogin alfa

This drug is contraindicated in patients who are hypersensitive to the drug or any of its components. It's also contraindicated in patients with active internal bleeding and those who have had hemorrhagic stroke in the past 3 months or intracranial or intraspinal surgery in the past 2 months. In addition, the drug is contraindicated in patients with severe head trauma, trauma with increased risk of life-threatening bleeding, an epidural catheter, an intracranial neoplasm or mass lesion, or cerebral herniation.

*Warning!*

## Adverse reactions to drotrecogin alfa

The most common adverse reaction to drotrecogin alfa is bleeding. Bleeding seen with this drug most often occurs as ecchymosis or GI bleeding.

## Pharmacotherapeutics

Drotrecogin alfa is used to treat adults who have severe sepsis associated with acute organ dysfunction and who have a high risk of death. The drug has antithrombotic, anti-inflammatory, and fibrinolytic properties.

## Drug interactions

Drotrecogin alfa may interact with another drug that affects hemostasis, such as an anticoagulant, antiplatelet drug, or thrombolytic, possibly increasing the risk of bleeding. (See *Adverse reactions to drotrecogin alfa* and *Contraindications for drotrecogin alfa*.)

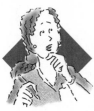

# Quick quiz

**1.** Which rationale best justifies administering different antitubercular drugs concurrently in treating active tuberculosis?

 A. They're second-line drugs and effective only together.
 B. Rifampin increases the activity of isoniazid.
 C. Combination therapy can prevent or delay bacterial resistance.
 D. Single therapy isn't effective.

*Answer:* C. Combination therapy can prevent or delay bacterial resistance to antitubercular drugs.

**2.** Which adverse reaction do most patients experience when receiving I.V. amphotericin B?

 A. Anuria
 B. Coagulation defects
 C. Shortness of breath
 D. Normochromic or normocytic anemia

*Answer:* D. Normochromic or normocytic anemia is a common adverse effect of I.V. amphotericin B.

**3.** What's the I.V. drug of choice for serious resistant staphylococcal infections in the patient who's allergic to penicillin?

 A. Vancomycin
 B. Erythromycin
 C. Azithromycin
 D. Streptomycin

*Answer:* A. Vancomycin is the I.V. drug of choice for methicillin-resistant *S. aureus* infections.

## Scoring

☆☆☆  If you answered all three items correctly, extraordinary! You're more than a match for unwanted microbes!

☆☆  If you answered two items correctly, congratulations. You're winning the battle against bacteria.

☆  If you answered fewer than two items correctly, dig in! The war with drugs continues for five more chapters!

# Anti-inflammatory, anti-allergy, and immunosuppressant drugs

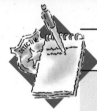

## Just the facts

In this chapter, you'll learn:

♦ classes of drugs that modify immune or inflammatory responses

♦ uses and varying actions of these drugs

♦ how these drugs are absorbed, distributed, metabolized, and excreted

♦ drug interactions and adverse reactions to these drugs.

## Drugs and the immune system

Immune and inflammatory responses protect the body from invading foreign substances. These responses can be modified by certain classes of drugs:

• Antihistamines block the effects of histamine on target tissues.

• Corticosteroids suppress immune responses and reduce inflammation.

• Noncorticosteroid immunosuppressants prevent rejection of transplanted organs and can be used to treat auto immune disease.

• Uricosurics prevent or control the frequency of gouty arthritis attacks.

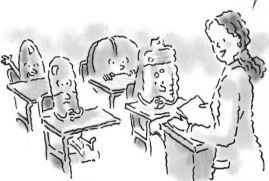

Quiet down, class! Today's lesson includes information about drug classes that can modify responses.

# Antihistamines

*Antihistamines* primarily act to block histamine effects that occur in an immediate (type I) hypersensitivity reaction, commonly called an *allergic reaction*. They're available alone or in combination products by prescription or over-the-counter.

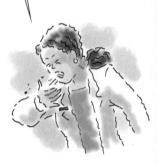

Antihistamines relieve symptoms of an allergy; however, they don't give the body immunity to the allergen itself.

## Histamine-1 receptor antagonists

The term *antihistamine* refers to drugs that act as histamine-1 ($H_1$) receptor antagonists; that is, they compete with histamine for binding to $H_1$-receptor sites throughout the body. However, they don't displace histamine already bound to the receptor.

### It's all about chemistry

Based on chemical structure, antihistamines are categorized into five major classes:
• Ethanolamines include clemastine fumarate, dimenhydrinate, and diphenhydramine hydrochloride.
• Alkylamines include brompheniramine maleate, chlorpheniramine maleate, and dexchlorpheniramine maleate.
• Phenothiazines include promethazine hydrochloride.
• Piperidines include azatadine maleate, cetirizine hydrochloride, cyproheptadine hydrochloride, desloratadine, fexofenadine hydrochloride, loratadine, and meclizine hydrochloride.
• Miscellaneous drugs, such as hydroxyzine hydrochloride and hydroxyzine pamoate, also act as antihistamines.

### Pharmacokinetics (how drugs circulate)

$H_1$-receptor antagonists are well absorbed after oral or parenteral administration. Some can also be given rectally.

#### Distribution

With the exception of loratadine and desloratadine, antihistamines are distributed widely throughout the body and central nervous system (CNS).

### Less penetration, fewer effects

Fexofenadine, desloratadine, and loratadine, which are nonsedating antihistamines, minimally penetrate the blood-brain barrier so that little of the drug is distributed in the CNS, producing fewer effects there than other antihistamines.

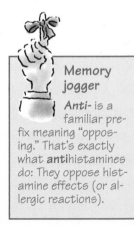

**Memory jogger**

*Anti-* is a familiar prefix meaning "opposing." That's exactly what **anti**histamines do: They oppose histamine effects (or allergic reactions).

### *Metabolism and excretion*

Antihistamines are metabolized by liver enzymes and excreted in urine; small amounts appear in breast milk. Fexofenadine, mainly excreted in stool, is an exception. Cetirizine undergoes limited hepatic metabolism.

## Pharmacodynamics (how drugs act)

$H_1$-receptor antagonists compete with histamine for $H_1$ receptors on effector cells (the cells that cause allergic symptoms), blocking histamine from producing its effects. (See *How chlorpheniramine stops an allergic response*, page 296.)

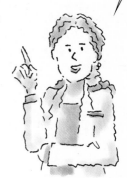

Keep in mind that although histamine binding is blocked, the overall release of histamine continues.

### Antagonizing tactics

$H_1$-receptor antagonists produce their effects by:
- blocking the action of histamine on the small blood vessels
- decreasing dilation of arterioles and engorgement of tissues
- reducing the leakage of plasma proteins and fluids out of the capillaries (capillary permeability), thereby lessening edema
- inhibiting most smooth-muscle responses to histamine (in particular, blocking the constriction of bronchial, GI, and vascular smooth muscle)
- relieving symptoms by acting on the terminal nerve endings in the skin that flare and itch when stimulated by histamine
- suppressing adrenal medulla stimulation, autonomic ganglia stimulation, and exocrine gland secretion, such as lacrimal and salivary secretion.

### Straight to the head

Several antihistamines have a high affinity for $H_1$ receptors in the brain and are used for their CNS effects. These drugs include diphenhydramine, dimenhydrinate, promethazine, and various piperidine derivatives.

### No stomach for this

$H_1$-receptor antagonists don't affect parietal cell secretion in the stomach because their receptors are $H_2$ receptors, not $H_1$.

## Pharmacotherapeutics (how drugs are used)

Antihistamines are used to treat the symptoms of type I hypersensitivity reactions, such as:
- allergic rhinitis (runny nose and itchy eyes caused by a local sensitivity reaction)
- vasomotor rhinitis (rhinitis not caused by allergy or infection)
- allergic conjunctivitis (inflammation of the membranes of the eye)

*Now I get it!*

# How chlorpheniramine stops an allergic response

Although chlorpheniramine can't reverse symptoms of an allergic response, it can stop the progression of the response. Here's what happens.

**Release the mediators**

When sensitized to an antigen, a mast cell reacts to repeated antigen exposure by releasing chemical mediators. One of these mediators, histamine, binds to histamine-1 ($H_1$) receptors found on effector cells (the cells responsible for allergic symptoms). This initiates the allergic response that affects the respiratory, cardiovascular, GI, endocrine, and integumentary systems.

**The first one there wins**

Chlorpheniramine competes with histamine for $H_1$-receptor sites on the effector cells. By attaching to these sites first, the drug prevents more histamine from binding to the effector cells.

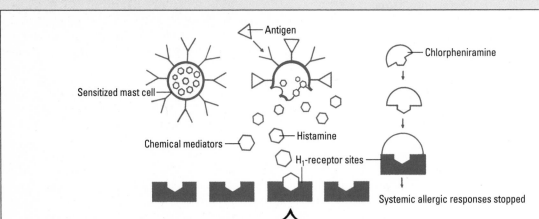

**Effector cells**

*Respiratory responses*
• Bronchial constriction and bronchospasm
• Decreased vital capacity
• Itchy nose and throat
• Rhinorrhea (runny nose)
• Sneezing

*Cardiovascular responses*
• Decreased blood pressure
• Elevated heart rate
• Increased vasodilation
• More capillary permeability

*GI responses*
• Increased parietal cell secretion
• Increased smooth-muscle contraction

*Endocrine responses*
• Increased release of epinephrine and norepinephrine

*Integumentary responses*
• Angioedema (hives and swelling of skin, mucous membranes, or internal organs)
• Flushing
• Itching

- urticaria (hives)
- angioedema (submucosal swelling in the hands, face, and feet).

## Not just for allergies

Antihistamines can have other therapeutic uses:
- Many are used primarily as antiemetics (to control nausea and vomiting).
- They can also be used as adjunctive therapy to treat an anaphylactic reaction after the serious symptoms are controlled.
- Diphenhydramine can help treat Parkinson's disease and drug-induced extrapyramidal reactions (abnormal involuntary movements).
- Because of its antiserotonin qualities, cyproheptadine may be used to treat Cushing's disease, serotonin-associated diarrhea, vascular cluster headaches, and anorexia nervosa.

## Drug interactions

Antihistamines may interact with many drugs, sometimes with life-threatening consequences:
- They may block or reverse the vasopressor effects of epinephrine, producing vasodilation, increased heart rate, and very low blood pressure.
- They may mask the toxic signs and symptoms of ototoxicity (a detrimental effect on hearing) associated with aminoglycosides or large dosages of salicylates.
- They may increase the sedative and respiratory depressant effects of CNS depressants, such as tranquilizers or alcohol.
- Loratadine may cause serious cardiac effects when taken with macrolide antibiotics (such as erythromycin), fluconazole, ketoconazole, itraconazole, miconazole, cimetidine, ciprofloxacin, and clarithromycin. (See *Adverse reactions to antihistamines*.)

# Corticosteroids

*Corticosteroids* suppress immune responses and reduce inflammation. They're available as natural or synthetic steroids.

## There's no improving on nature

Natural corticosteroids are hormones produced by the adrenal cortex; most corticosteroids are synthetic forms of these hormones. Natural and synthetic corticosteroids are classified according to their biological activities:
- Glucocorticoids, such as cortisone acetate and dexamethasone, affect carbohydrate and protein metabolism.

*Warning!*

## Adverse reactions to antihistamines

The most common adverse reaction to antihistamines (with the exceptions of fexofenadine and loratadine) is central nervous system (CNS) depression. Other CNS reactions include:
- dizziness
- lassitude and fatigue
- disturbed coordination
- muscle weakness.

**Gut reactions**
GI reactions may include:
- epigastric distress
- loss of appetite
- nausea and vomiting
- constipation
- diarrhea
- dryness of the mouth, nose, and throat.

**They can get the heart racing**
Cardiovascular reactions may include:
- hypotension
- hypertension
- rapid heart rate
- arrhythmias.

**A sensitive issue**
Sensitivity reactions can also occur.

* Mineralocorticoids, such as aldosterone and fludrocortisone acetate, regulate electrolyte and water balance.

# Glucocorticoids

Most *glucocorticoids* are synthetic analogues of hormones secreted by the adrenal cortex. They exert anti-inflammatory, metabolic, and immunosuppressant effects. Drugs in this class include:
* beclomethasone
* betamethasone
* cortisone
* dexamethasone
* hydrocortisone
* methylprednisolone
* prednisolone
* prednisone
* triamcinolone.

## Pharmacokinetics

Glucocorticoids are well absorbed when administered orally. After I.M. administration, they're absorbed completely.

### Distribution

Glucocorticoids are bound to plasma proteins and distributed through the blood.

### Metabolism and excretion

Glucocorticoids are metabolized in the liver and excreted by the kidneys.

## Pharmacodynamics

Glucocorticoids suppress hypersensitivity and immune responses through a process that isn't entirely understood. Researchers believe that glucocorticoids inhibit immune responses by:
* suppressing or preventing cell-mediated immune reactions
* reducing levels of leukocytes, monocytes, and eosinophils
* decreasing the binding of immunoglobulins to cell surface receptors
* inhibiting interleukin synthesis.

### Taking the red (and more) out

Glucocorticoids suppress the redness, edema, heat, and tenderness associated with the inflammatory response. They start on the cellular level by stabilizing the lysosomal membrane (a structure

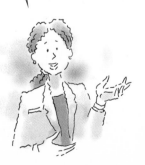

Unfortunately, when glucocorticoids inhibit the immune response they may also simultaneously mask the signs and symptoms of serious infections.

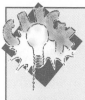

*Now I get it!*

## How methylprednisolone works

Tissue trauma normally leads to tissue irritation, edema, inflammation, and production of scar tissue. Methylprednisolone counteracts the initial effects of tissue trauma, promoting healing.

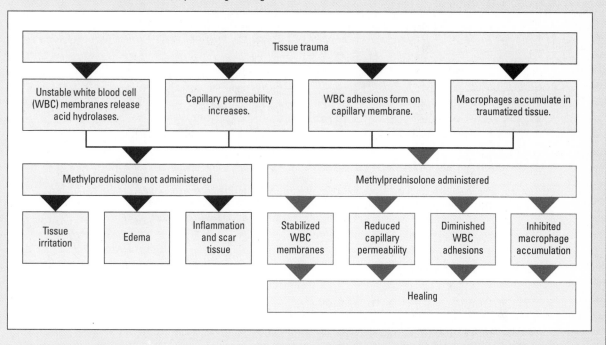

within the cell that contains digestive enzymes) so that it doesn't release its store of hydrolytic enzymes into the cells.

## No leaks, no drips

As corticosteroids, glucocorticoids prevent the leakage of plasma from capillaries, suppress the migration of polymorphonuclear leukocytes (cells that kill and digest microorganisms), and inhibit phagocytosis (ingestion and destruction).

To ensure a job well done, glucocorticoids decrease antibody formation in injured or infected tissues and disrupt histamine synthesis, fibroblast development, collagen deposition, capillary dilation, and capillary permeability. (See *How methylprednisolone works*.)

**Warning!**

## Adverse reactions to corticosteroids

Corticosteroids affect almost all body systems. Their wide-spread adverse effects include:
• insomnia
• increased sodium and water retention
• increased potassium excretion

• suppressed immune and inflammatory responses
• osteoporosis
• intestinal perforation
• peptic ulcers
• impaired wound healing.

**Diabetes and more**
Endocrine system reactions may include:

• diabetes mellitus
• hyperlipidemia
• adrenal atrophy
• hypothalamic-pituitary axis suppression
• cushingoid signs and symptoms (such as buffalo hump, moon face, and elevated blood glucose levels).

## Pharmacotherapeutics

Besides their use as replacement therapy for patients with adreno-cortical insufficiency, glucocorticoids are prescribed for immuno-suppression and reduction of inflammation and for their effects on the blood and lymphatic systems.

## Drug interactions

Many drugs interact with corticosteroids:
• Aminoglutethimide, barbiturates, phenytoin, and rifampin may reduce the effects of corticosteroids.
• Their potassium-wasting effects may be enhanced by amphotericin B, chlorthalidone, ethacrynic acid, furosemide, and thiazide diuretics.
• Erythromycin and troleandomycin may increase their effects by reducing their metabolism.
• They reduce the serum concentration and effects of salicylates.
• The risk of peptic ulcers associated with nonsteroidal anti-inflammatory drugs and salicylates increases when these agents are taken with corticosteroids.
• The response to vaccines and toxoids may be reduced in a patient taking corticosteroids.
• Estrogen and hormonal contraceptives that contain estrogen increase the effects of corticosteroids.
• The effects of antidiabetic drugs may be reduced, resulting in increased blood glucose levels. (See *Adverse reactions to corticosteroids.*)

# Mineralocorticoids

*Mineralocorticoids* affect electrolyte and water balance. These drugs include:
• fludrocortisone acetate, a synthetic analogue of hormones secreted by the adrenal cortex
• aldosterone, a natural mineralocorticoid (the use of which has been curtailed by high cost and limited availability).

## Pharmacokinetics

Fludrocortisone acetate is absorbed well and distributed to all parts of the body.

### Metabolism and excretion

Fludrocortisone acetate is metabolized in the liver to inactive metabolites. The drug is excreted by the kidneys, primarily as inactive metabolites.

## Pharmacodynamics

Fludrocortisone acetate affects fluid and electrolyte balance by acting on the distal renal tubule to increase sodium reabsorption and potassium and hydrogen secretion.

## Pharmacotherapeutics

Fludrocortisone acetate is used as replacement therapy for patients with adrenocortical insufficiency (reduced secretion of glucocorticoids, mineralocorticoids, and androgens).

*Seasoning reasoning*

Fludrocortisone acetate may also be used to treat salt-losing congenital adrenogenital syndrome (characterized by a lack of cortisol and deficient aldosterone production) after the patient's electrolyte balance has been restored.

## Drug interactions

As is the case with adverse reactions, the drug interactions associated with mineralocorticoids are similar to those associated with glucocorticoids.

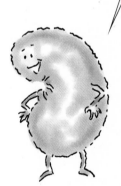

Fludrocortisone acetate gets me working harder to increase sodium reabsorption and potassium and hydrogen secretion.

# Other immunosuppressants

Several drugs used for their immunosuppressant effects in patients undergoing allograft transplantation (transplantation between two people who aren't identical twins) are also used experimentally to treat autoimmune diseases (diseases resulting from an inappropriate immune response directed against the self). They include:

- azathioprine
- basiliximab
- cyclosporine
- daclizumab
- lymphocyte immune globulin (ATG [equine])
- muromonab-CD3
- mycophenolate mofetil
- sirolimus
- tacrolimus
- thymoglobulin (antithymocyte globulin [rabbit]).

*Also these*

Cyclophosphamide, classified as an alkylating drug, is also used as an immunosuppressant; however, it's primarily used to treat cancer.

Anakinra is an immunosuppressant used to treat adults with moderate to severe active rheumatoid arthritis who haven't responded to at least one disease-modifying antirheumatic drug.

## Pharmacokinetics

Immunosuppressants take different paths through the body.

### Absorption

When administered orally, azathioprine and mycophenolate are readily absorbed from the GI tract, whereas absorption of cyclosporine, tacrolimus, and sirolimus is varied and incomplete.

*Only I.V.*

Anakinra, ATG, basiliximab, daclizumab, muromonab-CD3, and thymoglobulin are administered only by I.V. injection.

### Distribution

The distribution of azathioprine, basiliximab, and daclizumab isn't fully understood. Cyclosporine and muromonab-CD3 are distributed widely throughout the body. Azathioprine and cyclosporine cross the placental barrier. The distribution of ATG isn't clear, but it may appear in breast milk. Distribution of tacrolimus depends on several factors; 75% to 99% is protein-bound. Sirolimus is 97% protein-bound.

### Metabolism and excretion

Azathioprine and cyclosporine are metabolized in the liver. Muromonab-CD3 is consumed by T cells circulating in the blood. The metabolism of ATG is unknown.

Mycophenolate is metabolized in the liver to mycophenolate acid, an active metabolite, and then further metabolized to an inactive metabolite, which is excreted in urine and bile. Concentrations of mycophenolate and acyclovir may increase in the presence of nephrotoxicity.

Azathioprine, anakinra, and ATG are excreted in urine; cyclosporine is excreted principally in bile. It's unknown how muromonab-CD3 is excreted.

Tacrolimus is extensively metabolized and excreted primarily in bile; less than 1% is excreted unchanged in urine. Sirolimus is metabolized by the mixed function oxidase system, primarily cytochrome P-450 (CYP3A4); 91% is excreted in stool and 2.2% in urine. Metabolism and excretion of basiliximab and daclizumab aren't understood.

## Pharmacodynamics

How certain immunosuppressants achieve their desired effects has yet to be determined.

### What's going on here?

The exact mechanism of action of azathioprine, cyclosporine, and ATG is unknown, but may be explained by these theories:
• Azathioprine antagonizes metabolism of the amino acid purine and, therefore, may inhibit ribonucleic acid and deoxyribonucleic acid structure and synthesis. It also may inhibit coenzyme formation and function.
• Cyclosporine is thought to inhibit helper T cells and suppressor T cells.
• ATG may eliminate antigen-reactive T cells in the blood, alter T-cell function, or both.

### They do know this much...

In patients receiving kidney allografts, azathioprine suppresses cell-mediated hypersensitivity reactions and produces various alterations in antibody production. Muromonab-CD3, a monoclonal antibody, is understood to block the function of T cells.

Anakinra, basiliximab, and daclizumab block the activity of interleukin. Mycophenolate inhibits responses of T and B lympho-

> Cyclosporine may inhibit helper T cells, but we aren't really sure.

cytes, suppresses antibody formation by B lymphocytes, and may inhibit recruitment of leukocytes into sites of inflammation and graft rejection.

Sirolimus is an immunosuppressant that inhibits T-lymphocyte activation and proliferation that occur in response to antigenic and cytokine stimulation; it also inhibits antibody formation.

## Pharmacotherapeutics

Immunosuppressants are used mainly to prevent rejection in patients who undergo organ transplantation. (See *Cyclosporine: Miracle drug or death sentence?*)

## Drug interactions

Most drug interactions with this class of drugs involve other immunosuppressant and anti-inflammatory drugs and various antibiotic and antimicrobial drugs. (See *Adverse reactions to noncorticosteroid immunosuppressants.*)
• Allopurinol increases the blood levels of azathioprine.
• Verapamil increases blood levels of sirolimus.
• Voriconazole shouldn't be given with sirolimus because the combination inhibits CYP3A4 enzymes, resulting in increased sirolimus levels.
• When mycophenolate is taken with antacids or cholestyramine, mycophenolate levels decrease.

*Warning!*

# Adverse reactions to noncorticosteroid immunosuppressants

All noncorticosteroid immunosuppressants can cause hypersensitivity reactions. Here are adverse reactions to individual drugs.

**Azathioprine**
- Bone marrow suppression
- Nausea and vomiting
- Liver toxicity

**Cyclosporine**
- Kidney toxicity
- Hyperkalemia
- Infection
- Liver toxicity
- Nausea and vomiting

**Daclizumab**
- GI disorders
- Hypertension
- Hypotension
- Chest pain
- Tachycardia
- Edema
- Dyspnea

- Pulmonary edema
- Thrombosis
- Bleeding
- Renal tubular necrosis

**Lymphocyte immune globulin**
- Fever and chills
- Reduced white blood cell (WBC) or platelet count
- Infection
- Nausea and vomiting

**Muromonab-CD3**
- Fever and chills
- Nausea and vomiting
- Tremor
- Pulmonary edema
- Infection

**Mycophenolate mofetil**
- Nausea
- Diarrhea
- Leukopenia
- Headache
- Weakness
- Urinary frequency
- Leg cramps or pain
- Liver function test result abnormalities
- Rash

**Sirolimus**
- Anemia
- Thrombocytopenia
- Hyperlipidemia
- Hypertension

**Tacrolimus**
- Nausea and vomiting

- Diarrhea
- Constipation
- Tremor
- Leukopenia
- Hypertension
- Nephrotoxicity
- Hepatotoxicity

**Thymoglobulin**
- Abdominal pain
- Diarrhea
- Dyspnea
- Fever and chills
- Headache
- Infection
- Nausea and vomiting
- Reduced WBC or platelet count
- Systemic infections
- Dizziness

---

- Coadministration of mycophenolate with acyclovir, especially in patients with renal impairment, may increase concentrations of both drugs.
- Cyclosporine levels may increase if cyclosporine is taken with ketoconazole, calcium channel blockers, cimetidine, anabolic steroids, hormonal contraceptives, erythromycin, or metoclopramide.
- The risk of toxicity to the kidneys increases when cyclosporine or sirolimus is taken with acyclovir, aminoglycosides, or amphotericin B.
- Taking anakinra, ATG, basiliximab, cyclosporine, daclizumab, muromonab-CD3, sirolimus, or thymoglobulin with other immunosuppressants (except corticosteroids) increases the risk of infection and lymphoma (neoplasm of the lymph tissue; typically malignant).
- Barbiturates, rifampin, phenytoin, sulfonamides, and trimethoprim decrease plasma cyclosporine and sirolimus levels.

• Serum digoxin levels may increase when cyclosporine is taken with digoxin.
• Anakinra shouldn't be given to patients with active infections or neutropenia.

# Uricosurics and other antigout drugs

*Uricosurics*, along with other antigout drugs, exert their effects through their anti-inflammatory actions.

## Uricosurics

The two major uricosurics are:

 probenecid

 sulfinpyrazone.

### Getting the gout out

Uricosurics act by increasing uric acid excretion in urine. The primary goal in using uricosurics is to prevent or control the frequency of gouty arthritis attacks.

### Pharmacokinetics

Uricosurics are absorbed from the GI tract.

#### Distribution

Distribution of the two drugs is similar, with 75% to 95% of probenecid and 98% of sulfinpyrazone being protein-bound.

#### Metabolism and excretion

Metabolism of the drugs occurs in the liver, and excretion is primarily by the kidneys. Only small amounts of these drugs are excreted in stool.

### Pharmacodynamics

Probenecid and sulfinpyrazone reduce the reabsorption of uric acid at the proximal convoluted tubules of the kidneys. This results in excretion of uric acid in urine, reducing serum urate levels.

### Pharmacotherapeutics

Probenecid and sulfinpyrazone are indicated for the treatment of:

- chronic gouty arthritis
- tophaceous gout (the deposition of tophi or urate crystals under the skin and into joints).

## A part-time promoter

Probenecid is also used to promote uric acid excretion in patients experiencing hyperuricemia.

## Substitute when acute

Probenecid and sulfinpyrazone shouldn't be given during an acute gouty attack. If taken at that time, these drugs prolong inflammation. Because these drugs may increase the chance of an acute gouty attack when therapy begins and whenever the serum urate level changes rapidly, colchicine is administered during the first 3 to 6 months of probenecid or sulfinpyrazone therapy.

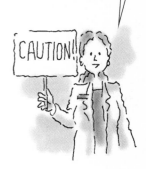

Probenecid and sulfinpyrazone shouldn't be used to treat an acute gouty attack.

### Drug interactions

Many drug interactions, some potentially serious, can occur with uricosuric drugs:
- Probenecid significantly increases or prolongs the effects of cephalosporins, penicillins, and sulfonamides.
- Serum urate levels may increase when probenecid is taken with antineoplastic drugs.
- Probenecid increases the serum concentration of dapsone, aminosalicylic acid, and methotrexate, causing toxic reactions.
- Sulfinpyrazone increases the effectiveness of warfarin, increasing the risk of bleeding.
- Salicylates reduce the effects of sulfinpyrazone.
- Sulfinpyrazone may potentiate the effects of oral antidiabetic drugs, increasing the risk of hypoglycemia. (See *Adverse reactions to uricosurics.*)

# Other antigout drugs

*Allopurinol* is used to reduce production of uric acid, preventing gouty attacks, and *colchicine* is used to treat acute gouty attacks.

## Pharmacokinetics

Allopurinol and colchicine take somewhat different paths through the body.

## All aboard allopurinol

When given orally, allopurinol is absorbed from the GI tract. Allopurinol and its metabolite oxypurinol are distributed throughout the body except in the brain, where drug concentrations are 50%

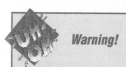

*Warning!*

## Adverse reactions to uricosurics

Adverse reactions to uricosurics include uric acid stone formation and blood abnormalities.

**Probenecid**
- Headache
- Anorexia
- Nausea and vomiting
- Hypersensitivity reactions

**Sulfinpyrazone**
- Nausea
- Indigestion
- GI pain
- GI blood loss

of those found in the rest of the body. It's metabolized by the liver and excreted in urine.

### Following colchicine's course

Colchicine is absorbed from the GI tract and is partially metabolized in the liver. The drug and its metabolites then reenter the intestinal tract through biliary secretions. After reabsorption from the intestines, colchicine is distributed to various tissues. It's excreted primarily in stool and to a lesser degree in urine.

## Pharmacodynamics

Allopurinol and its metabolite oxypurinol inhibit xanthine oxidase, the enzyme responsible for the production of uric acid. By reducing uric acid formation, allopurinol eliminates the hazards of hyperuricuria.

### Migration control

Colchicine appears to reduce the inflammatory response to monosodium urate crystals deposited in joint tissues. Colchicine may produce its effects by inhibiting migration of white blood cells (WBCs) to the inflamed joint. This reduces phagocytosis and lactic acid production by WBCs, decreasing urate crystal deposits and reducing inflammation.

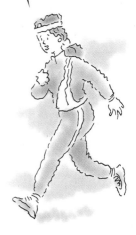

Colchicine relieves a painful gouty attack by going to work right in the joint. It can have you running smoothly again.

## Pharmacotherapeutics

Allopurinol treats primary gout, hopefully preventing acute gouty attacks. It can be prescribed with uricosurics when smaller dosages of each drug are directed. It's used to treat:
• gout or hyperuricemia that may occur with blood abnormalities and during treatment of tumors or leukemia
• primary or secondary uric acid nephropathy (with or without the accompanying symptoms of gout)
• patients who respond poorly to maximum dosages of uricosurics or who have allergic reactions or intolerance to uricosuric drugs (it's also used to prevent recurrent uric acid stone formation).

### Acute alert

Colchicine is used to relieve the inflammation of acute gouty arthritis attacks. If given promptly, it's especially effective in relieving pain. In addition, giving colchicine during the first several months of allopurinol, probenecid, or sulfinpyrazone therapy may prevent the acute gouty attacks that sometimes accompany the use of these drugs.

## Drug interactions

Colchicine doesn't interact significantly with other drugs. When allopurinol is used with other drugs, the resulting interactions can be serious:

• Allopurinol potentiates the effect of oral anticoagulants.
• Allopurinol increases the serum concentrations of mercaptopurine and azathioprine, increasing the risk of toxicity.
• Angiotensin-converting enzyme inhibitors increase the risk of hypersensitivity reactions to allopurinol.
• Allopurinol increases serum theophylline levels.
• The risk of bone marrow depression increases when cyclophosphamide is taken with allopurinol. (See *Adverse reactions to other antigout drugs*.)

*Warning!*

### Adverse reactions to other antigout drugs

Allopurinol and colchicine commonly cause nausea, vomiting, diarrhea, and intermittent abdominal pain.

**Allopurinol**
The most common adverse reaction to allopurinol is a rash.

**Colchicine**
Prolonged administration of colchicine may cause bone marrow suppression.

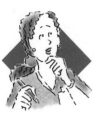

# *Quick quiz*

**1.** How does diphenhydramine work?
  A. It blocks production of histamine.
  B. It prevents binding of histamine to receptors.
  C. It reverses the effects of histamine.
  D. It increases levels of histamine.

*Answer:* B. Diphenhydramine prevents binding of histamine to receptors.

**2.** What's the most common adverse reaction for most antihistamines, with the exceptions of fexofenadine and loratadine?
  A. Drug fever
  B. GI distress
  C. Respiratory distress
  D. Sedation

*Answer:* D. Sedation, or CNS depression, is the most common adverse reaction to most antihistamines.

**3.** Which signs and symptoms suggest that a patient is experiencing Cushing's syndrome?
  A. Buffalo hump, elevated blood glucose levels, and moon face
  B. Low blood pressure, rapid heart rate, and difficulty breathing
  C. Low blood glucose levels and reduced platelet count
  D. Increased thirst, increased urination, and increased appetite

*Answer:*   A. Buffalo hump, elevated blood glucose levels, and moon face are all signs and symptoms of Cushing's syndrome. This condition can occur as an adverse reaction to corticosteroids.

**4.**   Which condition indicates that a patient is experiencing an adverse reaction to azathioprine?
  - A.   Kidney failure
  - B.   Peptic ulcer
  - C.   Bone marrow suppression
  - D.   Heart failure

*Answer:*   C. Bone marrow suppression indicates that a patient is experiencing an adverse reaction to azathioprine.

**5.**   Which sign is an adverse reaction to probenecid?
  - A.   Edema
  - B.   Vomiting
  - C.   Vertigo
  - D.   Decreased urine output

*Answer:*   B. Vomiting is an adverse reaction to probenecid.

## Scoring

☆☆☆   If you answered all five items correctly, extraordinary! You certainly aren't allergic to smarts!

☆☆   If you answered three or four items correctly, congratulations! You're taking the sting out of learning!

☆   If you answered fewer than three items correctly, keep trying! With continued improvement, the next chapter should have you feeling better!

# Psychotropic drugs

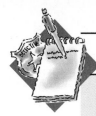

## Just the facts

In this chapter, you'll learn:

♦ classes of drugs that alter psychogenic behavior and promote sleep

♦ uses and varying actions of these drugs

♦ how these drugs are absorbed, distributed, metabolized, and excreted

♦ drug interactions and adverse reactions to these drugs.

## Drugs and psychiatric disorders

This chapter presents drugs that are used to treat various sleep and psychogenic disorders, such as anxiety, depression, and psychotic disorders.

## Sedative and hypnotic drugs

*Sedatives* reduce anxiety, tension, or excitement. Some degree of drowsiness commonly accompanies sedative use.

### You're getting very sleepy...

When given in large doses, sedatives are considered hypnotics, which induce a state resembling natural sleep. The three main classes of synthetic drugs used as sedatives and hypnotics are:

 benzodiazepines

 barbiturates

 nonbenzodiazepine-nonbarbiturate drugs.

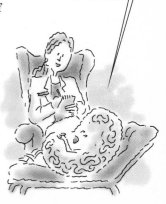

Just talking about hypnotics makes me sleepy.

## And if that doesn't put you to sleep...

Other sedatives may include sedating antidepressants, such as trazodone, and over-the-counter sleep aids.

# Benzodiazepines

*Benzodiazepines* produce many therapeutic effects, including:
- sedation before anesthesia
- sleep inducement
- relief of anxiety and tension
- skeletal muscle relaxation
- anticonvulsant activity.

## Keep your eye on the hypnotic ones

Benzodiazepines are used in various clinical situations and exert either a primary or a secondary sedative or hypnotic effect. Benzodiazepines used primarily for their sedative or hypnotic effects include:
- estazolam
- flurazepam
- lorazepam
- quazepam
- temazepam
- triazolam.

## When some calm is needed

Benzodiazepines used primarily for the treatment of anxiety include:
- alprazolam
- chlordiazepoxide
- clonazepam
- clorazepate
- diazepam
- lorazepam
- oxazepam.

### Pharmacokinetics (how drugs circulate)

Benzodiazepines are absorbed rapidly and completely from the GI tract and are distributed widely in the body. Penetration into the brain also occurs rapidly. Some benzodiazepines, such as diazepam and lorazepam, may also be given parenterally.

## How fast?

The rate of absorption determines how quickly the drug will work; flurazepam and triazolam have the fastest onset.

## How long?

The duration of effect is determined by the extent of distribution. Triazolam binds quickly to fat and is widely distributed; therefore, it has a short duration of action.

### Metabolism and excretion

All benzodiazepines are metabolized in the liver and excreted primarily in urine. Some benzodiazepines have active metabolites, which may give these drugs a longer period of action.

## Pharmacodynamics (how drugs act)

Researchers believe that benzodiazepines work by stimulating gamma-aminobutyric acid (GABA) receptors in the ascending reticular activating system (RAS) of the brain. The RAS is associated with wakefulness and attention and includes the cerebral cortex and limbic, thalamic, and hypothalamic levels of the central nervous system (CNS). (See *How benzodiazepines work*, page 314.)

### Low will ease your mind

At low dosages, benzodiazepines decrease anxiety by acting on the limbic system and other areas of the brain that help regulate emotional activity. The drugs can usually calm or sedate the patient without causing drowsiness.

### High will ease you into sleep

At higher dosages, benzodiazepines induce sleep, probably because they depress the RAS of the brain.

### Zzzzzzzzzzzz...

Benzodiazepines increase total sleep time and reduce the number of awakenings. In most cases, benzodiazepines don't decrease the time spent in rapid-eye-movement (REM) sleep, the state of sleep in which brain activity resembles the activity it shows when awake; the body's muscles relax, and the eyes move rapidly. Because benzodiazepines don't decrease the duration of REM sleep, they have a significant advantage over barbiturates.

During each sleep cycle the sleeping person progresses from stage 1, which is drowsiness, to stages 3 and 4, which are deep-sleep stages. Benzodiazepines reduce the amount of time spent in stages 3 and 4. The decrease in stage 4 sleep is accompanied by a reduction in nightmares.

## Pharmacotherapeutics (how drugs are used)

Clinical indications for benzodiazepines include:

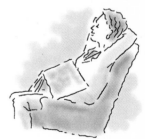

At low dosages, benzodiazepines decrease anxiety without causing drowsiness.

*Now I get it!*

# How benzodiazepines work

These illustrations show how benzodiazepines work at the cellular level.

## Speed and passage

The speed of impulses from a presynaptic neuron across a synapse is influenced by the number of chloride ions in the postsynaptic neuron. The passage of chloride ions into the postsynaptic neuron depends on the inhibitory neurotransmitter called *gamma-aminobutyric acid,* or GABA.

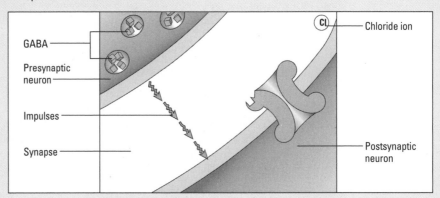

## It binds

When GABA is released from the presynaptic neuron, it travels across the synapse and binds to GABA receptors on the postsynaptic neuron. This binding opens the chloride channels, allowing chloride ions to flow into the postsynaptic neuron and causing the nerve impulses to slow down.

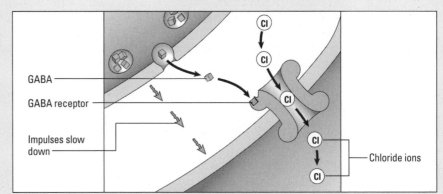

## The result is another kind of depression

Benzodiazepines bind to receptors on or near the GABA receptor, enhancing the effect of GABA and allowing more chloride ions to flow into the postsynaptic neuron. This depresses the nerve impulses, causing them to slow down or stop.

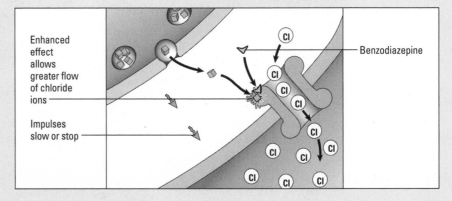

- relaxing the patient during the day of or before surgery
- treating insomnia
- producing I.V. anesthesia
- treating alcohol withdrawal symptoms
- treating anxiety and seizure disorders
- producing skeletal muscle relaxation.

## Drug interactions

Except for other CNS depressants such as alcohol, few drugs interact with benzodiazepines.

*Deep sleep*

When benzodiazepines are taken with other CNS depressants (including alcohol and anticonvulsants), the result is enhanced sedative and CNS depressant effects, including reduced level of consciousness, reduced muscle coordination, respiratory depression, and death.

*Possible problems with the pill*

Hormonal contraceptives may reduce the metabolism of flurazepam hydrochloride, increasing the risk of toxicity.

Triazolam may be affected by inhibitors of the CYP3A system (such as erythromycin and ketoconazole). (See *Adverse reactions to benzodiazepines.*)

---

**Warning!**

## Adverse reactions to benzodiazepines

Benzodiazepines may cause:
- amnesia
- fatigue
- muscle weakness
- mouth dryness
- nausea and vomiting
- dizziness
- ataxia (impaired ability to coordinate movement).

**Getting groggy**
Unintentional daytime sedation, hangover effect (residual drowsiness and impaired reac-

tion time on awakening), and rebound insomnia may also occur.

**One more may be one too many**
These drugs have a potential for abuse, tolerance, and physical dependence. Benzodiazepines with a long half-life or active metabolites may accumulate and cause adverse effects in elderly patients. In general, lower starting doses, with gradual dosage increases, should be used in elderly patients who are taking benzodiazepines.

# Barbiturates

The major pharmacologic action of *barbiturates* is to reduce overall CNS alertness. Barbiturates used primarily as sedatives and hypnotics include:

- amobarbital
- butabarbital
- mephobarbital
- pentobarbital
- phenobarbital
- secobarbital.

## On the dose

Low doses of barbiturates depress the sensory and motor cortex in the brain, causing drowsiness. High doses may cause respiratory depression and death because of their ability to depress all levels of the CNS.

## Pharmacokinetics

Barbiturates are well absorbed from the GI tract, distributed rapidly, metabolized by the liver, and excreted in urine.

## Pharmacodynamics

As sedative-hypnotics, barbiturates depress the sensory cortex of the brain, decrease motor activity, alter cerebral function, and produce drowsiness, sedation, and hypnosis.

## We interrupt this transmission...

These drugs appear to act throughout the CNS; however, the RAS of the brain, which is responsible for wakefulness, is a particularly sensitive site.

## Pharmacotherapeutics

Barbiturates have many clinical indications, including:

- daytime sedation (for short periods only, typically less than 2 weeks)
- hypnotic effects for patients with insomnia
- preoperative sedation and anesthesia
- relief of anxiety
- anticonvulsant effects.

## Popularity plunge

Patients develop tolerance to barbiturates more quickly than to benzodiazepines, and physical dependence on barbiturates

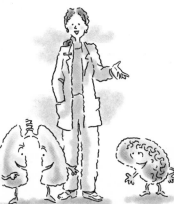

Low doses of barbiturates depress parts of the brain. High doses cause respiratory depression.

may occur even with a small daily dosage. In comparison, benzo-diazepines are relatively effective and safe and, for these reasons, have replaced barbiturates as the sedatives and hypnotics of choice.

## Drug interactions

Barbiturates may interact with many other drugs:
• They may reduce the effects of beta-adrenergic blockers (meto-prolol, propranolol), chloramphenicol, corticosteroids, doxycy-cline, oral anticoagulants, hormonal contraceptives, quinidine, tri-cyclic antidepressants (TCAs), metronidazole, theophylline, and cyclosporine.
• Hydantoins, such as phenytoin, reduce the metabolism of phe-nobarbital, resulting in increased toxic effects.
• Their use with methoxyflurane may stimulate production of metabolites that are toxic to the kidneys.
• Their use with other CNS depressants (especially alcohol) may cause excessive CNS depression.
• Valproic acid may increase barbiturate levels.
• Monoamine oxidase inhibitors (MAOIs) inhibit the metabolism of barbiturates, increasing their sedative effects.
• When barbiturates are taken with acetaminophen, the risk of liver toxicity increases. (See *Adverse reactions to barbiturates*.)

# Nonbenzodiazepines-nonbarbiturates

*Nonbenzodiazepine-nonbarbiturates* act as hypnotics for treat-ment of simple insomnia. These drugs, which offer no special ad-vantages over other sedatives, include:
• chloral hydrate
• eszopiclone
• ramelton
• zaleplon
• zolpidem.

## Diminishing returns

Chloral hydrate and zaleplon lose their effectiveness by the end of the second week. Zolpidem is usually effective for up to 35 days. Eszopiclone and ramelton are approved for long-term treatment of insomnia.

## Pharmacokinetics

Nonbenzodiazepines-nonbarbiturates are absorbed rapidly from the GI tract, metabolized in the liver, and excreted in urine.

**Warning!**

## Adverse reactions to barbiturates

Barbiturates may have widespread adverse ef-fects.

### S.O.S. for CNS

Central nervous system (CNS) reactions include:
• drowsiness
• lethargy
• headache
• depression.

### Heart of the matter

Cardiovascular and res-piratory effects include:
• mild bradycardia
• hypotension
• hypoventilation
• spasm of the larynx (voice box) and bronchi
• reduced rate of breathing
• severe respiratory de-pression.

### All the rest

Other reactions include:
• vertigo
• nausea and vomiting
• diarrhea
• epigastric pain
• allergic reactions.

*Safe and sound*

## Warning about sleep agents

The U.S. Food and Drug Administration requires that all sedative-hypnotic drugs include a warning on the drug label about the risk of complex sleep-related behaviors. Complex sleep-related behaviors include preparing and eating food, making phone calls, and even driving when not fully awake, while having no memory of the event.

*Warning!*

## Adverse reactions to nonbenzodiazepines-nonbarbiturates

The most common dose-related adverse reactions involving nonbenzodiazepines-nonbarbiturates include:
• nausea and vomiting
• gastric irritation
• hangover effects (possibly leading to respiratory depression or even respiratory failure).

### Pharmacodynamics

The mechanism of action for nonbenzodiazepines-nonbarbiturates isn't fully known; however, they produce depressant effects similar to barbiturates.

### Pharmacotherapeutics

Nonbenzodiazepines-nonbarbiturates are typically used for:
• treatment of simple insomnia
• sedation before surgery
• sedation before EEG studies.

### Drug interactions

When nonbenzodiazepines-nonbarbiturates are used with other CNS depressants, additive CNS depression occurs, resulting in drowsiness, respiratory depression, stupor, coma, or death. (See *Warning about sleep agents.*)

*A chlorus of interactions*

Chloral hydrate may increase the risk of bleeding in patients taking oral anticoagulants. Use with I.V. furosemide may produce sweating, flushing, variable blood pressure, and uneasiness. (See *Adverse reactions to nonbenzodiazepines-nonbarbiturates.*)

# Antianxiety drugs

*Antianxiety drugs*, also called *anxiolytics*, include some of the most commonly prescribed drugs in the United States. They are used primarily to treat anxiety disorders. The three main types of antianxiety drugs are benzodiazepines (discussed in a previous section), barbiturates (also discussed in a previous section), and buspirone.

# Buspirone

*Buspirone* is the first antianxiety drug in a class of drugs known as *azaspirodecanedione derivatives*. This drug's structure and mechanism of action differ from those of other antianxiety drugs.

## Advantage, buspirone

Buspirone has several advantages, including:
• less sedation
• no increase in CNS depressant effects when taken with alcohol or sedative-hypnotics
• lower abuse potential.

## Pharmacokinetics

Buspirone is absorbed rapidly, undergoes extensive first-pass effect, and is metabolized in the liver to at least one active metabolite. The drug is eliminated in urine and stool.

## Pharmacodynamics

Although the mechanism of action of buspirone isn't known, it's known that buspirone doesn't affect GABA receptors like the benzodiazepines do.

## Midbrain modulator

Buspirone seems to produce various effects in the midbrain and acts as a midbrain modulator, possibly due to its high affinity for serotonin receptors.

## Pharmacotherapeutics

Buspirone is used to treat generalized anxiety states. Patients who haven't received benzodiazepines seem to respond better to buspirone.

## In case of panic

Because of its slow onset of action, buspirone is ineffective when quick relief from anxiety is needed.

## Drug interactions

Unlike other antianxiety drugs, buspirone doesn't interact with alcohol or other CNS depressants. When buspirone is given with MAOIs, hypertensive reactions may occur. (See *Adverse reactions to buspirone*.)

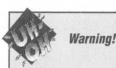

**Warning!**

## Adverse reactions to buspirone

The most common reactions to buspirone include:
• dizziness
• light-headedness
• insomnia
• rapid heart rate
• palpitations
• headache.

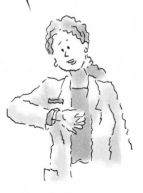

Buspirone has a slow onset, so it isn't useful for panic attacks.

# Antidepressant and mood stabilizer drugs

*Antidepressant* and *mood stabilizer drugs* are used to treat affective disorders—disturbances in mood, characterized by depression or elation.

## Pole positions

Unipolar disorders, characterized by periods of clinical depression, are treated with:
- selective serotonin reuptake inhibitors (SSRIs)
- MAOIs
- TCAs
- miscellaneous antidepressants.

Bipolar disorders, characterized by alternating periods of manic behavior and clinical depression, are treated with lithium and anticonvulsant drugs.

Other mood stabilizers include divalproex, carbamazepine, and olanzapine.

## Putting a new stress on SSRIs

The Food and Drug Administration approved sertraline (Zoloft) and paroxetine (Paxil) as the drugs of choice for treating posttraumatic stress disorder. In order for these drugs to be used, the patient must have symptoms, such as intense fear, helplessness, and horror that exist for at least 1 month and cause significant impaired functioning.

# Selective serotonin reuptake inhibitors

Developed to treat depression with fewer adverse reactions, *SSRIs*, are chemically different from MAOIs and TCAs. (See *Putting a new stress on SSRIs.*)

Some of the SSRIs currently available are:
- citalopram
- duloxetine
- escitalopram
- fluoxetine
- fluvoxamine
- paroxetine
- sertraline
- venlafaxine. (See *Stopping SSRIs.*)

## Pharmacokinetics

SSRIs are absorbed almost completely after oral administration and are highly protein-bound.

### Metabolism and excretion

SSRIs are primarily metabolized in the liver and are excreted in urine.

*Safe and sound*

## Stopping SSRIs

Abruptly stopping selective serotonin reuptake inhibitor (SSRI) therapy may result in SSRI discontinuation syndrome, with dizziness, vertigo, ataxia, nausea, vomiting, muscle pains, fatigue, tremor, and headache. Psychological symptoms, such as anxiety, crying spells, irritability, feeling sad, memory problems, and vivid dreams, may also occur.

This syndrome is more common in SSRIs with a shorter half-life, such as paroxetine and venlafaxine, and occurs in up to one-third of patients receiving SSRI therapy.

**Go slow**

Tapering the dosage of the drug slowly over several weeks can prevent SSRI discontinuation syndrome. Fluoxetine is the least likely to cause this problem because of its extremely long half-life. The syndrome is self-limiting (over 2 to 3 weeks with treatment).

## Pharmacodynamics

SSRIs inhibit the neuronal reuptake of the neurotransmitter serotonin.

## Pharmacotherapeutics

SSRIs are used to treat the same major depressive episodes as TCAs and have the same degree of effectiveness. Fluvoxamine, fluoxetine, sertraline, and paroxetine are also used to treat obsessive-compulsive disorder. Fluoxetine has also been approved for the treatment of bulimia. Paroxetine is also indicated for social anxiety disorder.

Venlafaxine is an antidepressant drug that's chemically different from other antidepressants and has unique properties in terms of absorption and mechanism of action. It has been particularly effective in patients with very severe depression.

*Don't panic, but there's more...*

SSRIs may also be useful in treating panic disorders, eating disorders, personality disorders, impulse control disorders, and anxiety disorders. Several SSRIs are approved for premenstrual (dysphoric) disorder.

## Drug interactions

Drug interactions associated with SSRIs involve their ability to competitively inhibit a liver enzyme that's responsible for oxidation of numerous drugs, including TCAs, carbamazepine, metoprolol, flecainide, encainide, and antipsychotics, such as clozapine and thioridazine.

## They don't mix with MAOIs

The use of SSRIs with MAOIs can cause serious, potentially fatal reactions. Individual SSRIs also have their own particular interactions. (See *Adverse reactions to SSRIs*.)
• Use of citalopram and paroxetine with warfarin may lead to increased bleeding.
• Carbamazepine may increase clearance of citalopram.
• Fluoxetine increases the half-life of diazepam and displaces highly protein-bound drugs, leading to toxicity.
• Fluvoxamine use with diltiazem hydrochloride may cause bradycardia.
• Paroxetine shouldn't be used with tryptophan because this combination can cause headache, nausea, sweating, and dizziness.
• Paroxetine may increase procyclidine levels, causing increased anticholinergic effects.
• Cimetidine, phenobarbital, and phenytoin may reduce paroxetine metabolism by the liver, increasing the risk of toxicity.
• Paroxetine and sertraline may interact with other highly protein-bound drugs, causing adverse reactions to either drug. (See *Risks of antidepressants*.)

# Tricyclic antidepressants

*TCAs* are used to treat depression. They include:
• amitriptyline
• amoxapine
• clomipramine
• desipramine
• doxepin

- imipramine
- nortriptyline
- protriptyline
- trimipramine.

## Pharmacokinetics

All of the TCAs are active pharmacologically, and some of their metabolites are also active. They're absorbed completely when taken orally but undergo first-pass effect.

### Distribution, metabolism, and excretion

With first-pass effect, a drug passes from the GI tract to the liver, where it's partially metabolized before entering the circulation. TCAs are metabolized extensively in the liver and eventually excreted as inactive compounds (only small amounts of active drug are excreted) in urine.

### They just melt in fat

The extreme fat solubility of these drugs accounts for their wide distribution throughout the body, slow excretion, and long half-lives.

## Pharmacodynamics

Researchers believe that TCAs increase the amount of norepinephrine, serotonin, or both in the CNS by preventing their reuptake into the storage granules in the presynaptic nerves. They also block acetylcholine and histamine receptors.

### The upside to preventing reuptake

After a neurotransmitter has performed its job, several fates are possible, including rapidly reentering the neuron from which it was released (or reuptake). Preventing reuptake results in increased levels of these neurotransmitters in the synapses, relieving depression.

## Pharmacotherapeutics

TCAs are used to treat episodes of major depression. They're especially effective in treating depression of insidious onset accompanied by weight loss, anorexia, or insomnia. Physical signs and symptoms may respond after 1 to 2 weeks of therapy; psychological symptoms, after 2 to 4 weeks.

**Warning!**

## Adverse reactions to TCAs

Adverse reactions to TCAs include:
- orthostatic hypotension (a drop in blood pressure on standing)
- sedation
- jaundice
- rashes
- photosensitivity reactions
- a fine resting tremor
- decreased sexual desire
- inhibited ejaculation
- transient eosinophilia
- reduced white blood cell count
- manic episodes (in patients with or without bipolar disorder)

- exacerbation of psychotic symptoms in susceptible patients.

**Special effects**
Although rare, TCA therapy may also lead to:
- granulocytopenia
- palpitations
- conduction delays
- rapid heartbeat
- impaired cognition, cardiovascular adverse reactions (in elderly patients).

Sudden death has occurred in children and adolescents taking desipramine. For this reason a baseline electrocardiogram is recommended before giving a TCA to patients in this age-group.

## Problem patients

TCAs are much less effective in patients with hypochondriasis, atypical depression, or depression accompanied by delusions. When given with a mood stabilizer, they may be helpful in treating acute episodes of depression in bipolar I disorder.

## Migraines and more

TCAs are also used for preventing migraine headaches and in treating phobias (panic disorder with agoraphobia), urinary incontinence, attention deficit disorder, obsessive-compulsive disorder, neuropathic pain (chronic pain that can occur with peripheral neuropathies, herpes zoster infections, traumatic nerve injuries, and some types of cancer or cancer treatments), diabetic neuropathy, and enuresis.

## Drug interactions

TCAs interact with several commonly used drugs:
- They increase the catecholamine effects of amphetamines and sympathomimetics, leading to hypertension.
- Barbiturates increase the metabolism of TCAs and decrease their blood levels.

• Cimetidine impairs metabolism of TCAs by the liver, increasing the risk of toxicity.
• Concurrent use of TCAs with MAOIs may cause an extremely elevated body temperature, excitation, and seizures.
• An increased anticholinergic effect, such as dry mouth, urine retention, and constipation, is seen when anticholinergic drugs are taken with TCAs.
• TCAs reduce the antihypertensive effects of clonidine and guanethidine. (See *Adverse reactions to TCAs.*)

# Monoamine oxidase inhibitors

*MAOIs* are divided into two classifications based on chemical structure:
• hydrazines, which include phenelzine sulfate
• nonhydrazines, consisting of a single drug, tranylcypromine sulfate.

## Pharmacokinetics

MAOIs are absorbed rapidly and completely from the GI tract and are metabolized in the liver to inactive metabolites. These metabolites are excreted mainly by the GI tract and, to a lesser degree, by the kidneys.

## Pharmacodynamics

MAOIs appear to work by inhibiting MAO, an enzyme that's widely distributed throughout the body and that normally metabolizes many neurotransmitters, including norepinephrine, dopamine, and serotonin. This leaves more norepinephrine, dopamine, and serotonin available to the receptors, thereby relieving the symptoms of depression.

## Pharmacotherapeutics

The indications for MAOIs are similar to those for other antidepressants. MAOIs are particularly effective for treating panic disorder with agoraphobia, eating disorders, posttraumatic stress disorder, and pain disorders.

MAOIs may be more effective than other antidepressants in the treatment of atypical depression. Atypical depression produces signs opposite to those of typical depression. For example, the patient gains weight, sleeps more, and has a higher susceptibility to rejection.

If other
therapies don't
work, MAOIs may
be prescribed.

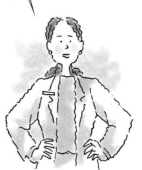

## It tackles typical depression, too

MAOIs may be used to treat typical depression resistant to other
therapies or when other therapies are contraindicated. For example, tranylcypromine is the preferred MAOI for patients with depression who have liver disease. Other uses include treatment for:
• phobic anxieties
• neurodermatitis (an itchy skin disorder seen in anxious, nervous people)
• hypochondriasis (abnormal concern about health)
• refractory narcolepsy (sudden sleep attacks).

## Drug interactions

MAOIs interact with a wide variety of drugs:
• Taking MAOIs with amphetamines, methylphenidate, levodopa,
sympathomimetics, and nonamphetamine appetite suppressants
may increase catecholamine release, causing hypertensive crisis.
• Using them with fluoxetine, TCAs, citalopram, clomipramine,
trazodone, sertraline, paroxetine, and fluvoxamine may result in
an elevated body temperature, excitation, and seizures.
• When taken with doxapram, MAOIs may cause hypertension
and arrhythmias and may increase the adverse reactions to
doxapram.
• MAOIs may enhance the hypoglycemic effects of antidiabetic
drugs.
• Administering MAOIs with meperidine may result in excitation,
hypertension or hypotension, extremely elevated body temperature, and coma. (See *Moving from MAOIs.*)

### Moving from MAOIs

Monoamine oxidase in-
hibitors (MAOIs) should
be discontinued 2 weeks
before starting an alter-
native antidepressant. A
2-week waiting period
(5 weeks for fluoxetine)
should also elapse when
discontinuing an anti-
depressant and starting
an MAOI.

## Forbidden fruit (and other foods)

Certain foods can interact with MAOIs and produce severe reactions. The most serious reactions involve tyramine-rich foods, such as red wines, aged cheese, and fava beans. Foods with moderate tyramine contents—for example, yogurt and ripe bananas—may be eaten occasionally, but with care. (See *Adverse reactions to MAOIs*.)

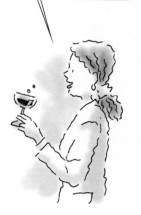

Tyramine-rich foods, such as red wine, can produce severe reactions if taken with MAOIs.

# Miscellaneous antidepressants

Other *antidepressants* in use today include:
• maprotiline and mirtazapine, tetracyclic antidepressants
• bupropion, a dopamine reuptake blocking agent
• venlafaxine, a serotonin-norepinephrine reuptake inhibitor
• trazodone, a triazolopyridine agent
• nefazodone, a phenylpiperazine agent.

## Pharmacokinetics

The paths these antidepressants take through the body may vary:
• Maprotiline and mirtazapine are absorbed from the GI tract, distributed widely in the body, metabolized by the liver, and excreted by the kidneys.
• Bupropion is well absorbed from the GI tract and metabolized by the liver. Its metabolites are excreted by the kidneys. It appears to be highly bound to plasma proteins.
• Venlafaxine is rapidly absorbed after oral administration, partially bound to plasma proteins, metabolized in the liver, and excreted in urine.
• Trazodone is well absorbed from the GI tract, distributed widely in the body, and metabolized by the liver. About 75% is excreted in urine; the remainder is excreted in stool.
• Nefazodone is rapidly and completely absorbed but, because of extensive metabolism, only about 20% of the drug is available. The drug is almost completely bound to plasma proteins and is excreted in urine.

## Pharmacodynamics

Much about how these drugs work has yet to be fully understood:
• Maprotiline and mirtazapine probably increase the amount of norepinephrine, serotonin, or both in the CNS by blocking their reuptake by presynaptic neurons (nerve terminals).

- Bupropion was once thought to inhibit the reuptake of the neurotransmitter dopamine; however, it more likely acts on nonadrenergic receptors.
- Venlafaxine is thought to potentiate neurotransmitter activity in the CNS by inhibiting the neural reuptake of serotonin and norepinephrine.
- Trazodone, although its action is unknown, is thought to exert antidepressant effects by inhibiting the reuptake of norepinephrine and serotonin in the presynaptic neurons.
- Nefazodone's action isn't precisely defined. It inhibits neuronal uptake of serotonin and norepinephrine. It's also a serotonin antagonist, which explains its effectiveness in treating anxiety.

## Pharmacotherapeutics

These miscellaneous drugs are all used to treat depression. Trazodone may also be effective in treating aggressive behavior and panic disorder.

## Drug interactions

All of these antidepressants may have serious, potentially fatal, effects when combined with MAOIs. Each of these drugs also carries its own specific risks when used with other drugs:
- Maprotiline and mirtazapine interact with CNS depressants to cause an additive effect.
- Bupropion combined with levodopa, phenothiazines, or TCAs increases the risk of adverse reactions, including seizures.

---

*Warning!*

## Adverse reactions to miscellaneous antidepressants

These antidepressants may produce various adverse reactions.

| Maprotiline | Mirtazapine | Bupropion | Venlafaxine and nefazodone | Trazodone |
|---|---|---|---|---|
| • Seizures | • Tremors | • Headache | • Headache | • Drowsiness |
| • Orthostatic hypotension | • Confusion | • Confusion | • Somnolence | • Dizziness |
| • Tachycardia | • Nausea | • Tremor | • Dizziness | |
| • Electrocardiographic changes | • Constipation | • Agitation | • Nausea | |
| | | • Tachycardia | | |
| | | • Anorexia | | |
| | | • Nausea and vomiting | | |

• Trazodone may increase serum levels of digoxin and phenytoin. Its use with antihypertensive agents may increase hypotensive effects. CNS depression may be enhanced if trazodone is administered with other CNS depressants.

• Nefazodone may increase the digoxin level if administered with digoxin. It increases CNS depression when combined with CNS depressants. (See *Adverse reactions to miscellaneous antidepressants.*)

# Lithium

*Lithium carbonate* and *lithium citrate* are used to prevent or treat mania. The discovery of lithium was a milestone in treating mania and bipolar disorders.

## Pharmacokinetics

When taken orally, lithium is absorbed rapidly and completely and is distributed to body tissues.

### Metabolism and excretion

An active drug, lithium isn't metabolized and is excreted from the body unchanged.

## Pharmacodynamics

It's theorized that in mania, the patient experiences excessive catecholamine stimulation. In bipolar disorder, the patient is affected by swings between the excessive catecholamine stimulation of mania and the diminished catecholamine stimulation of depression.

### Returning to normal

Lithium's exact mechanism of action is unknown. It may regulate catecholamine release in the CNS by:

• increasing norepinephrine and serotonin uptake
• reducing the release of norepinephrine from the synaptic vesicles (where neurotransmitters are stored) in the presynaptic neuron
• inhibiting norepinephrine's action in the postsynaptic neuron.

### Getting more of the message

Researchers are also examining lithium's effects on electrolyte and ion transport. Lithium may also modify the actions of second messengers such as cyclic adenosine monophosphate.

### Pharmacotherapeutics

Lithium is used primarily to treat acute episodes of mania and to prevent relapses of bipolar disorders.

## Under investigation

Other uses of lithium being researched include preventing unipolar depression and migraine headaches and treating depression, alcohol dependence, anorexia nervosa, syndrome of inappropriate antidiuretic hormone, and neutropenia.

## No margin for error

Lithium has a narrow therapeutic margin of safety. A blood level that is even slightly higher than the therapeutic level can be dangerous.

### Drug interactions

Serious interactions with other drugs can occur because of lithium's narrow therapeutic range:
• The risk of lithium toxicity increases when lithium is taken with thiazide and loop diuretics and nonsteroidal anti-inflammatory drugs.
• Administration of lithium with haloperidol, phenothiazines, or carbamazepine may increase the risk of neurotoxicity.
• Lithium may increase the hypothyroid effects of potassium iodide.
• Sodium bicarbonate may increase lithium excretion, reducing its effects.
• Lithium's effects are reduced when lithium is taken with theophylline.

## Take this with a grain (or more) of salt

A patient on a severe salt-restricted diet is susceptible to lithium toxicity. On the other hand, an increased intake of sodium may reduce the therapeutic effects of lithium. (See *Adverse reactions to lithium*.)

### Warning!

## Adverse reactions to lithium

Common adverse reactions to lithium include:
• reversible electrocardiogram changes
• thirst
• polyuria
• elevated white blood cell count.

**A flood in the blood**
Elevated toxic blood levels of lithium may produce:
• confusion
• lethargy
• slurred speech
• increased reflex reactions
• seizures.

# Antipsychotic drugs

A regular salt intake helps to maintain steady lithium levels.

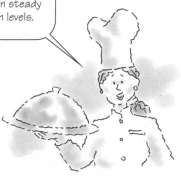

*Antipsychotic drugs* can control psychotic symptoms, such as delusions and hallucinations, and thought disorders that can occur with schizophrenia, mania, and other psychoses.

## By any other name

Drugs used to treat psychoses have several different names, including:
• antipsychotic, because they can eliminate signs and symptoms of psychoses
• major tranquilizer, because they can calm an agitated patient
• neuroleptic, because they have an adverse neurobiologic effect that causes abnormal body movements.

## Two major groups

Regardless of what they're called, all antipsychotic drugs belong to one of two major groups:

atypical antipsychotics, which include aripiprazole, clozapine, olanzapine, paliperidone, quetiapine, risperidone, and ziprasidone

typical antipsychotics, which include phenothiazines and nonphenothiazines.

# Atypical antipsychotics

*Atypical antipsychotic drugs* are agents designed to treat schizophrenia. They include aripiprazole, clozapine, olanzapine, paliperidone, quetiapine, risperidone, and ziprasidone.

## Pharmacokinetics

Atypical antipsychotics are absorbed after oral administration.

### Metabolism and excretion

Atypical antipsychotics are metabolized by the liver. Metabolites of clozapine, olanzapine, quetiapine, and ziprasidone are inactive, whereas risperidone and paliperidone have active metabolites. They're highly plasma protein-bound and eliminated in urine, with a small portion eliminated in stool.

## Pharmacodynamics

Atypical antipsychotics typically block the dopamine receptors, but to a lesser extent than the typical antipsychotics, resulting in far fewer extrapyramidal adverse effects. Additionally, atypical antipsychotics block serotonin receptor activity.

## Putting it together

These combined actions account for their effectiveness against the positive and negative symptoms of schizophrenia with minimal extrapyramidal effects.

## Pharmacotherapeutics

Atypical antipsychotics are considered the first line of treatment for patients with schizophrenia because of equal or improved effectiveness combined with improved tolerability.

## Lower doses do for dementia

Atypical antipsychotics are commonly used to treat behavioral and psychotic symptoms in patients with dementia. Dosages are significantly lower for these patients than for patients with schizophrenia.

## Drug interactions

Drugs that alter the P-450 enzyme system alter the metabolism of some atypical antipsychotics.

## The straight "dopa"

Atypical antipsychotics counteract the effects of levodopa and other dopamine agonists. (See *Adverse reactions to atypical antipsychotics.*)

---

*Warning!*

## Adverse reactions to atypical antipsychotics

Atypical antipsychotics have fewer extrapyramidal effects than typical antipsychotics and carry a minimal risk for seizures (except for clozapine).

**Aripiprazole**
Aripiprazole is a newer atypical antipsychotic and may produce mild sedation.

**Clozapine**
Clozapine is associated with agranulocytosis (an abnormal decrease in white blood cells). Weight gain is common, and seizures may also occur.

**Olanzapine**
Olanzapine places the patient at minimal risk for extrapyramidal effects. Weight gain is common.

**Quetiapine**
Quetiapine is associated with sedation.

**Risperidone and paliperidone**
Risperidone and paliperidone have a higher risk of extrapyramidal effects than other atypical antipsychotics, especially when prescribed at doses at the higher range of normal.

**Ziprasidone**
Because ziprasidone may cause electrocardiogram changes, it's usually recommended as an alternative therapy only after the patient has failed to respond to other atypical antipsychotics.

# Typical antipsychotics

*Typical antipsychotics*, which include phenothiazines and non-phenothiazines, can be broken down into smaller classifications.

## Different adverse reactions

Many clinicians believe that the phenothiazines should be treated as three distinct drug classes because of the differences in the adverse reactions they cause:
• Aliphatics primarily cause sedation and anticholinergic effects. They're low potency drugs that include chlorpromazine.
• Piperazines primarily cause extrapyramidal reactions and include fluphenazine decanoate, fluphenazine enanthate, fluphenazine hydrochloride, perphenazine, and trifluoperazine.
• Piperidines primarily cause sedation and anticholinergic and cardiac effects; they include mesoridazine and thioridazine.

## Different chemical structure

Based on their chemical structure, nonphenothiazine antipsychotics can be divided into several drug classes, including:
• butyrophenones, such as haloperidol and haloperidol decanoate
• dibenzoxazepines such as loxapine
• dihydroindolones such as molindone
• diphenylbutylpiperidines such as pimozide
• thioxanthenes, such as thiothixene and thiothixene hydrochloride.

## Pharmacokinetics

Although phenothiazines are absorbed erratically, they're very lipid-soluble and highly protein-bound. Therefore, they're distributed to many tissues and are highly concentrated in the brain.

Like phenothiazines, nonphenothiazines are absorbed erratically, are lipid-soluble, and are highly protein-bound. They're also distributed throughout the tissues and are highly concentrated in the brain.

### Metabolism and excretion

All phenothiazines are metabolized in the liver and excreted in urine and bile. Because fatty tissues slowly release accumulated phenothiazine metabolites into the plasma, phenothiazines may produce effects up to 3 months after they're stopped.

Nonphenothiazines are also metabolized in the liver and excreted in urine and bile.

## Pharmacodynamics

Although the mechanism of action of phenothiazines isn't fully understood, researchers believe that these drugs work by blocking postsynaptic dopaminergic receptors in the brain.

The mechanism of action of nonphenothiazines resembles that of phenothiazines.

### Erecting a blockade

The antipsychotic effect of phenothiazines is due to receptor blockade in the limbic system. Their antiemetic effect is due to receptor blockade in the chemoreceptor trigger zone located in the brain's medulla.

### Sending a charge

Phenothiazines also stimulate the extrapyramidal system (motor pathways that connect the cerebral cortex with the spinal nerve pathways).

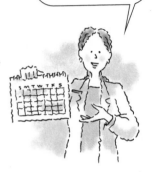

Phenothiazines may produce effects up to 3 months after they're stopped.

## Pharmacotherapeutics

Phenothiazines are used primarily to:
• treat schizophrenia
• calm anxious or agitated patients
• improve a patient's thought processes
• alleviate delusions and hallucinations.

### Working overtime

Other therapeutic uses have been found for phenothiazines:
• They're administered to treat other psychiatric disorders, such as brief reactive psychosis, atypical psychosis, schizoaffective psychosis, autism, and major depression with psychosis.
• In combination with lithium, they're used in the treatment of patients with bipolar disorder, until the slower-acting lithium produces its therapeutic effect.
• They're prescribed to quiet mentally challenged children and agitated geriatric patients, particularly those with dementia.
• The preoperative effects of analgesics may be boosted with their addition.
• They're helpful in the management of pain, anxiety, and nausea in patients with cancer.

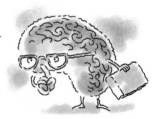

Phenothiazines are sometimes prescribed to quiet mentally challenged children and agitated geriatric patients.

### Solo solutions

As a group, nonphenothiazines are used to treat psychotic disorders. Thiothixene is also used to control acute agitation. Haloperidol and pimozide may also be used to treat Tourette syndrome.

## Drug interactions

Phenothiazines interact with many different types of drugs and may have serious effects:
• Increased CNS depressant effects, such as stupor, may occur when phenothiazines are taken with CNS depressants.
• CNS depressants may reduce phenothiazine effectiveness, resulting in increased psychotic behavior or agitation.
• Taking anticholinergic drugs with phenothiazines may result in increased anticholinergic effects, such as dry mouth and constipation. By increasing phenothiazine metabolism, anticholinergic drugs may also reduce the antipsychotic effects of phenothiazines.
• Phenothiazines may reduce the antiparkinsonian effects of levodopa.
• Concurrent use with lithium increases the risk of neurotoxicity.
• Concurrent use with droperidol increases the risk of extrapyramidal effects.
• The threshold for seizures is lowered when phenothiazines are used with anticonvulsants.
• Phenothiazines may increase the serum levels of TCAs and beta-adrenergic blockers. Thioridazine can cause serious, even fatal, cardiac arrhythmias when combined with such drugs as fluvoxamine, propranolol, pindolol, and fluoxetine that inhibit the cytochrome P-450 2D6 isoenzyme, or drugs known to prolong the QTc interval. (See *Adverse reactions to typical antipsychotics*.)

*Warning!*

## Adverse reactions to typical antipsychotics

Neurologic reactions are the most common and serious adverse reactions associated with phenothiazines.

### Extrapyramidal symptoms
Extrapyramidal symptoms (EPS) may appear after the first few days of therapy; tardive dyskinesia may occur after several years of treatment.

### S.O.S.! Extreme EPS!
Neuroleptic malignant syndrome is a potentially fatal condition that produces muscle rigidity, extreme EPS, severely elevated body temperature, hypertension, and rapid heart rate. If left untreated, it can result in respiratory failure and cardiovascular collapse.

### Little difference
Most nonphenothiazines cause the same adverse reactions as phenothiazines.

### Special caution
Antipsychotics with anticholinergic properties should be avoided in elderly patients.

## Fewer interactions

Nonphenothiazines interact with fewer drugs than phenothiazines. Their dopamine-blocking activity can inhibit levodopa and may cause disorientation in patients receiving both medications. Haloperidol may boost the effects of lithium, producing encephalopathy (brain dysfunction).

# Stimulants

Stimulants are used to treat attention deficit hyperactivity disorder (ADHD), a condition characterized by inattention, impulsivity, and hyperactivity. They include:
- dextroamphetamine
- lisdexamfetamine
- methylphenidate
- mixed amphetamine salts
- modafinil.

## Pharmacokinetics

Stimulants are well absorbed from the GI tract and are distributed widely in the body. Methylphenidate undergoes significant first pass effect.

### Metabolism and excretion

Stimulants are metabolized in the liver and excreted primarily in urine.

## Pharmacodynamics

These drugs are believed to work by increasing levels of dopamine and norepinephrine in one of three ways: by blocking the reuptake of dopamine and norepinephrine, by enhancing the presynaptic release, or by inhibiting MAO.

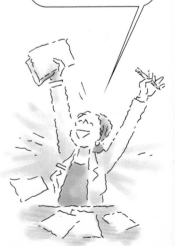

Stimulants are used to help patients with ADHD improve school and work performance.

## Pharmacotherapeutics

Stimulants are the treatment of choice for ADHD. They're helpful in improving attention, leading to improved school or work performance, and decreasing impulsivity and hyperactivity, if present. Pemoline, however, is no longer a first line choice for treatment of ADHD because it can cause hepatotoxicity.

Dextroamphetamine and methylphenidate are also used in the treatment of narcolepsy.

**Warning!**

## Adverse reactions to stimulants

Adverse reactions to stimulants are listed below.

**Dextroamphetamine and lisdexamfetamine**
- Restlessness
- Tremor
- Insomnia
- Tachycardia
- Palpitations
- Arrhythmias
- Dry mouth
- Unpleasant taste
- Diarrhea

**Methylphenidate**
- Dizziness
- Insomnia
- Seizures
- Palpitations
- Arrhythmias
- Abdominal pain
- Rash
- Thrombocytopenia

**Mixed amphetamine salts**
- Restlessness
- Insomnia
- Hyperexcitability
- Palpitations
- Arrhythmias
- Tremor
- Abdominal pain
- Dry mouth
- Unpleasant taste

**Measure up**
Stimulants may affect growth; children should be monitored closely for height and weight changes.

**Take a holiday**
Drug holidays are recommended every year to assess the continued need for a stimulant.

### Drug interactions
- Methylphenidate may decrease the effect of guanethidine and may increase the effects of TCAs, warfarin, and some anticonvulsant drugs.
- Stimulants shouldn't be used within 14 days of discontinuing therapy with an MAOI.
- Stimulants are highly abused substances, and close monitoring is required. (See *Adverse reactions to stimulants*.)

# Quick quiz

1. What's the difference between a sedative and a hypnotic?
   A. Sedatives produce physical dependence; hypnotics don't.
   B. Sedatives reduce anxiety or excitement; hypnotics induce sleep.
   C. Sedatives require larger doses than hypnotics to produce desired effects.
   D. Sedatives increase anxiety; hypnotics reduce anxiety.

*Answer:* B. Sedatives reduce anxiety or excitement; hypnotics induce sleep.

**2.**    With the use of the nonbenzodiazepine-nonbarbiturate chloral hydrate, what adverse reactions are most likely?

    A.    Severe withdrawal symptoms

    B.    Hypersensitivity reactions

    C.    Cardiac adverse effects

    D.    GI symptoms and hangover effects

*Answer:*    D. GI symptoms and hangover effects are common adverse reactions to chloral hydrate.

**3.**    Which medication should a patient treated with lithium avoid?

    A.    Hormonal contraceptives

    B.    Loop diuretics

    C.    Oral antidiabetic drugs

    D.    Antihypertensive drugs

*Answer:*    B. Lithium shouldn't be prescribed with loop diuretics.

## Scoring

★★★    If you answered all three items correctly, extraordinary! You definitely aren't psyched out by pharmacology!

★★    If you answered two items correctly, congratulations! Your knowledge should have you feeling elated!

★    If you answered fewer than two items correctly, there's no need for anxiety! By the end of the next chapter, you'll probably have your head on straight!

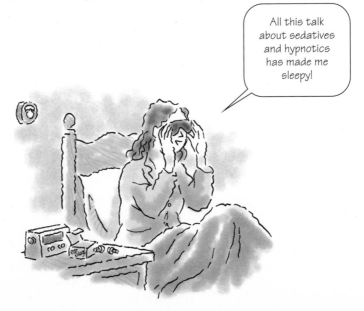

All this talk about sedatives and hypnotics has made me sleepy!

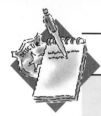

# 13

## Endocrine drugs

### Just the facts

In this chapter, you'll learn:

♦ classes of drugs that affect the endocrine system

♦ uses and varying actions of these drugs

♦ how these drugs are absorbed, distributed, metabolized, and excreted

♦ drug interactions and adverse reactions to these drugs.

## Drugs and the endocrine system

The endocrine system consists of *glands*, which are specialized cell clusters, and *hormones*, the chemical transmitters secreted by the glands in response to stimulation.

### Keeping well balanced

Together with the central nervous system, the endocrine system regulates and integrates the body's metabolic activities and maintains homeostasis (the body's internal equilibrium). The drug classes that treat endocrine system disorders include:
• natural hormones and their synthetic analogues
• hormonelike substances
• drugs that stimulate or suppress hormone secretion.

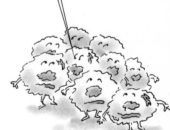

We're special. We help make up glands, which are a part of the endocrine system.

## Antidiabetic drugs and glucagon

Insulin, a pancreatic hormone, and oral antidiabetic drugs are classified as *hypoglycemic drugs* because they lower blood glucose levels. Glucagon, another pancreatic hormone, is classified as a *hyperglycemic drug* because it raises blood glucose levels.

## Sugar surplus

Diabetes mellitus, or simply diabetes, is a chronic disease of insulin deficiency or resistance. It's characterized by disturbances in carbohydrate, protein, and fat metabolism. This leads to elevated levels of the sugar glucose in the body. The disease appears in two primary forms:

☝ type 1, previously referred to as insulin-dependent diabetes mellitus

✌ type 2, previously referred to as non-insulin-dependent diabetes mellitus.

# Insulin

Patients with type 1 diabetes require an external source of *insulin* to control blood glucose levels. Insulin may also be given to patients with type 2 diabetes.

Types of insulin include:
- rapid-acting: lispro
- short-acting: regular
- intermediate-acting: NPH
- long-acting: Ultralente.

## Pharmacokinetics (how drugs circulate)

Insulin isn't effective when taken orally because the GI tract breaks down the protein molecule before it reaches the bloodstream.

### Under the skin

All insulins, however, may be given by subcutaneous (subQ) injection. Absorption of subQ insulin varies according to the injection site, the blood supply, and degree of tissue hypertrophy at the injection site.

### In the I.V. league

Regular insulin may also be given by I.V. infusion as well as in dialysate fluid infused into the peritoneal cavity for patients on peritoneal dialysis therapy.

### Distribution, metabolism, and excretion

After absorption into the bloodstream, insulin is distributed throughout the body. Insulin-responsive tissues are located in the liver, adipose tissue, and muscle. Insulin is metabolized primarily in the liver and to a lesser extent in the kidneys and muscle, and it's excreted in stool and urine.

*Now I get it!*

## How insulin aids glucose uptake

These illustrations show how insulin allows a cell to use glucose for energy.

Glucose can't enter the cell without the aid of insulin.

Normally produced by the beta cells of the pancreas, insulin binds to the receptors on the surface of the target cell. Insulin and its receptor first move to the inside of the cell, which activates glucose transporter channels to move to the surface of the cell.

These channels allow glucose to enter the cell. The cell can then use the glucose for metabolism.

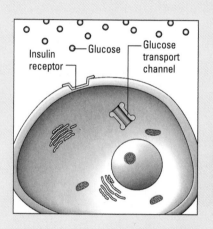

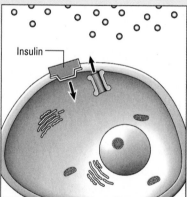

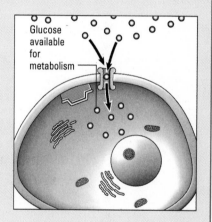

## Pharmacodynamics (how drugs act)

Insulin is an anabolic, or building, hormone that helps:
- promote storage of glucose as glycogen
- increase protein and fat synthesis
- slow the breakdown of glycogen, protein, and fat
- balance fluids and electrolytes.

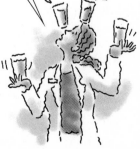

*Insulin can help balance fluids and electrolytes!*

### Insulin's special effects

Although it has no antidiuretic effect, insulin can correct the polyuria (excessive urination) and polydipsia (excessive thirst) associated with the osmotic diuresis that occurs in hyperglycemia by decreasing the blood glucose level. Insulin also facilitates the movement of potassium from the extracellular fluid into the cell. (See *How insulin aids glucose uptake.*)

## Pharmacotherapeutics (how drugs are used)

Insulin is indicated for:
- type 1 diabetes
- type 2 diabetes when other methods of controlling blood glucose levels have failed or are contraindicated
- type 2 diabetes when blood glucose levels are elevated during periods of emotional or physical stress (such as infection and surgery)
- type 2 diabetes when oral antidiabetic drugs are contraindicated because of pregnancy or hypersensitivity
- gestational diabetes.

### When things get complicated

Insulin is also used to treat two complications of diabetes: diabetic ketoacidosis, more common with type 1 diabetes, and hyperosmolar hyperglycemic nonketotic syndrome, which is more common with type 2 diabetes.

### What? But I don't have diabetes...

Insulin is also used to treat severe hyperkalemia (elevated serum potassium levels) in patients without diabetes. Potassium moves with glucose from the bloodstream into the cell, lowering serum potassium levels.

## Drug interactions

Some drugs interact with insulin, altering its ability to decrease the blood glucose level; other drugs directly affect glucose levels:
- Anabolic steroids, salicylates, alcohol, and monoamine oxidase inhibitors (MAOIs) may increase the hypoglycemic effect of insulin.
- Corticosteroids, sympathomimetic drugs, thiazide diuretics, and dextrothyroxine sodium may reduce the effects of insulin, resulting in hyperglycemia.
- Beta-adrenergic blockers may prolong the hypoglycemic effect of insulin and may mask signs and symptoms of hypoglycemia. (See *Adverse reactions to insulin.*)

---

# Oral antidiabetic drugs

Many types of *oral antidiabetic drugs* are approved for use in the United States. Types of available oral antidiabetic drugs include:
- first-generation sulfonylureas, which include acetohexamide, chlorpropamide, tolazamide, and tolbutamide
- second-generation sulfonylureas, which include gliclazide, glipizide, glimepiride, and glyburide.

**Warning!**

## Adverse reactions to insulin

Adverse reactions to insulin include:
- hypoglycemia (below-normal blood glucose levels)
- Somogyi effect (hypoglycemia followed by rebound hyperglycemia)
- hypersensitivity reactions
- lipodystrophy (disturbance in fat deposition)
- insulin resistance.

- thiazolidinediones, which include pioglitazone and rosiglitazone
- a biguanide drug, metformin
- alpha-glucosidase inhibitors, which include acarbose and miglitol
- a meglitinide drug, repaglinide
- an amino acid derivative, nateglinide
- combination therapies, which include glipizide and metformin, glyburide and metformin, and rosiglitazone and metformin.

## Pharmacokinetics

Oral antidiabetic drugs are well absorbed from the GI tract and distributed via the bloodstream throughout the body. Because repaglinide has a short duration of action, it's given before meals.

### Metabolism and excretion

Oral antidiabetic drugs are metabolized primarily in the liver and are excreted mostly in urine, with some excreted in bile. Glyburide is excreted equally in urine and stool; rosiglitazone and pioglitazone are largely excreted in both.

## Pharmacodynamics

It's believed that oral antidiabetic drugs produce actions both within and outside the pancreas (extrapancreatic) to regulate blood glucose.

### Pancreas partners

Oral antidiabetic drugs probably stimulate pancreatic beta cells to release insulin in a patient with a minimally functioning pancreas. Within a few weeks to a few months of starting sulfonylureas, pancreatic insulin secretion drops to pretreatment levels, but blood glucose levels remain normal or near-normal. Most likely, it's the actions of the oral antidiabetic agents outside of the pancreas that maintain this glucose control.

### Working beyond the pancreas

Oral antidiabetic drugs provide several extrapancreatic actions to decrease and control blood glucose. They can go to work in the liver and decrease glucose production (gluconeogenesis) there. Also, by increasing the number of insulin receptors in the peripheral tissues, they provide more opportunities for the cells to bind sufficiently with insulin, initiating the process of glucose metabolism.

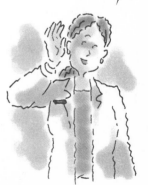

What's that? Aha! Oral antidiabetic drugs work in and out of the pancreas to regulate glucose levels.

## Getting in on the action

Other oral antidiabetic agents produce specific actions:

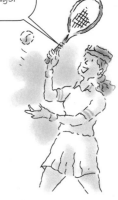

If diet and exercise don't work, it might be time for oral antidiabetic drugs.

• Pioglitazone and rosiglitazone improve insulin sensitivity and lower glucose production by the liver.
• Metformin decreases liver production and intestinal absorption of glucose and improves insulin sensitivity.
• Acarbose and miglitol inhibit enzymes, delaying glucose absorption.
• Repaglinide and nateglinide increase insulin secretion.

## Pharmacotherapeutics

Oral antidiabetic drugs are indicated for patients with type 2 diabetes if diet and exercise can't control blood glucose levels. These drugs aren't effective in patients with type 1 diabetes because the patients' pancreatic beta cells aren't functioning at a minimal level.

### The old 1-2 punch

Combinations of multiple oral antidiabetic drugs or an oral antidiabetic drug with insulin therapy may be indicated for some patients who don't respond to either therapy alone. (See *Cautionary tales*.)

## Drug interactions

Hypoglycemia and hyperglycemia are the main risks when oral antidiabetic drugs interact with other drugs.

### Getting too low

Hypoglycemia may occur when sulfonylureas are combined with alcohol, anabolic steroids, chloramphenicol, cimetidine, clofibrate, coumadin, fluconazole, gemfibrozil, MAOIs, phenylbutazone, ranitidine, salicylates, or sulfonamides. It may also occur when metformin is combined with cimetidine, nifedipine, procainamide, ranitidine, or vancomycin. Hypoglycemia is less likely to occur when metformin is used as a single agent.

### Going too high

Hyperglycemia may occur when sulfonylureas are taken with corticosteroids, dextrothyroxine, rifampin, sympathomimetics, and thiazide diuretics.

Because metformin given with iodinated contrast dyes can cause acute renal failure, metformin doses should be withheld in patients undergoing procedures that require I.V. contrast dye and

**Safe and sound**

## Cautionary tales

To maintain blood glucose levels as close to normal as possible, pregnant women should avoid oral antidiabetic agents. Insulin therapy is recommended instead.

Because aging is commonly associated with a decline in kidney function, and because the kidneys substantially excrete metformin, metformin should be used with caution in elderly patients. Patients with renal and hepatic impairment should also avoid metformin.

not restarted for at least 48 hours after the procedure. (See *Adverse reactions to oral antidiabetic drugs.*)

# Glucagon

*Glucagon,* a hyperglycemic drug that raises blood glucose levels, is a hormone normally produced by the alpha cells of the islets of Langerhans in the pancreas. (See *How glucagon raises glucose levels,* page 346.)

## Pharmacokinetics

After subQ, I.M., or I.V. injection, glucagon is absorbed rapidly. Glucagon is distributed throughout the body, although its effect occurs primarily in the liver.

### Metabolism and excretion

Glucagon is degraded extensively by the liver, kidneys, and plasma, and at its tissue receptor sites in plasma membranes. It's removed from the body by the liver and the kidneys.

## Pharmacodynamics

Glucagon regulates the rate of glucose production through:
• glycogenolysis, the conversion of glycogen back into glucose by the liver
• gluconeogenesis, the formation of glucose from free fatty acids and proteins
• lipolysis, the release of fatty acids from adipose tissue for conversion to glucose.

## Pharmacotherapeutics

Glucagon is used for emergency treatment of severe hypoglycemia. It's also used during radiologic examination of the GI tract to reduce GI motility.

## Drug interactions

Glucagon interacts adversely only with oral anticoagulants, increasing the tendency to bleed. Adverse reactions to glucagon are rare.

*Warning!*

**Adverse reactions to oral antidiabetic drugs**

Hypoglycemia is a major adverse reaction to oral antidiabetic drugs, especially when combination therapy is used. Here are some common adverse reactions to individual oral antidiabetic drugs.

**Sulfonylureas**
• Nausea
• Epigastric fullness
• Blood abnormalities
• Water retention
• Rash
• Hyponatremia
• Photosensitivity

**Metformin**
• Metallic taste
• Nausea and vomiting
• Abdominal discomfort

**Acarbose**
• Abdominal pain
• Diarrhea
• Flatulence

**Thiazolidinediones**
• Weight gain
• Swelling

*Now I get it!*

# How glucagon raises glucose levels

When adequate stores of glycogen are present, glucagon can raise glucose levels in patients with severe hypoglycemia. What happens is easy to follow:
• Initially, glucagon stimulates the formation of adenylate cyclase in the liver cell.
• Adenylate cyclase then converts adenosine triphosphate (ATP) to cyclic adenosine monophosphate (cAMP).

• This product initiates a series of reactions that result in an active phosphorylated glucose molecule.
• In this phosphorylated form, the large glucose molecule can't pass through the cell membrane.
• Through glycogenolysis (the breakdown of glycogen, the stored form of glucose), the liver removes the phosphate group and allows the glucose to enter the bloodstream, raising blood glucose levels for short-term energy needs.

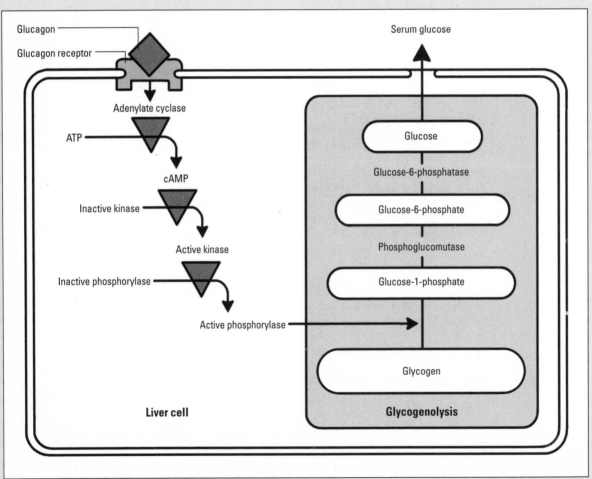

# Estrogens

*Estrogens* mimic the physiologic effects of naturally occurring female sex hormones.

## To serve and protect

Estrogens are used to correct estrogen-deficient states and, along with hormonal contraceptives, prevent pregnancy.

## Natural and synthetic estrogen

Estrogens that treat endocrine system disorders include:
• natural products, such as conjugated estrogenic substances, estradiol, and estropipate
• synthetic estrogens, such as esterified estrogens, estradiol cypionate, estradiol valerate, and ethinyl estradiol.

I take care of excretion...

...and I'm in charge of metabolism.

### Pharmacokinetics

Estrogens are well absorbed and distributed throughout the body. Metabolism occurs in the liver, and the metabolites are excreted primarily by the kidneys.

### Pharmacodynamics

The exact mechanism of action of estrogen isn't clearly understood, but it's believed to increase synthesis of deoxyribonucleic acid, ribonucleic acid, and protein in estrogen-responsive tissues in the female breast, urinary tract, and genital organs.

### Pharmacotherapeutics

Estrogens are prescribed:
• primarily for hormone replacement therapy in postmenopausal women to relieve symptoms caused by loss of ovarian function (see *Hormone replacement therapy and heart disease*, page 348)
• less commonly for hormonal replacement therapy in women with primary ovarian failure or female hypogonadism (reduced hormonal secretion by the ovaries), for prevention and treatment of osteoporosis in postmenopausal women, and in patients who have undergone surgical castration
• palliatively to treat advanced, inoperable breast cancer in postmenopausal women and prostate cancer in men.

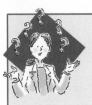

*Yea or nay?*

## Hormone replacement therapy and heart disease

Following a 5-year study, the Women's Health Initiative reported increased risks of myocardial infarction, stroke, breast cancer, pulmonary emboli, and deep vein thrombosis in women being treated with conjugated equine estrogens and progesterone as compared to those taking a placebo.

The U.S. Preventive Services Task Force recommends against the use of estrogen and progestin to prevent coronary heart disease in healthy women.

**What to do?**

Because the long-term safety of short-term therapy has yet to be determined, the Food and Drug Administration and American College of Obstetricians and Gynecologists recommend that women who choose to take hormone replacement therapy for menopausal symptoms use these drugs for the shortest duration possible and in the lowest possible dosages.

*Warning!*

## Adverse reactions to estrogens

Adverse reactions to estrogens include:
• hypertension
• thromboembolism (blood vessel blockage caused by a blood clot)
• thrombophlebitis (vein inflammation associated with clot formation).

## Drug interactions

Relatively few drugs interact with estrogens:
• Estrogens may decrease the effects of anticoagulants, increasing the risk of blood clots.
• Antibiotics, barbiturates, carbamazepine, phenytoin, primidone, and rifampin reduce estrogen effectiveness.
• Estrogens interfere with the absorption of dietary folic acid, which may result in a folic acid deficiency. (See *Adverse reactions to estrogens*.)

# Pituitary drugs

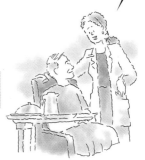

Estrogens can be used to treat prostate cancer in men.

*Pituitary drugs* are natural or synthetic hormones that mimic the hormones produced by the pituitary gland. The pituitary drugs consist of two groups:
• Anterior pituitary drugs may be used diagnostically or therapeutically to control the function of other endocrine glands, such as the thyroid gland, adrenals, ovaries, and testes.
• Posterior pituitary drugs may be used to regulate fluid volume and stimulate smooth-muscle contraction in selected clinical situations.

# Anterior pituitary drugs

The protein hormones produced in the anterior pituitary gland regulate growth, development, and sexual characteristics by stimulating the actions of other endocrine glands. *Anterior pituitary drugs* include:
- adrenocorticotropics, which include corticotropin, corticotropin repository, corticotropin zinc hydroxide, and cosyntropin
- somatrem and somatropin, growth hormones
- gonadotropics, which include chorionic gonadotropin and menotropins
- thyrotropics, which include thyroid-stimulating hormone, thyrotropin, and protirelin.

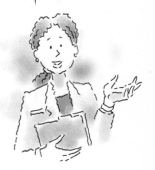

Anterior pituitary drugs act on endocrine glands to control their functions.

## Pharmacokinetics

Anterior pituitary drugs aren't given orally because they're destroyed in the GI tract. Some of these hormones can be administered topically, but most require injection.

### Absorption, distribution, and metabolism

Usually, natural hormones are absorbed, distributed, and metabolized rapidly. Some analogues, however, are absorbed and metabolized more slowly. Anterior pituitary hormone drugs are metabolized at the receptor site and in the liver and kidneys. The hormones are excreted primarily in urine.

## Pharmacodynamics

Anterior pituitary drugs exert a profound effect on the body's growth and development. The hypothalamus controls secretions of the pituitary gland. In turn, the pituitary gland secretes hormones that regulate secretions or functions of other glands.

## Concentrate on this formula

The concentration of hormones in the blood helps determine hormone production rate. Increased hormone levels inhibit hormone production; decreased levels raise production and secretion.

## Pharmacotherapeutics

Anterior pituitary hormone drugs are used for diagnostic and therapeutic purposes:
- Corticotropin and cosyntropin are used diagnostically to differentiate between primary and secondary failure of the adrenal cortex.
- Corticotropin is also used to treat adrenal insufficiency.
- Somatrem is used to treat growth hormone deficiency.

## Drug interactions

Anterior pituitary drugs interact with several types of drugs:
• Administering immunizations to a person receiving corticotropin increases the risk of neurologic complications and may reduce the antibody response.
• Corticotropin reduces salicylate levels.
• Enhanced potassium loss may occur when diuretics are taken with corticotropins.
• Barbiturates, phenytoin, and rifampin increase the metabolism of corticotropin, reducing its effects.

### Estrogen effects

• Estrogen increases the effect of corticotropin.
• Taking estrogens, amphetamines, and lithium with cosyntropin can alter results of adrenal function tests.
• Concurrent use of amphetamines and androgens with somatrem may promote epiphyseal closure (closure of the cartilaginous bone growth plate).
• Concurrent use of somatrem and corticosteroids inhibits the growth-promoting action of somatrem. (See *Adverse reactions to anterior pituitary drugs.*)

# Posterior pituitary drugs

*Posterior pituitary hormones* are synthesized in the hypothalamus and stored in the posterior pituitary, which, in turn, secretes the hormones into the blood. These drugs include:
• all forms of antidiuretic hormone (ADH), such as desmopressin acetate and vasopressin
• the oxytocic drug oxytocin.

## Pharmacokinetics

Because enzymes in the GI tract can destroy all protein hormones, these drugs can't be given orally. Posterior pituitary drugs may be given by injection or intranasal spray.

### Absorption, distribution, and metabolism

Like other natural hormones, oxytocic drugs are usually absorbed, distributed, and metabolized rapidly. Parenterally administered oxytocin is absorbed rapidly; however, when it's administered intranasally, absorption is erratic.

**Warning!**

## Adverse reactions to anterior pituitary drugs

The major adverse reactions to pituitary drugs are hypersensitivity reactions.

**Over the long haul**
Long-term use of corticotropin can cause Cushing's syndrome.

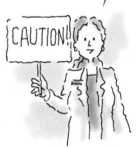

When giving certain drugs, you need to be careful to avoid some diuretics.

## Pharmacodynamics

Under neural control, posterior pituitary hormones affect:
- smooth-muscle contraction in the uterus, bladder, and GI tract
- fluid balance through kidney reabsorption of water
- blood pressure through stimulation of the arterial wall muscles.

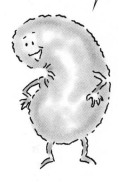

Without ADH, I can't reabsorb fluid.

### Going to cAMP

ADH increases cyclic adenosine monophosphate (cAMP), which increases the permeability of the tubular epithelium in the kidneys, promoting reabsorption of water. High dosages of ADH stimulate contraction of blood vessels, increasing the blood pressure.

Desmopressin reduces diuresis and promotes clotting by increasing the plasma level of factor VIII (antihemophilic factor).

### Baby talk

In pregnant women, oxytocin may stimulate uterine contractions by increasing the permeability of uterine cell membranes to sodium ions. It also can stimulate lactation through its effect on mammary glands.

## Pharmacotherapeutics

ADH is prescribed for hormone replacement therapy in patients with neurogenic diabetes insipidus (an excessive loss of urine caused by a brain lesion or injury that interferes with ADH synthesis or release). However, it doesn't effectively treat nephrogenic diabetes insipidus (caused by renal tubular resistance to ADH).

### The ABC's of ADH treatment

Desmopressin is the drug of choice for chronic ADH deficiency and is administered intranasally. It's also indicated for primary nocturnal enuresis. Desmopressin has a long duration of action and relatively few adverse effects.

Short-term ADH treatment is indicated for patients with transient diabetes insipidus after head injury or surgery; therapy may be lifelong for patients with idiopathic hormone deficiencies. Used for short-term therapy, vasopressin elevates blood pressure in patients with hypotension caused by lack of vascular tone. It also relieves postoperative gaseous distention.

### They help with deliveries (before, during, and after)

Oxytocics are used to:
- induce labor and complete incomplete abortions
- treat preeclampsia, eclampsia, and premature rupture of membranes
- control bleeding and uterine relaxation after delivery
- hasten uterine shrinking after delivery
- stimulate lactation.

## Warning!

## Adverse reactions to posterior pituitary drugs

Hypersensitivity reactions are the most common adverse reactions to posterior pituitary drugs.

**Natural ADH**
Anaphylaxis may occur after injection. Natural antidiuretic hormone (ADH) can also cause:
• ringing in the ears
• anxiety

• hyponatremia (low serum sodium levels)
• proteins in urine
• eclamptic attacks
• pupil dilation
• transient edema.

**Synthetic ADH**
Adverse reactions to synthetic ADH are rare.

### Drug interactions

A variety of drugs can cause interactions with posterior pituitary drugs:
• Alcohol, demeclocycline, epinephrine, and lithium may decrease the ADH activity of desmopressin and vasopressin.
• Chlorpropamide, clofibrate, carbamazepine, and cyclophosphamide increase ADH activity.
• Synergistic effects may occur when barbiturates or cyclopropane anesthetics are used concurrently with ADH, leading to coronary insufficiency or arrhythmias.
• Cyclophosphamide may increase the effect of oxytocin.
• Concurrent use of vasopressors (anesthetics, ephedrine, methoxamine) and oxytocin increases the risk of hypertensive crisis and postpartum rupture of cerebral blood vessels. (See *Adverse reactions to posterior pituitary drugs*.)

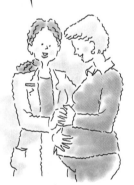

Oxytocin is used to induce labor and can also help with postdelivery problems.

# Thyroid and antithyroid drugs

*Thyroid* and *antithyroid drugs* function to correct thyroid hormone deficiency (hypothyroidism) and thyroid hormone excess (hyperthyroidism).

## Thyroid drugs

*Thyroid drugs* can be natural or synthetic hormones and may contain triiodothyronine ($T_3$), thyroxine ($T_4$), or both.

## All natural

Natural thyroid drugs are made from animal thyroid and include:
- thyroid USP (desiccated), which contains both $T_3$ and $T_4$
- thyroglobulin, which also contains both $T_3$ and $T_4$.

## Man-made

Synthetic thyroid drugs are actually the sodium salts of the L-isomers of the hormones. These synthetic hormones include:
- levothyroxine sodium, which contains $T_4$
- liothyronine sodium, which contains $T_3$
- liotrix, which contains both $T_3$ and $T_4$.

## Pharmacokinetics

Thyroid hormones are absorbed variably from the GI tract, distributed in plasma, and bound to serum proteins.

### Metabolism and excretion

Thyroid drugs are metabolized through deiodination, primarily in the liver, and excreted unchanged in stool.

## Pharmacodynamics

The principal pharmacologic effect is an increased metabolic rate in body tissues. Thyroid hormones affect protein and carbohydrate metabolism and stimulate protein synthesis. They promote gluconeogenesis (the formation of glucose from free fatty acids and proteins) and increase the use of glycogen stores.

## They get the heart pumping...

Thyroid hormones increase heart rate and cardiac output (the amount of blood pumped by the heart each minute). They may even increase the heart's sensitivity to catecholamines and increase the number of beta-adrenergic receptors in the heart (stimulation of beta receptors in the heart increases heart rate and contractility).

## ...and the blood flowing

Thyroid hormones may increase blood flow to the kidneys and increase the glomerular filtration rate (the amount of plasma filtered through the kidney each minute) in hypothyroid patients, producing diuresis.

## Pharmacotherapeutics

Thyroid drugs act as replacement or substitute hormones in these situations:

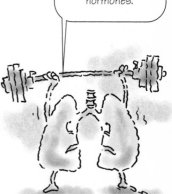

I can pump more and more with thyroid hormones.

**Warning!**

# Adverse reactions to thyroid drugs

Most adverse reactions to thyroid drugs result from toxicity.

**GI impact**
Adverse reactions in the GI system include:
• diarrhea
• abdominal cramps
• weight loss
• increased appetite.

**Heart of the matter**
Adverse reactions in the cardiovascular system include:
• palpitations
• sweating
• rapid heart rate
• increased blood pressure
• angina
• arrhythmias.

**Toxic topics**
General manifestations of toxic doses include:
• headache
• tremor
• insomnia
• nervousness
• fever
• heat intolerance
• menstrual irregularities.

• to treat the many forms of hypothyroidism
• with antithyroid drugs to prevent goiter formation (an enlarged thyroid gland) and hypothyroidism
• to differentiate between primary and secondary hypothyroidism during diagnostic testing
• to treat papillary or follicular thyroid carcinoma.

## The drug of choice

Levothyroxine is the drug of choice for thyroid hormone replacement and thyroid-stimulating hormone suppression therapy.

## Drug interactions

Thyroid drugs interact with several common medications. (See *Adverse reactions to thyroid drugs.*)
• They increase the effects of oral anticoagulants, increasing the tendency to bleed.
• Cholestyramine and colestipol reduce the absorption of thyroid hormones.
• Phenytoin may displace thyroxine from plasma-binding sites, temporarily increasing levels of free thyroxine.
• Taking thyroid drugs with digoxin may reduce serum digoxin levels, increasing the risk of arrhythmias or heart failure.
• Carbamazepine, phenytoin, phenobarbital, and rifampin increase metabolism of thyroid hormones, reducing their effectiveness.
• Serum theophylline levels may increase when theophylline is administered with thyroid drugs.

# Antithyroid drugs

A number of drugs act as *antithyroid drugs*, or *thyroid antagonists*. Used for patients with hyperthyroidism (thyrotoxicosis), these drugs include:
- thioamides, which include propylthiouracil and methimazole
- iodides, which include stable iodine and radioactive iodine.

## Pharmacokinetics

Thioamides and iodides are absorbed through the GI tract, concentrated in the thyroid, metabolized by conjugation, and excreted in urine.

## Pharmacodynamics

Drugs used to treat hyperthyroidism work in different ways.

### The antithesis to synthesis

Thioamides block iodine's ability to combine with tyrosine, thereby preventing thyroid hormone synthesis.

### In Wolff (-Chaikoff)'s clothing

Stable iodine inhibits hormone synthesis through the Wolff-Chaikoff effect, in which excess iodine decreases the formation and release of thyroid hormone.

### Warning: Radioactive material

Radioactive iodine reduces hormone secretion by destroying thyroid tissue through induction of acute radiation thyroiditis (inflammation of the thyroid gland) and chronic gradual thyroid atrophy. Acute radiation thyroiditis usually occurs 3 to 10 days after administering radioactive iodine. Chronic thyroid atrophy may take several years to appear.

> In the Wolff-Chaikoff effect, excess iodine decreases the formation and release of thyroid hormone.

## Pharmacotherapeutics

Antithyroid drugs are commonly used to treat hyperthyroidism, especially in the form of Graves' disease (hyperthyroidism caused by autoimmunity), which accounts for 85% of all cases.

### In case of removal

To treat hyperthyroidism, the thyroid gland may be removed by surgery or destroyed by radiation. Before surgery, stable iodine is used to prepare the gland for surgical removal by firming it and decreasing its vascularity.

Stable iodine is also used after radioactive iodine therapy to control symptoms of hyperthyroidism while the radiation takes effect.

### If it gets too severe

Propylthiouracil, which lowers serum $T_3$ levels faster than methimazole, is usually used for rapid improvement of severe hyperthyroidism.

### When taking them for two

Propylthiouracil is preferred over methimazole in pregnant women because its rapid action reduces transfer across the placental barrier and it doesn't cause aplasia cutis (a severe skin disorder) in the fetus.

Propylthiouracil and methimazole appear in breast milk, so it's recommended that mothers taking these drugs shouldn't breast-feed. If a breast-feeding woman must take one of these drugs, propylthiouracil is the preferred drug.

### One a day keeps the trouble away

Because methimazole blocks thyroid hormone formation for a longer time, it's better suited for administration once per day to patients with mild to moderate hyperthyroidism. Therapy may continue for 12 to 24 months before remission occurs.

## Drug interactions

Iodide preparations may react synergistically with lithium, causing hypothyroidism. Other interactions aren't clinically significant. (See *Adverse reactions to antithyroid drugs.*)

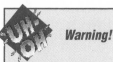

**Warning!**

## Adverse reactions to antithyroid drugs

The most serious adverse reaction to thioamide therapy is granulocytopenia. Hypersensitivity reactions may also occur.

**In bad taste**
The iodides can cause an unpleasant brassy taste and burning sensation in the mouth, increased salivation, and painful swelling of the parotid glands.

**Too sensitive**
Rarely, I.V. iodine administration can cause an acute hypersensitivity reaction. Radioactive iodine also can cause a rare—but acute—reaction 3 to 14 days after administration.

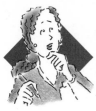

# Quick quiz

**1.** How does insulin lower the blood glucose level?
  A.   It prevents glucose absorption from the GI tract.
  B.   It increases glucose excretion from the GI tract.
  C.   It increases glucose absorption.
  D.   It promotes the transport of glucose into cells.

*Answer:*   D. Insulin promotes the transport of glucose into cells.

**2.** Why can't glucagon be given orally?
  A.   It works too slowly when given orally.
  B.   It's destroyed by the GI tract.
  C.   It's absorbed unpredictably.
  D.   It's too caustic to the GI tract.

*Answer:*   B. Glucagon is destroyed by the GI tract.

**3.** Which signs indicate that a patient taking levothyroxine is experiencing thyroid toxicity?
  A.   Diarrhea and weight loss
  B.   Weight gain and constipation
  C.   Slow heart rate and low blood pressure
  D.   Irregular heart rate and low blood pressure

*Answer:*   A. Diarrhea and weight loss are signs of thyroid toxicity in a patient taking levothyroxine.

**4.** The posterior pituitary drug used to stimulate uterine contractions is:
  A.   vasopressin.
  B.   oxytocin.
  C.   desmopressin.
  D.   estrogen.

*Answer:*   B. Oxytocin stimulates uterine contractions by increasing permeability of uterine cell membranes to sodium ions. It can also stimulate lactation.

**5.** Estrogens are sometimes prescribed to treat which condition in men?
  A.   Renal cancer
  B.   Testicular cancer
  C.   Colorectal cancer
  D.   Prostate cancer

*Answer:*   D. Estrogens are sometimes prescribed for palliative treatment of prostate cancer.

## Scoring

☆☆☆ If you answered all five items correctly, extraordinary! You're hyper-knowledgeable about hyperglycemic drugs and more!

☆☆ If you answered four items correctly, congratulations! You have a well-balanced understanding of pharmacology!

☆ If you answered fewer than four items correctly, keep trying! You have two more Quick quizzes to go!

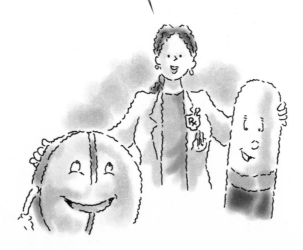

# Drugs for fluid and electrolyte balance

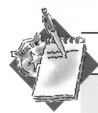

## Just the facts

In this chapter, you'll learn:

♦ classes of drugs that affect fluid and electrolyte balance

♦ uses and varying actions of these drugs

♦ how these drugs are absorbed, distributed, metabolized, and excreted

♦ drug interactions and adverse reactions to these drugs.

## Drugs and homeostasis

Illness can easily disturb the homeostatic mechanisms that help maintain normal fluid and electrolyte balance. Such occurrences as loss of appetite, medication administration, vomiting, diarrhea, surgery, and diagnostic tests can also alter this delicate balance. Fortunately, numerous drugs can be used to correct these imbalances and help bring the body back to homeostasis.

## Electrolyte replacement drugs

An electrolyte is a compound or element that carries an electrical charge when dissolved in water. *Electrolyte replacement drugs* are inorganic or organic salts that increase depleted or deficient electrolyte levels, helping to maintain homeostasis, the stability of body fluid composition and volume. They include:

• potassium, the primary intracellular fluid (ICF) electrolyte

• calcium, a major extracellular fluid (ECF) electrolyte

• magnesium, an electrolyte essential for homeostasis found in ICF

• sodium, the principal electrolyte in ECF necessary for homeostasis.

> Look out! An electrolyte carries an electrical charge when it's dissolved in water.

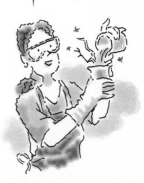

# Potassium

*Potassium* is the major positively charged ion (cation) in ICF. Because the body can't store potassium, adequate amounts must be ingested daily. If this isn't possible, potassium replacement can be accomplished orally or I.V. with potassium salts, such as:

- potassium acetate
- potassium bicarbonate
- potassium chloride
- potassium gluconate
- potassium phosphate.

## Pharmacokinetics (how drugs circulate)

Oral potassium is absorbed readily from the GI tract.

### Absorption, metabolism, and excretion

After absorption into the ECF, almost all of the potassium passes into the ICF. There, the enzyme adenosinetriphosphatase maintains the concentration of potassium by pumping sodium out of the cell in exchange for potassium.

Normal serum levels of potassium are maintained by the kidneys, which excrete most excess potassium intake. The rest is excreted in stool and sweat.

## Pharmacodynamics (how drugs act)

Potassium moves quickly into ICF to restore depleted potassium levels and reestablish balance. It's an essential element in determining cell membrane potential and excitability.

### Feel nervous about potassium?

Potassium is necessary for proper functioning of all nerve and muscle cells and for nerve impulse transmission. It's also essential for tissue growth and repair and for maintenance of acid-base balance.

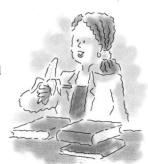

Because the body can't store potassium, I make sure I eat adequate amounts every day. This banana is a good source of potassium.

## Pharmacotherapeutics (how drugs are used)

Potassium replacement therapy corrects hypokalemia, low levels of potassium in the blood. Hypokalemia is a common occurrence in conditions that increase potassium excretion or depletion, such as:

- vomiting, diarrhea, or nasogastric suction
- excessive urination
- some kidney diseases
- cystic fibrosis
- burns

- excess of antidiuretic hormone or therapy with a potassium-depleting diuretic
- laxative abuse
- alkalosis
- insufficient potassium intake from starvation, anorexia nervosa, alcoholism, or clay ingestion
- administration of a glucocorticoid, I.V. amphotericin B, vitamin $B_{12}$, folic acid, granulocyte-macrophage colony–stimulating factor, or I.V. solutions that contain insufficient potassium.

## Be still my heart

Potassium decreases the toxic effects of digoxin. Because potassium inhibits the excitability of the heart, normal potassium levels moderate the action of digoxin, reducing the chances of toxicity.

## Drug interactions

Potassium should be used cautiously in patients receiving potassium-sparing diuretics (such as amiloride, spironolactone, and triamterene) or angiotensin-converting enzyme inhibitors (such as captopril, enalapril, and lisinopril) to avoid hyperkalemia. (See *Adverse reactions to potassium*.)

# Calcium

*Calcium* is a major cation in ECF. Almost all of the calcium in the body (99%) is stored in bone, where it can be mobilized, if necessary. When dietary intake isn't enough to meet metabolic needs, calcium stores in bone are reduced.

## Bound, complexed, ionized

Extracellular calcium exists in three forms—it's bound to plasma protein (mainly albumin); complexed with such substances as phosphate, citrate, or sulfate; and ionized. Ionized calcium is the physiologically active form and plays a role in cellular functions.

## Salting the body

Chronic insufficient calcium intake can result in bone demineralization. Calcium is replaced orally or I.V. with calcium salts, such as:
- calcium carbonate
- calcium chloride
- calcium citrate
- calcium glubionate
- calcium gluceptate
- calcium gluconate
- calcium lactate.

**Warning!**

## Adverse reactions to potassium

Most adverse reactions to potassium are related to the method of administration.

### Oral history
Oral potassium sometimes causes nausea, vomiting, abdominal pain, and diarrhea. Enteric-coated tablets may cause small-bowel ulceration, stenosis, hemorrhage, and obstruction.

### I.V. issues
I.V. infusion of potassium preparations can cause pain at the injection site and phlebitis (vein inflammation). Given rapidly, I.V. administration may cause cardiac arrest. Infusion of potassium in patients with decreased urine production increases the risk of hyperkalemia.

## Pharmacokinetics

Oral calcium is absorbed readily from the duodenum and proximal jejunum. A pH of 5 to 7, parathyroid hormone, and vitamin D all aid calcium absorption.

### Absorbed with absorption

Absorption also depends on dietary factors, such as calcium binding to fiber, phytates, and oxalates, and on fatty acids, with which calcium salts form insoluble soaps.

### Distribution and excretion

Calcium is distributed primarily in bone. Calcium salts are eliminated unchanged primarily in stool; the remainder is excreted in urine.

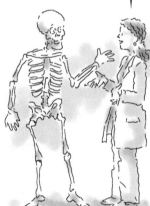

Just about all the calcium in the body can be found in the bones.

## Pharmacodynamics

Calcium moves quickly into ECF to restore calcium levels and reestablish balance. Calcium has several important roles in the body:
• Extracellular ionized calcium plays an essential role in normal nerve and muscle excitability.
• Calcium is integral to normal functioning of the heart, kidneys, and lungs, and it affects the blood coagulation rate as well as cell membrane and capillary permeability.
• Calcium is a factor in neurotransmitter and hormone activity, amino acid metabolism, vitamin $B_{12}$ absorption, and gastrin secretion.
• Calcium plays a major role in normal bone and tooth formation.

## Pharmacotherapeutics

Calcium is helpful in treating magnesium intoxication. It also helps strengthen myocardial tissue after defibrillation (electric shock to restore normal heart rhythm) or a poor response to epinephrine during resuscitation. Pregnancy and breast-feeding increase calcium requirements, as do periods of bone growth during childhood and adolescence.

### In the I.V. league

The major clinical indication for I.V. calcium is acute hypocalcemia (low serum calcium levels), which necessitates a rapid increase in serum calcium levels, as in tetany, cardiac arrest, vitamin D deficiency, parathyroid surgery, and alkalosis. I.V. calcium is also used to prevent a hypocalcemic reaction during exchange transfusions.

## Oral history

Oral calcium is commonly used to supplement a calcium-deficient diet and prevent osteoporosis. Chronic hypocalcemia from such conditions as chronic hypoparathyroidism (a deficiency of parathyroid hormones), osteomalacia (softening of bones), long-term glucocorticoid therapy, and plicamycin and vitamin D deficiency is also treated with oral calcium.

### Drug interactions

Calcium has few significant interactions with other drugs.
• Preparations administered with digoxin may cause cardiac arrhythmias.
• Calcium replacement drugs may reduce the response to calcium channel blockers.
• Calcium replacements may inactivate tetracyclines.
• Calcium supplements may decrease the amount of atenolol available to the tissues, resulting in decreased effectiveness of the drug.
• When given in total parenteral nutrition, calcium may react with phosphorus present in the solution to form insoluble calcium phosphate granules, which may find their way into pulmonary arterioles, causing emboli and possibly death. (See *Adverse reactions to calcium*.)

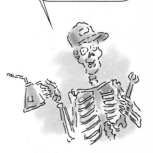

Always oil the ol' bones with some calcium!

# Magnesium

*Magnesium* is the most abundant cation in ICF after potassium. It's essential in transmitting nerve impulses to muscle and activating enzymes necessary for carbohydrate and protein metabolism. About 65% of all magnesium is in bone, and 20% is in muscle.

## Officiating in the ICF

Magnesium stimulates parathyroid hormone secretion, thus regulating ICF calcium levels.

## Traffic control

Magnesium also aids in cell metabolism and the movement of sodium and potassium across cell membranes.

## A run on magnesium

Magnesium stores may be depleted by:
• malabsorption
• chronic diarrhea
• prolonged treatment with diuretics

**Warning!**

## Adverse reactions to calcium

Calcium preparations may produce hypercalcemia (elevated serum calcium levels). Early signs include:
• drowsiness
• lethargy
• muscle weakness
• headache
• constipation
• metallic taste.

**Take this to heart**
Electrocardiogram changes that occur with elevated serum calcium levels include a shortened QT interval and heart block. Severe hypercalcemia can cause cardiac arrhythmias, cardiac arrest, and coma.

- nasogastric suctioning
- prolonged therapy with parenteral fluids not containing magnesium
- hyperaldosteronism
- hypoparathyroidism or hyperparathyroidism
- excessive release of adrenocortical hormones
- acute and chronic alcohol consumption
- drugs, such as cisplatin, aminoglycosides, cyclosporine, and amphotericin B.

## Restocking the mineral stores

Magnesium is typically replaced in the form of magnesium sulfate when administered I.V. or in the form of magnesium oxide if given orally.

## Pharmacokinetics

Magnesium sulfate is distributed widely throughout the body. I.V. magnesium sulfate acts immediately, whereas the drug acts within 30 minutes after I.M. administration. However, I.M. injections can be painful, can induce sclerosis, and need to be repeated frequently.

### Metabolism and excretion

Magnesium sulfate isn't metabolized and is excreted unchanged in urine and stool; some appears in breast milk.

## Pharmacodynamics

Magnesium sulfate replenishes and prevents magnesium deficiencies. It also prevents or controls seizures by blocking neuromuscular transmission.

## Pharmacotherapeutics

I.V. magnesium sulfate is the drug of choice for replacement therapy in symptomatic magnesium deficiency (hypomagnesemia). It's widely used to treat or prevent preeclamptic and eclamptic seizure activity and is used to treat ventricular arrhythmias such as torsades de pointes. It's also used to treat seizures, severe toxemia, and acute nephritis in children.

## Drug interactions

Magnesium has few significant interactions with other drugs.
- Magnesium used with digoxin may lead to heart block.
- Magnesium sulfate combined with alcohol, narcotics, antianxiety drugs, barbiturates, antidepressants, hypnotics, antipsychotic

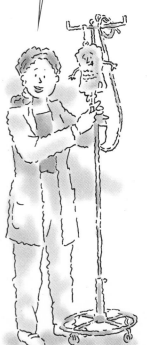

I.V. magnesium sulfate is the drug of choice for hypomagnesemia.

drugs, or general anesthetics may increase central nervous system depressant effects.
• Magnesium sulfate combined with succinylcholine or tubocurarine potentiates and prolongs the neuromuscular blocking action of these drugs. (See *Adverse reactions to magnesium*.)

# Sodium

*Sodium* is the major cation in ECF. Sodium performs many functions:
• It maintains the osmotic pressure and concentration of ECF, acid-base balance, and water balance.
• It contributes to nerve conduction and neuromuscular function.
• It plays a role in glandular secretion.

## Don't sweat it

Sodium replacement is necessary in conditions that rapidly deplete sodium, such as anorexia, excessive loss of GI fluids, and excessive perspiration. Diuretics and tap water enemas can also deplete sodium, particularly when fluids are replaced by plain water.

## The salt flats

Sodium also can be lost in trauma or wound drainage, adrenal gland insufficiency, cirrhosis of the liver with ascites, syndrome of inappropriate antidiuretic hormone, and prolonged I.V. infusion of dextrose in water without other solutes.

## Calling all chlorides

Sodium is typically replaced in the form of sodium chloride.

## Pharmacokinetics

Oral and parenteral sodium chloride are quickly absorbed and distributed widely throughout the body.

### Metabolism and excretion

Sodium chloride isn't significantly metabolized. It's eliminated primarily in urine but also in sweat, tears, and saliva.

## Pharmacodynamics

Sodium chloride solution replaces deficiencies of the sodium and chloride ions in the blood plasma.

## Adverse reactions to magnesium

Adverse reactions to magnesium sulfate, which can be life-threatening, include:
• hypotension
• circulatory collapse
• flushing
• depressed reflexes
• respiratory paralysis
• cardiac arrest.

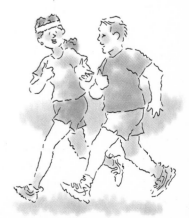

When I'm out jogging, I lose important fluids. Sodium can help me replace depleted fluids and maintain water balance.

### Pharmacotherapeutics

Sodium chloride is used for water and electrolyte replacement in patients with hyponatremia from electrolyte loss or severe sodium chloride depletion.

## A welcome infusion

Severe symptomatic sodium deficiency may be treated by I.V. infusion of a solution containing sodium chloride.

### Drug interactions

No significant drug interactions have been reported with sodium chloride. (See *Adverse reactions to sodium*.)

**Warning!**

## Adverse reactions to sodium

Adverse reactions to sodium include:
• pulmonary edema (if given too rapidly or in excess)
• hypernatremia
• potassium loss.

# Alkalinizing and acidifying drugs

*Alkalinizing* and *acidifying drugs* act to correct acid-base imbalances in the blood. These acid-base imbalances include:
• *metabolic acidosis,* a decreased serum pH caused by excess hydrogen ions in the ECF, which is treated with alkalinizing drugs
• *metabolic alkalosis,* an increased serum pH caused by excess bicarbonate in the ECF, which is treated with acidifying drugs.

## Odd couple

Alkalinizing and acidifying drugs have opposite effects:
• An alkalinizing drug will increase the pH of the blood and decrease the concentration of hydrogen ions.
• An acidifying drug will decrease the pH of the blood and increase the concentration of hydrogen ions.

## Rx for o.d.

Some of these drugs also alter urine pH, making them useful in treating some urinary tract infections and drug overdoses.

# Alkalinizing drugs

*Alkalinizing drugs* are used to treat metabolic acidosis and to increase blood pH. These include:
• sodium bicarbonate
• sodium citrate
• sodium lactate
• tromethamine.

## Increasing another pH

Sodium bicarbonate is also used to increase urine pH.

### Pharmacokinetics

All of the alkalinizing drugs are absorbed well when given orally.

#### *Metabolism and excretion*

Sodium citrate and sodium lactate are metabolized to the active ingredient, bicarbonate. Sodium bicarbonate isn't metabolized. Tromethamine undergoes little or no metabolism and is excreted unchanged in urine.

### Pharmacodynamics

Sodium bicarbonate separates in the blood, providing bicarbonate ions that are used in the blood buffer system to decrease the hydrogen ion concentration and raise blood pH. (Buffers prevent extreme changes in pH by taking or giving up hydrogen ions to neutralize acids or bases.) As the bicarbonate ions are excreted in urine, urine pH rises. Sodium citrate and lactate, after conversion to bicarbonate, alkalinize the blood and urine in the same way.

## Hitching up with hydrogen

Tromethamine acts by combining with hydrogen ions to alkalinize the blood; the resulting tromethamine–hydrogen ion complex is excreted in urine.

### Pharmacotherapeutics

Alkalinizing drugs are commonly used to treat metabolic acidosis. Other uses include raising urine pH to help remove certain substances, such as phenobarbital, after an overdose.

### Drug interactions

The alkalinizing drugs sodium bicarbonate, sodium citrate, and sodium lactate can interact with a wide range of drugs to increase or decrease their pharmacologic effects.
• They may increase excretion and reduce the effects of chlorpropamide, ketoconazole, lithium, and salicylates.
• They may reduce the excretion and increase the effects of amphetamines, flecainide, quinidine, and pseudoephedrine.
• The antibacterial effects of methenamine are reduced when taken with alkalinizing drugs. (See *Adverse reactions to alkalinizing drugs*, page 368.)

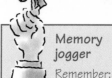

**Memory jogger**

Remember: A low pH means a solution is acidic, and a high pH means it's alkaline. Therefore, to raise the pH, you use an alkalinizing drug and, likewise, to lower the pH, you use an acidifying drug.

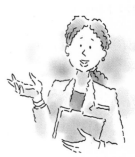

Alkalinizing drugs treat metabolic acidosis by increasing blood pH.

**Warning!**

## Adverse reactions to alkalinizing drugs

Adverse reactions to alkalinizing drugs vary.

**Sodium bicarbonate**
• Bicarbonate overdose
• Cerebral dysfunction, tissue hypoxia, and lactic acidosis (with rapid administration for diabetic ketoacidosis)
• Water retention and edema

**Sodium citrate**
• Metabolic alkalosis, tetany, or aggravation of existing heart disease (with overdose)
• Laxative effect (with oral administration)

**Sodium lactate**
• Metabolic alkalosis (with overdose)
• Extravasation
• Water retention or edema (in patient with kidney disease or heart failure)

**Tromethamine**
• Hypoglycemia
• Respiratory depression
• Extravasation
• Hyperkalemia
• Toxic drug levels (if given for more than 24 hours)

# Acidifying drugs

*Acidifying drugs* are used to correct metabolic alkalosis. These include:
• acetazolamide (used in treatment of acute mountain sickness)
• ammonium chloride.
    Ascorbic acid, along with ammonium chloride, serves as a urinary acidifier.

## Pharmacokinetics

The action of most acidifying drugs is immediate.

### Absorption, metabolism, and excretion

Orally administered ammonium chloride is absorbed completely in 3 to 6 hours. It's metabolized in the liver to form urea, which is excreted by the kidneys.

Break it down

Acetazolamide inhibits the enzyme carbonic anhydrase, which blocks hydrogen ion secretion in the renal tubule, resulting in increased excretion of bicarbonate and a lower pH. Acetazolamide also acidifies urine but may produce metabolic acidosis in normal patients.

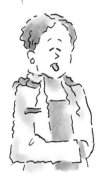

When your stomach doesn't feel quite right, you might need some acidifying drugs!

## Pharmacodynamics

Acidifying drugs have several actions:
• Ammonium chloride lowers the blood pH after being metabolized to urea and to hydrochloric acid, which provides hydrogen ions to acidify the blood or urine.
• Ascorbic acid directly acidifies urine, providing hydrogen ions and lowering urine pH.
• Acetazolamide increases the excretion of bicarbonate, lowering blood pH.

## Pharmacotherapeutics

A patient with metabolic alkalosis requires therapy with an acidifying drug that provides hydrogen ions; such a patient may need chloride ion therapy as well.

### Safe and easy

Most patients receive both types of ions in oral or parenteral doses of ammonium chloride, a safer drug that's easy to prepare.

### Kidney concerns

In patients with renal dysfunction, acetazolamide may be ineffective and cause loss of potassium in urine.

## Drug interactions

Acidifying drugs don't cause clinically significant drug interactions. However, concurrent use of ammonium chloride and spironolactone may cause increased systemic acidosis. (See *Adverse reactions to acidifying drugs.*)

**Warning!**

## Adverse reactions to acidifying drugs

Adverse reactions to acidifying drugs are usually mild, such as GI distress. Overdose may lead to acidosis.

**Acetazolamide**
• Drowsiness
• Seizures
• Anorexia
• Nausea and vomiting
• Diarrhea
• Altered taste
• Aplastic anemia

**Ammonium chloride**
• Metabolic acidosis and loss of electrolytes, especially potassium (with large doses)

**Ascorbic acid**
• GI distress (with high doses)
• Hemolytic anemia (in a patient with glucose-6-phosphate dehydrogenase deficiency)

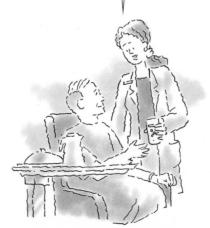

Oral forms of ammonium chloride are safer and easier to prepare.

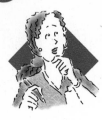

# Quick quiz

1. Which drug can cause hypokalemia?
   A. Digoxin
   B. Amphotericin B
   C. Spironolactone
   D. Lansoprazole

*Answer:* B. Hypokalemia is a common occurrence in conditions that increase potassium excretion or depletion, such as administration of glucocorticoid, I.V. amphotericin B, vitamin $B_{12}$, folic acid, granulocyte-macrophage colony–stimulating factor, or I.V. solutions that contain insufficient potassium.

2. Potassium should be used cautiously in patients receiving:
   A. amiloride.
   B. furosemide.
   C. digoxin.
   D. cetirizine.

*Answer:* A. Potassium should be used cautiously in patients receiving potassium-sparing diuretics, such as amiloride, to avoid hyperkalemia.

3. How does sodium bicarbonate correct metabolic acidosis?
   A. By lowering blood pH after being metabolized
   B. By increasing hydrogen ion concentration
   C. By combining with hydrogen ions to alkalinize the blood
   D. By decreasing hydrogen ion concentration

*Answer:* D. Sodium bicarbonate corrects acidosis by decreasing hydrogen ion concentration.

## Scoring

⭐⭐⭐ If you answered all three items correctly, extraordinary! You're one well-balanced individual!

⭐⭐ If you answered two items correctly, congratulations! You're moving closer to complete harmony!

⭐ If you answered fewer than two items correctly, keep trying! By the end of the book, you're sure to have all your levels up!

# Antineoplastic drugs

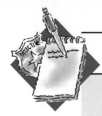

## Just the facts

In this chapter, you'll learn:

♦ classes of drugs used to treat cancer

♦ uses and varying actions of these drugs

♦ how these drugs are absorbed, distributed, metabolized, and excreted

♦ drug interactions and adverse reactions to these drugs.

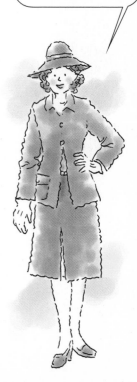

The 1940s saw the development of chemotherapeutic drugs.

# Drugs and cancer

In the 1940s, *antineoplastic* (chemotherapeutic) *drugs* were developed to treat cancer. However, these agents commonly had serious adverse effects.

### A brighter future

Today, many of these toxicities can be lessened so they aren't as devastating to the patient. With modern chemotherapy, childhood malignancies, such as acute lymphoblastic leukemia, and adult cancers, such as testicular cancer, are curable in most patients. New therapeutic strategies, such as using monoclonal antibodies or targeting specific proteins, are further improving the time that a patient's cancer can remain in remission. In addition, drugs such as interferons are being used to treat patients with cancer.

# Alkylating drugs

*Alkylating drugs*, given alone or with other drugs, effectively act against various malignant neoplasms. These drugs fall into one of six classes:
• nitrogen mustards
• alkyl sulfonates

- nitrosoureas
- triazenes
- ethylenimines
- alkylating-like drugs.

## Unfazed at any phase

All of these drugs produce their antineoplastic effects by damaging deoxyribonucleic acid (DNA). They halt DNA's replication process by cross-linking its strands so that amino acids don't pair up correctly. Alkylating drugs are cell cycle–phase nonspecific. This means that their alkylating actions may take place at any phase of the cell cycle.

# Nitrogen mustards

*Nitrogen mustards* represent the largest group of alkylating drugs. They include:
- chlorambucil
- cyclophosphamide
- estramustine
- ifosfamide
- mechlorethamine hydrochloride
- melphalan.

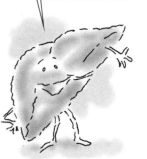

I see some nitrogen mustards headed my way. Time to get to work!

## First and fast

Mechlorethamine hydrochloride was the first nitrogen mustard introduced and is rapid-acting.

## Pharmacokinetics (how drugs circulate)

The absorption and distribution of nitrogen mustards, as with most alkylating drugs, vary widely.

### Metabolism and excretion

Nitrogen mustards are metabolized in the liver and excreted by the kidneys. Mechlorethamine undergoes metabolism so rapidly that no active drug remains after a few minutes. Most nitrogen mustards possess more intermediate half-lives than mechlorethamine.

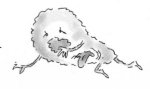

Alkylating drugs deactivate my DNA, cutting short my life.

## Pharmacodynamics (how drugs act)

Nitrogen mustards form covalent bonds with DNA molecules in a chemical reaction known as *alkylation*. Alkylated DNA can't replicate properly, thereby resulting in cell death. Unfortunately, cells

*Now I get it!*

## How alkylating drugs work

Alkylating drugs can attack deoxyribonucleic acid (DNA) in two ways, as shown in these illustrations.

**Bifunctional alkylation**

Some drugs become inserted between two base pairs in the DNA chain, forming an irreversible bond between them. This is called *bifunctional alkylation;* it causes cytotoxic effects capable of destroying or poisoning cells.

**Monofunctional alkylation**

Other drugs react with just one part of a pair, separating it from its partner and eventually causing it and its attached sugar to break away from the DNA molecule. This is called *monofunctional alkylation;* it eventually may cause permanent cell damage.

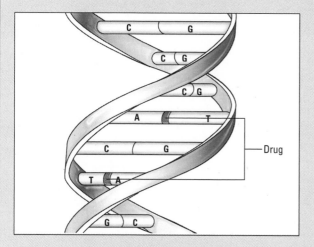

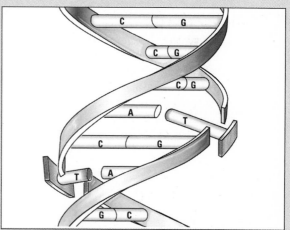

may develop resistance to the cytotoxic effects of nitrogen mustards. (See *How alkylating drugs work.*)

## Pharmacotherapeutics (how drugs are used)

Because they produce leukopenia (reduced number of white blood cells [WBCs]), the nitrogen mustards are effective in treating malignant neoplasms, such as Hodgkin's disease (cancer causing painless enlargement of the lymph nodes, spleen, and lymphoid tissues) and leukemia (cancer of the blood-forming tissues), that can have an associated elevated WBC count.

### Nitrogen bomb

Nitrogen mustards also prove effective against malignant lymphoma (cancer of the lymphoid tissue), multiple myeloma (cancer of the marrow plasma cells), melanoma (malignancy that arises from melanocytes), and cancers of the breast, ovaries, uterus, lung, brain, testes, bladder, prostate, and stomach.

## Drug interactions

Nitrogen mustards interact with a wide variety of other drugs:
• Calcium-containing drugs and foods, such as antacids and dairy products, reduce absorption of estramustine.
• Cyclophosphamide taken with cardiotoxic drugs produces additive cardiac effects.
• Cyclophosphamide may reduce serum digoxin levels.
• An increased risk of ifosfamide toxicity exists when the drug is taken with allopurinol, barbiturates, chloral hydrate, or phenytoin.
• Corticosteroids reduce the effects of ifosfamide.
• The lung toxicity threshold of carmustine may be reduced when taken with melphalan.
• Interferon alpha may reduce serum concentration of melphalan. (See *Adverse reactions to nitrogen mustards.*)

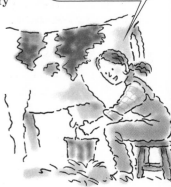

The calcium in dairy products reduces the absorption of estramustine.

# Alkyl sulfonates

*Busulfan*, an *alkyl sulfonate*, has historically been used to treat chronic myelogenous leukemia, polycythemia vera (increased red blood cell mass and increased number of WBCs and platelets), and other myeloproliferative (pertaining to an overactive bone marrow) disorders. It's also used for treatment of leukemia during bone marrow transplant procedures.

## Pharmacokinetics

Busulfan is rapidly well absorbed from the GI tract. Little is known about its distribution.

### Metabolism and excretion

Busulfan is extensively metabolized in the liver before urinary excretion. Its half-life is 2 to 3 hours.

## Pharmacodynamics

As an alkyl sulfonate, busulfan forms covalent bonds with the DNA molecules in alkylation.

## Pharmacotherapeutics

Busulfan primarily affects granulocytes (a type of WBC) and, to a lesser degree, platelets. Because of its action on granulocytes, it

*Warning!*

## Adverse reactions to nitrogen mustards

Many patients experience fatigue during nitrogen mustard therapy. Other adverse reactions include:
• severe leukopenia and thrombocytopenia
• nausea and vomiting
• stomatitis
• reversible hair loss
• severe skin reactions with direct contact
• severe tissue damage, if extravasation occurs.

has been used for treating chronic myelogenous leukemia and as adjunct therapy before and after bone marrow transplantation.

## A backup option

Busulfan is also effective in treating polycythemia vera, although other drugs are usually used to treat it because busulfan can cause severe myelosuppression (halting of bone marrow function).

### Drug interactions

There's an increased risk of bleeding when busulfan is taken with anticoagulants or aspirin. Concurrent use of busulfan and thioguanine may cause liver toxicity, esophageal varices (enlarged, swollen veins in the esophagus), or portal hypertension (increased pressure in the portal vein of the liver). (See *Adverse reactions to busulfan*.)

# Nitrosoureas

*Nitrosoureas* are alkylating agents that work by halting cancer cell reproduction. They include:
- carmustine
- lomustine
- streptozocin.

## Pharmacokinetics

When administered topically to treat mycosis fungoides (a rare skin malignancy), carmustine is 5% to 28% systemically absorbed. After oral administration, lomustine is absorbed adequately, though incompletely.

## I.V. is the way

Streptozocin and carmustine are administered I.V. because they're poorly absorbed orally.

### Metabolism and excretion

Nitrosoureas are lipophilic (attracted to fat), distributing to fatty tissues and cerebrospinal fluid. They're metabolized extensively before urine excretion.

## Pharmacodynamics

During a process called *bifunctional alkylation*, nitrosoureas interfere with amino acids, purines, and DNA needed for cancer cells to divide, thus halting their reproduction.

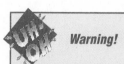

*Warning!*

### Adverse reactions to busulfan

The major adverse reaction to busulfan is bone marrow suppression, producing severe leukopenia, anemia, and thrombocytopenia (reduced white blood cells, red blood cells, and platelets, respectively). This reaction is usually dose-related and reversible.

## Pharmacotherapeutics

The nitrosoureas are highly lipid (fat) soluble, which allows them or their metabolites to easily cross the blood-brain barrier. Because of this ability, nitrosoureas are used to treat brain tumors and meningeal leukemias.

## Drug interactions

Each of the nitrosoureas has its own interactions with other drugs. Cimetidine may increase carmustine's bone marrow toxicity. Streptozocin prolongs the elimination half-life of doxorubicin, prolonging the leukopenia and thrombocytopenia. (See *Adverse reactions to nitrosoureas*.)

# Triazenes

*Dacarbazine*, a *triazene*, functions as an alkylating drug after being activated by the liver.

## Pharmacokinetics

After I.V. injection, dacarbazine is distributed throughout the body and metabolized in the liver. Within 6 hours, 30% to 46% of a dose is excreted by the kidneys (half is excreted unchanged, and half is excreted as one of the metabolites).

### Dysfunction junction

In patients with kidney or liver dysfunction, dacarbazine's half-life may increase to 7 hours.

## Pharmacodynamics

Dacarbazine must first be metabolized in the liver to become an active drug. It seems to inhibit ribonucleic acid (RNA) and protein synthesis. Like other alkylating drugs, dacarbazine is cell cycle–nonspecific.

## Pharmacotherapeutics

Dacarbazine is used primarily to treat patients with malignant melanoma but is also used with other drugs to treat patients with Hodgkin's disease.

**Warning!**

## Adverse reactions to nitrosoureas

All of the nitrosoureas can produce severe nausea and vomiting.

**Down to the bone**
Carmustine and lomustine produce bone marrow suppression that begins 4 to 6 weeks after treatment and lasts 1 to 2 weeks.

**Kidney concerns**
Kidney toxicity and kidney failure may also occur with patients taking nitrosoureas. High-dose carmustine may produce reversible liver toxicity.

**Pulmonary problems**
Carmustine may cause lung toxicity characterized by lung infiltrates or fibrosis (scarring).

## Drug interactions

No significant drug interactions have been reported with dacarbazine. (See *Adverse reactions to triazenes*.)

# Ethylenimines

*Thiotepa*, an *ethylenimine* derivative, is a multifunctional alkylating drug.

## Pharmacokinetics

After I.V. administration, thiotepa is 100% bioavailable. Significant systemic absorption may occur when thiotepa is administered into pleural (around the lungs) or peritoneal (abdominal) spaces to treat malignant effusions or is instilled into the bladder.

### Metabolism and excretion

Thiotepa crosses the blood-brain barrier and is metabolized extensively in the liver. Thiotepa and its metabolites are excreted in urine.

## Pharmacodynamics

Thiotepa exerts its cytotoxic activity by interfering with DNA replication and RNA transcription. Ultimately, it disrupts nucleic acid function and causes cell death.

## Pharmacotherapeutics

Thiotepa is used to treat bladder cancer. This alkylating drug is also prescribed for palliative (symptom-relief) treatment of lymphomas and ovarian or breast cancers.

Wait! There's more

Thiotepa is used for the treatment of intracavitary effusions (accumulation of fluid in a body cavity). It may also prove useful in the treatment of lung cancer.

## Drug interactions

Thiotepa may interact with other drugs.
• Concurrent use of thiotepa, anticoagulants, and aspirin may increase the risk of bleeding.
• Taking thiotepa with neuromuscular blocking drugs may prolong muscular paralysis.

*Warning!*

## Adverse reactions to triazenes

Dacarbazine use may cause some adverse reactions, including:
• leukopenia
• thrombocytopenia
• nausea and vomiting (which begin within 1 to 3 hours after administration in most patients and may last up to 48 hours)
• phototoxicity
• flulike symptoms
• hair loss.

• Concurrent use of thiotepa and other alkylating drugs or radiation therapy may intensify toxicity rather than enhance the therapeutic response.

## It'll take your breath away

When used with succinylcholine, thiotepa may cause prolonged respirations and apnea (periods of not breathing). Thiotepa appears to inhibit the activity of cholinesterase, the enzyme that deactivates succinylcholine. (See *Adverse reactions to thiotepa*.)

# Alkylating-like drugs

*Carboplatin*, *cisplatin*, and *oxaliplatin* are heavy metal complexes that contain platinum. Because their action resembles that of a bifunctional alkylating drug, they are referred to as *alkylating-like drugs*.

## Pharmacokinetics

The distribution and metabolism of carboplatin aren't defined clearly. After I.V. administration, carboplatin is eliminated primarily by the kidneys. The elimination of carboplatin is biphasic. It has an initial half-life of 1 to 2 hours and a terminal half-life of 2½ to 6 hours. In patients with decreased renal function, the terminal half-life of carboplatin may last from 30 to 300 hours.Oxaliplatin is 70% to 90% bound to plasma proteins, and the protein-binding increases over time. It's widely distributed into most body tissues and is eliminated in phases.

## Into the lungs and peritoneum

When administered intrapleurally (into the pleural space around the lung) or intraperitoneally (into the peritoneum), cisplatin may exhibit significant systemic absorption. Highly protein bound, cisplatin reaches high concentrations in the kidneys, liver, intestines, and testes but has poor central nervous system (CNS) penetration. The drug undergoes some liver metabolism, followed by excretion through the kidney.

## Going platinum

Platinum is detectable in tissue for at least 4 months after administration.

## Pharmacodynamics

Like alkylating drugs, carboplatin, cisplatin, and oxaliplatin are cell cycle–nonspecific and inhibit DNA synthesis. They act like bifunctional alkylating drugs by cross-linking strands of DNA and inhibiting DNA synthesis.

## Pharmacotherapeutics

These alkylating-like drugs are used in the treatment of several cancers.
• Carboplatin is used primarily to treat ovarian and lung cancer.
• Cisplatin is prescribed to treat bladder and metastatic ovarian cancer.
• Cisplatin is the drug of choice to treat metastatic testicular cancers.
• Cisplatin may also be used to treat head, neck, and lung cancer (although these indications are clinically accepted, they're currently unlabeled uses).
• Oxaliplatin is used in combination with other agents to treat colorectal cancer.

## Drug interactions

Alkylating-like drugs interact with a few other drugs:
• When carboplatin, oxaliplatin, or cisplatin is administered with an aminoglycoside, the risk of toxicity to the kidney increases.
• Carboplatin or cisplatin taken with bumetanide, ethacrynic acid, or furosemide increases the risk of ototoxicity (damaging the organs of hearing and balance).
• Cisplatin may reduce serum phenytoin levels. (See *Adverse reactions to alkylating-like drugs.*)

# Antimetabolite drugs

Because *antimetabolite drugs* structurally resemble DNA base pairs, they can become involved in processes associated with DNA base pairs—that is, the synthesis of nucleic acids and proteins.

## Getting specific

Antimetabolites differ sufficiently from DNA base pairs in how they interfere with this synthesis. Because the antimetabolites are cell cycle–specific and primarily affect cells that actively synthesize DNA, they're referred to as *S phase–specific.* Normal cells that are reproducing actively, as well as the cancer cells, are affected by the antimetabolites.

**Warning!**

## Adverse reactions to alkylating-like drugs

Alkylating-like drugs produce many of the same adverse reactions as the alkylating drugs.
• Carboplatin can produce bone marrow suppression.
• Kidney toxicity may occur with cisplatin, usually after multiple courses of therapy. Carboplatin is less toxic to the kidneys.
• Cisplatin produces marked nausea and vomiting. With long-term cisplatin therapy, neurotoxicity can occur. Neurotoxicity is less common with carboplatin.
• Tinnitus and hearing loss may occur with cisplatin and, less commonly, with carboplatin.
• Oxaliplatin may cause anaphylaxis, anemia, or increased risk of bleeding or infection.

## Each according to its metabolite

These drugs are subclassified according to the metabolite affected and include:
- folic acid analogues
- pyrimidine analogues
- purine analogues.

# Folic acid analogues

Although researchers have developed many *folic acid analogues*, the early compound *methotrexate* remains the most commonly used.

## Pharmacokinetics

Methotrexate is well absorbed and distributed throughout the body. It can accumulate in any fluid collection, such as ascites or pleural or pericardial effusion, possibly resulting in prolonged elimination and higher than expected toxicity, especially myelo-suppression. At usual dosages, it doesn't enter the CNS readily.

### Metabolism and excretion

Although methotrexate is metabolized partially, it's excreted primarily unchanged in urine.

## A disappearing act

Methotrexate exhibits a three-part disappearance from plasma; the rapid distributive phase is followed by a second phase, which reflects kidney clearance. The last phase, the terminal half-life, is 3 to 10 hours for a low dose and 8 to 15 hours for a high dose.

## Pharmacodynamics

Methotrexate reversibly inhibits the action of the enzyme dihydro-folate reductase, thereby blocking normal folic acid processing and thus inhibiting DNA and RNA synthesis. The result is cell death. Folinic acid is used in high-dose methotrexate therapy to help prevent cell death.

## Pharmacotherapeutics

Methotrexate is especially useful in treating:
- acute lymphoblastic leukemia (abnormal growth of lympho-cyte precursors, the lymphoblasts), the most common leukemia in children

> Methotrexate is especially useful in treating the most common childhood leukemia.

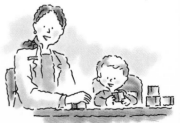

- acute lymphocytic leukemia (abnormal growth of lymphocytes); methotrexate may be given as treatment or prophylaxis for meningeal leukemia
- CNS diseases (given intrathecally, or through the spinal cord into the subarachnoid space)
- choriocarcinoma (cancer that develops from the chorionic portions of the products of conception)
- osteogenic sarcoma (bone cancer)
- malignant lymphomas
- cancers of the head, neck, bladder, testis, and breast.

## Unconventional treatment

The drug is also prescribed in low doses to treat such disorders as severe psoriasis, graft versus host disease, and rheumatoid arthritis that don't respond to conventional therapy.

## Drug interactions

Methotrexate interacts with several other drugs:
- Probenecid decreases methotrexate excretion, increasing the risk of methotrexate toxicity, including fatigue, bone marrow suppression, and stomatitis (mouth inflammation).
- Salicylates and nonsteroidal anti-inflammatory drugs, especially diclofenac, ketoprofen, indomethacin, and naproxen, also increase methotrexate toxicity.
- Cholestyramine reduces absorption of methotrexate from the GI tract.
- Concurrent use of alcohol and methotrexate increases the risk of liver toxicity.
- Taking co-trimoxazole with methotrexate may produce blood cell abnormalities.
- Penicillin decreases renal tubular secretion of methotrexate, increasing the risk of methotrexate toxicity. (See *Adverse reactions to methotrexate*.)

# Pyrimidine analogues

*Pyrimidine analogues* are a diverse group of drugs that inhibit production of pyrimidine nucleotides necessary for DNA synthesis. They include:
- capecitabine
- cytarabine
- floxuridine
- fluorouracil
- gemcitabine.

**Warning!**

## Adverse reactions to methotrexate

Adverse reactions to methotrexate include:
- bone marrow suppression
- stomatitis
- pulmonary toxicity, exhibited as pneumonitis or pulmonary fibrosis
- skin reactions, such as photosensitivity and hair loss.

### Kidney concerns
With high doses, kidney toxicity can also occur with methotrexate use. During high-dose therapy, leucovorin (folinic acid) may be used in a technique known as *leucovorin rescue* to minimize adverse reactions.

### The spine of the matter
Adverse reactions to intrathecal administration (through the dura into the subarachnoid space) of methotrexate may include seizures, paralysis, and death. Other less severe adverse reactions may also occur, including headaches, fever, neck stiffness, confusion, and irritability.

## How pyrimidine analogues work

To understand how pyrimidine analogues work, it helps to consider the basic structure of deoxyribonucleic acid (DNA).

**Climbing the ladder to understanding**
DNA resembles a ladder that has been twisted. The rungs of the ladder consist of pairs of nitrogenous bases: adenine always pairs with thymine, and guanine always pairs with cytosine. Cytosine and thymine are pyrimidines; adenine and guanine are purines.

**One part sugar...**
The basic unit of DNA is the nucleotide. A nucleotide is the building block of nucleic acids. It consists of a sugar, a nitrogen-containing base, and a phosphate group. It's on these components that pyrimidine analogues do their work.

**In the guise of a nucleotide**
After pyrimidine analogues are converted into nucleotides, they're incorporated into DNA, where they may inhibit DNA and ribonucleic acid synthesis as well as other metabolic reactions necessary for proper cell growth.

## Pharmacokinetics

Because pyrimidine analogues are poorly absorbed when they're given orally, they're usually administered by other routes.

### Distribution, metabolism, and excretion

With the exception of cytarabine, pyrimidine analogues are well distributed throughout the body, including in cerebrospinal fluid (CSF). They're metabolized extensively in the liver and are excreted in urine. Intrathecal cytarabine may be given with or without cranial radiation to treat CNS leukemia.

## Pharmacodynamics

Pyrimidine analogues kill cancer cells by interfering with the natural function of pyrimidine nucleotides. (See *How pyrimidine analogues work.*)

## Pharmacotherapeutics

Pyrimidine analogues may be used to treat many tumors. However, they're primarily indicated in the treatment of:
• acute leukemias
• GI tract adenocarcinomas, such as colorectal, pancreatic, esophageal, and stomach adenocarcinomas

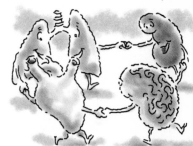

With pyrimidine analogues, we may all win!

• cancers of the breast and ovaries
• malignant lymphomas.

## Drug interactions

No significant drug interactions occur with most of the pyrimidine analogues; however, several drug interactions are possible with capecitabine.
• Antacids, when given with capecitabine, may increase absorption of capecitabine.
• Capecitabine can increase the pharmacodynamic effects of warfarin, thereby increasing the risk of bleeding.
• Capecitabine may increase serum phenytoin levels.
(See *Adverse reactions to pyrimidine analogues.*)

# Purine analogues

*Purine analogues* are incorporated into DNA and RNA, interfering with nucleic acid synthesis and replication. They include:
• fludarabine phosphate
• cladribine
• mercaptopurine
• pentostatin
• thioguanine.

## Pharmacokinetics

The pharmacokinetics of purine analogues aren't clearly defined. They're largely metabolized in the liver and excreted in urine.

## Pharmacodynamics

As with the other antimetabolites, fludarabine, mercaptopurine, and thioguanine first must be converted via phosphorylation (introduction to a phosphate) to the nucleotide level to be active. The resulting nucleotides are then incorporated into DNA, where they may inhibit DNA and RNA synthesis as well as other metabolic reactions necessary for proper cell growth. Cladribine responds in a similar fashion.

### Analogous to pyrimide analogues

This conversion to nucleotides is the same process that pyrimidine analogues go through but, in this case, it's purine nucleotides that are affected. Purine analogues are cell cycle–specific as well, exerting their effect during that same S phase.

### Death to T cells

Pentostatin inhibits adenosine deaminase (ADA), causing an increase in intracellular levels of deoxyadenosine triphosphate. This leads to cell damage and death. The greatest activity of ADA is in cells of the lymphoid system, especially malignant T cells.

## Pharmacotherapeutics

Purine analogues are used to treat acute and chronic leukemias and may be useful in the treatment of lymphomas.

## Drug interactions

No significant interactions occur with cladribine or thioguanine.

### A serious flub with fludarabine

- Taking fludarabine with pentostatin may cause severe pulmonary toxicity, which can be fatal.
- Taking pentostatin with allopurinol may increase the risk of rash.
- Taking pentostatin with vidarabine may enhance the effect of vidarabine and increase the risk of toxicity.

### Down to the bone

- Concomitant administration of mercaptopurine and allopurinol may increase bone marrow suppression by decreasing mercaptopurine metabolism. (See *Adverse reactions to purine analogues*.)

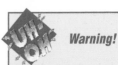

**Warning!**

## Adverse reactions to purine analogues

Purine analogues can cause:
- bone marrow suppression
- nausea and vomiting
- anorexia
- mild diarrhea
- stomatitis
- a rise in uric acid levels.

**High-dose horrors**
Fludarabine, when used at high doses, may cause severe neurologic effects, including blindness, coma, and death.

# Antibiotic antineoplastic drugs

*Antibiotic antineoplastic drugs* are antimicrobial products that produce tumoricidal (tumor-destroying) effects by binding with DNA. These drugs inhibit the cellular processes of normal and malignant cells. They include:
- anthracyclines (daunorubicin, doxorubicin, idarubicin)
- bleomycin
- dactinomycin
- mitomycin
- mitoxantrone.

## Pharmacokinetics

Antibiotic antineoplastic drugs are usually administered I.V.

### Direct deliveries

Some drugs are also administered directly into the body cavity being treated. Bleomycin, doxorubicin, and mitomycin are sometimes given as topical bladder instillations, resulting in minimal systemic absorption. When bleomycin is injected into the pleural space for malignant effusions, up to one-half of the dose is absorbed systemically.

### Distribution, metabolism, and excretion

Distribution of antibiotic antineoplastic drugs throughout the body varies; their metabolism and elimination also vary.

## Pharmacodynamics

With the exception of mitomycin, antibiotic antineoplastic drugs intercalate, or insert themselves, between adjacent base pairs of a DNA molecule, physically separating them.

### Taking the extra base

Remember, DNA looks like a twisted ladder with the rungs made up of pairs of nitrogenous bases. These drugs insert themselves between those nitrogenous bases. Then, when the DNA chain replicates, an extra base is inserted opposite the intercalated antibiotic, resulting in a mutant DNA molecule. The overall effect is cell death.

### Clean break

Mitomycin is activated inside the cell to a bifunctional or even trifunctional alkylating drug. Mitomycin produces single-strand breakage of DNA. It also cross-links DNA and inhibits DNA synthesis.

## Pharmacotherapeutics

Antibiotic antineoplastic drugs act against many cancers, including:
- acute leukemia
- breast, ovarian, bladder, and lung cancer
- cancers of the GI tract
- choriocarcinoma
- Ewing's sarcoma (a malignant tumor that originates in bone marrow, typically in long bones or the pelvis) and other soft-tissue sarcomas
- Hodgkin's disease and malignant lymphomas
- melanoma
- osteogenic sarcoma and rhabdomyosarcoma (malignant neoplasm composed of striated muscle cells)
- squamous cell carcinoma of the head, neck, and cervix
- testicular cancer
- Wilms' tumor (a malignant neoplasm of the kidney, occurring in young children).

## Drug interactions

Antibiotic antineoplastic drugs interact with many other drugs. (See *Adverse reactions to antibiotic antineoplastic drugs.*)
- Concurrent therapy with fludarabine and idarubicin isn't recommended because of the risk of fatal lung toxicity.
- Bleomycin may decrease serum digoxin and serum phenytoin levels.
- Doxorubicin may reduce serum digoxin levels.
- Combination chemotherapies enhance leukopenia and thrombocytopenia (reduced number of platelets).
- Mitomycin plus vinca alkaloids may cause acute respiratory distress.

**Warning!**

## Adverse reactions to antibiotic antineoplastic drugs

The primary adverse reaction to antibiotic antineoplastic drugs is bone marrow suppression. Irreversible cardiomyopathy and acute electrocardiogram changes can also occur as well as nausea and vomiting.

**Extra steps**
An antihistamine and an antipyretic should be given before bleomycin to prevent fever and chills. Anaphylactic reactions can occur in patients receiving bleomycin for lymphoma, so test doses should be given first.

**Seeing colors**
Doxorubicin may color urine red; mitoxantrone may color it blue-green.

# Hormonal antineoplastic drugs and hormone modulators

*Hormonal antineoplastic drugs* and *hormone modulators* are prescribed to alter the growth of malignant neoplasms or to manage and treat their physiologic effects.

## Hitting them where it hurts

Hormonal therapies and hormone modulators prove effective against hormone-dependent tumors, such as cancers of the prostate, breast, and endometrium. Lymphomas and leukemias are usually treated with therapies that include corticosteroids because of their potential for affecting lymphocytes.

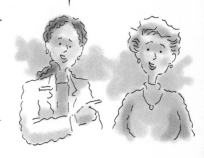

In postmenopausal women, estrogen is produced through aromatase.

# Aromatase inhibitors

In postmenopausal women, estrogen is produced through aromatase, an enzyme that converts hormone precursors into estrogen. *Aromatase inhibitors* prevent androgen from being converted into estrogen in postmenopausal women, thereby blocking estrogen's ability to activate cancer cells; limiting the amount of estrogen means that less estrogen is available to reach cancer cells and make them grow.

## Two types

There are two types of aromatase inhibitors. Type 1, or *steroidal*, inhibitors include exemestane; type 2, or *nonsteroidal*, inhibitors include anastrozole and letrozole.

## Pharmacokinetics

Aromatase inhibitors are taken orally (in pill form) and are usually well tolerated. Steady-state plasma levels after daily doses are reached in 2 to 6 weeks. Inactive metabolites are excreted in urine.

## Pharmacodynamics

Aromatase inhibitors work by lowering the body's production of estrogen. In about one-half of all patients with breast cancer, the tumors depend on estrogen to grow. Aromatase inhibitors are used only in postmenopausal women because they lower the amount of estrogen that's produced outside the ovaries, such as in muscle and fat tissue. Because these drugs induce estrogen deprivation, bone thinning and osteoporosis may develop over time.

## To reverse or not to reverse: That is the question

Type 1 inhibitors, such as exemestane, irreversibly inhibit the aromatase enzyme, whereas type 2 inhibitors, such as anastrozole, reversibly inhibit it. Type 1 aromatase inhibitors may still be effective after a type 2 aromatase inhibitor has failed.

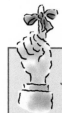

**Memory jogger**

Remember: Hormonal-dependent (gender specific) tumors are treated with hormonal therapies; tumors common to both genders are treated with corticosteroids.

## Competitive advantage

Anastrozale and letrozole work by competitively binding to heme of the cytochrome P450 subunit of aromatase, leading to decreased levels of estrogen in all tissues; they don't affect synthesis of adrenocorticosteroids, aldosterone, or thyroid hormones.

### Pharmacotherapeutics

Aromatase inhibitors are primarily used to treat postmenopausal women with metastatic breast cancer. They may be administered alone or with other agents such as tamoxifen.

### Drug interactions

Certain drugs may decrease the effectiveness of anastrozole, including tamoxifen and estrogen-containing drugs. (See *Adverse reactions to aromatase inhibitors*.)

# Antiestrogens

*Antiestrogens* bind to estrogen receptors and block estrogen action. The antiestrogens include *tamoxifen citrate*, *toremifene citrate*, and *fulvestrant*. Tamoxifen and toremifene are nonsteroidal estrogen agonist-antagonists, and fulvestrant is a pure estrogen antagonist.

### Pharmacokinetics

After oral administration, tamoxifen is well absorbed and undergoes extensive metabolism in the liver before being excreted in stool. Serum levels of fulvestrant, when given I.M., peak in 7 to 9 days. Its half-life is 40 days. Toremifene is well absorbed, and absorption isn't influencd by food.

### Pharmacodynamics

The exact antineoplastic action of these agents isn't known. However, they're known to act as estrogen antagonists. Estrogen receptors, found in the cancer cells of one-half of premenopausal and three-fourths of postmenopausal women with breast cancer, respond to estrogen to induce tumor growth.

## It's bound to inhibit growth

The antiestrogens fulvestrant, tamoxifen, and toremifene bind to the estrogen receptors and inhibit estrogen-mediated tumor growth in breast tissue. Tamoxifen may be able to do this because it binds to receptors at the nuclear level or because the binding re-

*Warning!*

## Adverse reactions to aromatase inhibitors

Adverse reactions to aromatase inhibitors are rare. They may include dizziness, mild nausea, mild muscle and joint aches, and hot flashes.

Occasionally, aromatase inhibitors can also affect cholesterol levels; anastrazole may elevate both high-density and low-density lipoprotein levels.

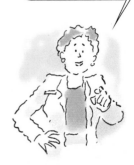

Aromatase inhibitors help treat metastatic breast cancer that occurs after menopause.

*Yea or nay?*

# Who benefits from tamoxifen?

The current indication for the use of tamoxifen is based on the 1998 results of the "Breast Cancer Prevention Trial," sponsored by the National Cancer Institute. Results indicated that tamoxifen reduced the rate of breast cancer in healthy high-risk women by one-half. However, tamoxifen has serious adverse effects that include potentially fatal blood clots and uterine cancer. The question is whether these risks are worth the benefits in healthy women.

### The National Cancer Institute's report

To help answer this question, the National Cancer Institute published a report in November of 1999. They concluded that most women older than age 60 would receive more harm than benefit from tamoxifen. Even though women younger than age 60 could benefit from taking tamoxifen, they were still at risk unless they had a hysterectomy, which eliminated the risk of uterine cancer or were in the very high-risk group for developing breast cancer.

### Breaking it down further

The report also concluded that the risks of tamoxifen were greater than the benefits for black women older than age 60 and almost all other women older than age 60 who still had a uterus. But for older women without a uterus and with a 3.5% chance of developing breast cancer over the next 5 years, the benefits may outweigh the risks.

### NSABP studies update

A report from the 2000 annual meeting of the American Society of Clinical Oncology, presented an analysis of data gathered from the National Surgical Adjuvant Breast and Bowel Project's (NSABP's) nine studies of adjuvant tamoxifen for breast cancer. The data analysis indicates that tamoxifen is as effective in Black women as in White women in reducing the occurrence of contralateral breast cancer (breast cancer that develops in the healthy breast after treatment in the opposite breast).

### Future findings

The Study of Tamoxifen and Raloxifene (STAR), is a clinical trial that was conducted to determine whether raloxifene can prevent breast cancer better and with fewer adverse effects than tamoxifen. The study began in 1999 and recently concluded. The results showed that the raloxifem-treated group had a lower incidence of uterine cancer and clotting events than the tamoxifen group.

duces the number of free receptors in the cytoplasm. Ultimately, DNA synthesis and cell growth are inhibited.

## Pharmacotherapeutics

Tamoxifen is used alone and as adjuvant treatment with radiation therapy and surgery in women with negative axillary lymph nodes and in postmenopausal women with positive axillary nodes. It's used for advanced breast cancer involving estrogen receptor–positive tumors in postmenopausal women and may be used in palliative treatment of advanced or metastatic breast cancer that's estrogen receptor–positive. Tumors in postmenopausal women are more responsive to tamoxifen than those in premenopausal women. Tamoxifen

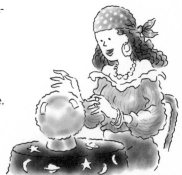

*I can see that the fates of some tumors are linked with the hormones they depend on. I predict hormonal therapies will put them in grave danger.*

may also be used to reduce the incidence of breast cancer in women at high risk.

Toremifene is used to treat metastatic breast cancer in postmenopausal women with estrogen receptor–positive tumors.

Fulvestrant is used in postmenopausal women with receptor-positive metastatic breast cancer with disease progression after treatment with tamoxifen. (See *Who benefits from tamoxifen?* page 389.)

## Drug interactions

There are no known drug interactions for fulvestrant. However, these reactions may occur with other antiestrogens:
• Tamoxifen and toremifene increase the effects of warfarin, increasing the risk of bleeding.
• Bromocriptine increases the effects of tamoxifen.
• Drugs that induce certain liver enzymes, such as phenytoin, rifampin, and carbamazepine, may increase tamoxifen metabolism, causing decreased serum levels. (See *Adverse reactions to antiestrogens.*)

# Androgens

The therapeutically useful *androgens* are synthetic derivatives of naturally occurring testosterone. They include:
• fluoxymesterone
• testolactone
• testosterone enanthate
• testosterone propionate.

## Pharmacokinetics

The pharmacokinetic properties of therapeutic androgens resemble those of naturally occurring testosterone.

### Absorption

The oral androgens—fluoxymesterone and testolactone—are well absorbed. The parenteral ones—testosterone enanthate and testosterone propionate—are designed specifically for slow absorption after I.M. injection.

### Distribution, metabolism, and excretion

Androgens are well distributed throughout the body, metabolized extensively in the liver, and excreted in urine.

*Warning!*

## Adverse reactions to antiestrogens

The most common adverse reactions to antiestrogens, such as tamoxifen, toremifene, and fulvestrant, include:
• hot flashes
• nausea
• vomiting.

**Tamoxifen**
• Diarrhea
• Fluid retention
• Vaginal bleeding

**Toremifene**
• Vaginal discharge or bleeding
• Edema

**Fulvestrant**
• Diarrhea
• Constipation
• Abdominal pain
• Headache
• Backache
• Pharyngitis

## Checking the suspension

The duration of the parenteral forms is longer because the oil suspension is absorbed slowly. Parenteral androgens are administered one to three times per week.

### Pharmacodynamics

Androgens probably act by one or more mechanisms. They may reduce the number of prolactin receptors or may bind competitively to those that are available.

## Keeping its sister hormone in check

Androgens may inhibit estrogen synthesis or competitively bind at estrogen receptors. These actions prevent estrogen from affecting estrogen-sensitive tumors.

### Pharmacotherapeutics

Androgens are indicated for the palliative treatment of advanced breast cancer, particularly in postmenopausal women with bone metastasis.

### Drug interactions

Androgens may alter dose requirement in patients receiving insulin, oral antidiabetic drugs, or oral anticoagulants. Taking them with drugs that are toxic to the liver increases the risk of liver toxicity. (See *Adverse reactions to androgens*.)

# Antiandrogens

*Antiandrogens* are used as an adjunct therapy with gonadotropin-releasing hormone analogues in treating advanced prostate cancer. These drugs include:
• flutamide
• nilutamide
• bicalutamide.

### Pharmacokinetics

After oral administration, antiandrogens are absorbed rapidly and completely.

#### Metabolism and excretion

Antiandrogens are metabolized rapidly and extensively and excreted primarily in urine.

**Warning!**

## Adverse reactions to androgens

Nausea and vomiting are the most common adverse reactions to androgens. Fluid retention caused by sodium retention may also occur.

**Just for women**
Women may develop:
• acne
• clitoral hypertrophy
• deeper voice
• increased facial and body hair
• increased sexual desire
• menstrual irregularity.

**Just for men**
Men may experience these effects as a result of conversion of steroids to female sex hormone metabolites:
• gynecomastia
• prostatic hyperplasia
• testicular atrophy.

**Just for kids**
Children may develop:
• premature epiphyseal closure
• secondary sex characteristic developments (especially in boys).

## Pharmacodynamics

Flutamide, nilutamide, and bicalutamide exert their antiandrogenic action by inhibiting androgen uptake or preventing androgen binding in cell nuclei in target tissues.

> Antiandrogens help treat metastatic prostate cancer.

## Pharmacotherapeutics

Antiandrogens are used with a gonadotropin-releasing hormone analogue, such as leuprolide, to treat metastatic prostate cancer.

### Special feature: no flareup

Concomitant administration of antiandrogens and a gonadotropin-releasing hormone analogue may help prevent the disease flare that occurs when the gonadotropin-releasing hormone analogue is used alone.

## Drug interactions

Antiandrogens don't interact significantly with other drugs. However, flutamide and bicalutamide may affect prothrombin time (a test to measure clotting factors) in a patient receiving warfarin. (See *Adverse reactions to antiandrogens*.)

# Progestins

*Progestins* are hormones used to treat various forms of cancer. These drugs include:
- hydroxyprogesterone caproate
- medroxyprogesterone acetate
- megestrol acetate.

## Pharmacokinetics

When taken orally, megestrol acetate is well absorbed. After I.M. injection in an aqueous or oil suspension, hydroxyprogesterone caproate and medroxyprogesterone are absorbed slowly from their deposit sites.

### Distribution, metabolism, and excretion

These drugs are well distributed throughout the body and may sequester in fatty tissue. Progestins are metabolized in the liver and excreted as metabolites in urine.

---

**Warning!**

## Adverse reactions to antiandrogens

When antiandrogens are used with gonadotropin-releasing hormone analogues, the most common adverse reactions are:
- hot flashes
- decreased sexual desire
- impotence
- diarrhea
- nausea
- vomiting
- breast enlargement.

## Pharmacodynamics

The mechanism of action of progestins in treating tumors isn't completely understood. Researchers believe the drugs bind to a specific receptor to act on hormonally sensitive cells.

### They aren't exhibitionists

Because progestins don't exhibit a cytotoxic activity (destroying or poisoning cells), they're considered cytostatic (they keep the cells from multiplying).

## Pharmacotherapeutics

Progestins are used for the palliative treatment of advanced endometrial, breast, prostate, and renal cancers. Of these drugs, megestrol is used most commonly.

## Drug interactions

No drug interactions have been identified for megestrol. However, other progestins do have significant interactions with other drugs.
• Barbiturates, carbamazepine, and rifampin reduce the progestin effects of hydroxyprogesterone.
• Hydroxyprogesterone and medroxyprogesterone may interfere with bromocriptine's effects, causing menstruation to stop.
• Hydroxyprogesterone taken with dantrolene and other liver-toxic drugs increases the risk of liver toxicity.
• Dose adjustments in oral anticoagulants may be needed when they're taken with hydroxyprogesterone.
• Aminoglutethimide and rifampin may reduce the progestin effects of medroxyprogesterone. (See *Adverse reactions to progestins*.)

**Warning!**

## Adverse reactions to progestins

Mild fluid retention is probably the most common reaction to progestins. Other adverse reactions include:
• thromboemboli
• breakthrough bleeding, spotting, and changes in menstrual flow
• breast tenderness
• liver function abnormalities.

### Oil issues

Patients who are hypersensitive to the oil carrier used for injection (usually sesame or castor oil) may experience a local or systemic hypersensitivity reaction.

# Gonadotropin-releasing hormone analogues

*Gonadotropin-releasing hormone analogues* are used for treatment of advanced prostate cancer. They include:
• goserelin
• leuprolide
• triptorelin.

## Pharmacokinetics

Goserelin is absorbed slowly for the first 8 days of therapy and rapidly and continuously thereafter. After subcutaneous injection, leuprolide is well absorbed. Neither drug's distribution, metabolism, or excretion is defined clearly.

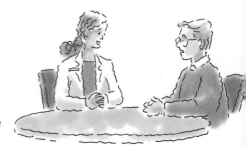

> Goserelin and leuprolide reduce the testosterone level, which can help inhibit tumor growth.

Triptorelin serum levels peak within 1 week of I.M. injection; the drug remains detectable in serum for 4 weeks.

## Pharmacodynamics

Goserelin and leuprolide act on the male's pituitary gland to increase luteinizing hormone (LH) secretion, which stimulates testosterone production. The peak testosterone level is reached about 72 hours after daily administration.

### Running the reverse

With long-term administration, however, goserelin and leuprolide inhibit LH release from the pituitary and subsequently inhibit testicular release of testosterone. Because prostate tumor cells are stimulated by testosterone, the reduced testosterone level inhibits tumor growth.

### Then there's triptorelin

Triptorelin is a potent inhibitor of gonadotropin secretion. After the first dose, levels of LH, follicle-stimulating hormone (FSH), testosterone, and estradiol surge transiently. After long-term continuous administration, LH and FSH secretion steadily declines and testicular and ovarian steroid production decreases. In men, testosterone declines to a level typically seen in surgically castrated men. As a result, tissues and functions that depend on these hormones become inactive.

## Pharmacotherapeutics

Goserelin, leuprolide, and triptorelin are used for the palliative treatment of metastatic prostate cancer. The drugs lower the testosterone level without the adverse psychological effects of castration or the adverse cardiovascular effects of diethylstilbestrol.

## Drug interactions

No drug interactions have been identified with goserelin, leuprolide, or triptorelin. (See *Adverse reactions to gonadotropin-releasing hormone analogues.*)

# Natural antineoplastic drugs

A subclass of antineoplastic drugs known as *natural products* includes:
- vinca alkaloids
- podophyllotoxins.

# Vinca alkaloids

*Vinca alkaloids* are nitrogenous bases derived from the periwinkle plant. These drugs are cell cycle–specific for the M phase and include:
- vinblastine
- vincristine
- vinorelbine.

## Pharmacokinetics

After I.V. administration, the vinca alkaloids are well distributed throughout the body.

### Metabolism and excretion

Vinca alkaloids undergo moderate liver metabolism before being eliminated through different phases, primarily in stool with a small percentage eliminated in urine.

## Pharmacodynamics

Vinca alkaloids may disrupt the normal function of the microtubules (structures within cells that are associated with the movement of DNA) by binding to the protein tubulin in the microtubules.

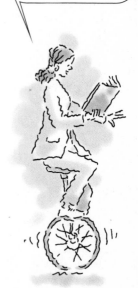

The vinca alkaloids are cell cycle–specific. They do their work during the M phase, which is the phase of mitosis, or cell division.

## Separation anxiety

With the microtubules unable to separate chromosomes properly, the chromosomes are dispersed throughout the cytoplasm or arranged in unusual groupings. As a result, formation of the mitotic spindle is prevented, and the cells can't complete mitosis (cell division).

## Under arrest

Cell division is arrested in metaphase, causing cell death. Therefore, vinca alkaloids are cell cycle–specific for the M phase. Interruption of the microtubule function may also impair some types of cellular movement, phagocytosis (engulfing and destroying microorganisms and cellular debris), and CNS functions.

### Pharmacotherapeutics

Vinca alkaloids are used in several therapeutic situations:
• Vinblastine is used to treat metastatic testicular cancer, lymphomas, Kaposi's sarcoma (the most common acquired immunodeficiency syndrome [AIDS]–related cancer), neuroblastoma (a highly malignant tumor originating in the sympathetic nervous system), breast cancer, and choriocarcinoma.
• Vincristine is used in combination therapy to treat Hodgkin's disease, non-Hodgkin's lymphoma, Wilms' tumor, rhabdomyosarcoma, and acute lymphocytic leukemia.
• Vinorelbine is used to treat non–small-cell lung cancer. It may also be used in the treatment of metastatic breast cancer, cisplatin-resistant ovarian cancer, and Hodgkin's disease.

### Drug interactions

Vinca alkaloids can interact with other drugs.
• Erythromycin may increase the toxicity of vinblastine.
• Vinblastine decreases the plasma levels of phenytoin.
• Vincristine reduces the effects of digoxin.
• Asparaginase decreases liver metabolism of vincristine, increasing the risk of toxicity.
• Calcium channel blockers enhance vincristine accumulation, increasing the tendency for toxicity. (See *Adverse reactions to vinca alkaloids*.)

# Podophyllotoxins

*Podophyllotoxins* are semisynthetic glycosides that are cell cycle–specific and act during the G2 and late S phases of the cell cycle. They include:

**Warning!**

## Adverse reactions to vinca alkaloids

Nausea, vomiting, constipation, and stomatitis may occur in patients taking vinca alkaloids. Tissue necrosis may also occur with extravasation.

**Toxic topics**
Vinblastine and vinorelbine toxicities occur primarily as bone marrow suppression.

**Muscle matters**
Neuromuscular abnormalities commonly occur with vincristine and vinorelbine and, occasionally, with vinblastine therapy.

**Tumor trouble**
Vinblastine may produce tumor pain described as an intense stinging or burning in the tumor bed, with an abrupt onset 1 to 3 minutes after drug administration. The pain usually lasts 20 minutes to 3 hours.

**Less hair there**
Reversible alopecia occurs in up to one-half of patients receiving vinca alkaloids; it's more likely to occur with vincristine than with vinblastine.

- etoposide
- teniposide.

## Outside activities

Etoposide is effective in the treatment of testicular cancer, non-Hodgkin's lymphoma, lung cancer, and acute leukemia. Teniposide has demonstrated some activity in treating Hodgkin's disease, lymphomas, and brain tumors.

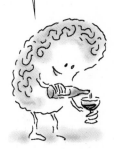

I may have a reason to celebrate! Teniposide shows some activity in treating brain tumors!

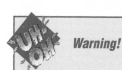

## Pharmacokinetics

When taken orally, podophyllotoxins are only moderately absorbed. Although the drugs are widely distributed throughout the body, they achieve poor CSF levels.

### Metabolism and excretion

Podophyllotoxins undergo liver metabolism and are excreted primarily in urine.

## Pharmacodynamics

Although their mechanism of action isn't completely understood, podophyllotoxins produce several biochemical changes in tumor cells.

## Arresting development

At low concentrations, these drugs block cells at the late S or G2 phase. At higher concentrations, they arrest the cells in the G2 phase.

## Breaking a rung on the ladder

Podophyllotoxins can also break one of the strands of the DNA molecule and can inhibit nucleotide transport and incorporation into nucleic acids.

## Pharmacotherapeutics

Etoposide is used to treat testicular cancer lymphomas, prostate cancer, and small-cell lung cancer. Teniposide is used to treat acute lymphoblastic leukemia.

## Drug interactions

Podophyllotoxins have few significant interactions with other drugs.
- Etoposide may increase the risk of bleeding in a patient taking warfarin.
- Teniposide may increase the clearance and intracellular levels of methotrexate. (See *Adverse reactions to podophyllotoxins*.)

---

**Warning!**

## Adverse reactions to podophyllotoxins

The majority of patients receiving podophyllotoxins experience hair loss. Other adverse reactions include:
- nausea and vomiting
- anorexia
- stomatitis
- bone marrow suppression, causing leukopenia and, less commonly, thrombocytopenia
- acute hypotension (if a podophyllotoxin is infused too rapidly I.V.).

# Monoclonal antibodies

Recombinant DNA technology has allowed for the development of *monoclonal antibodies* directed at such targets as other immune cells or cancer cells. Monoclonal antibodies include:
- alemtuzumab
- gemtuzumab ozogamicin
- ibritumomab tiuxetan
- rituximab
- trastuzumab.

## Pharmacokinetics

Because of their large protein molecule structure, monoclonal antibodies aren't absorbed orally. They may have a limited distribution as well as a long half-life, sometimes measured in weeks.

## Pharmacodynamics

Monoclonal antibodies bind to target receptors or cancer cells and cause tumor death via several mechanisms: They may induce programmed cell death; they may recruit other elements of the immune system to attack the cancer cell; or they may deliver a dose of a toxic chemotherapy drug (gemtuzumab) or radiation (ibritumomab) to the tumor site.

## Pharmacotherapeutics

Monoclonal antibodies have demonstrated activity in both solid tumors and hematologic malignancies, such as:
- non-Hodgkin's lymphoma—rituximab and ibritumomab (target CD20 or malignant B lymphocytes)
- chronic lymphocytic leukemia—alemtuzumab (target CD52 antigen or B cells)
- acute myeloid leukemia—gemtuzumab (target CD33 antigen in myeloid leukemic cells)
- breast cancer—trastuzumab (target HER-2 protein in breast cancer cells).

## Drug interactions

Although no interactions have been noted with alemtuzumab, multiple drug interactions are associated with other monoclonal antibodies.

These drugs sometimes work by recruiting the immune system to attack a cancer cell.

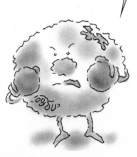

• Ibritumomab may interfere with the actions of such drugs as warfarin, aspirin, clopidogrel, ticlopidine, nonsteroidal anti-inflammatory drugs, azathioprine, cyclosporine, and corticosteroids.
• Trastuzumab increases the cardiac toxicity associated with anthracycline administration. (See *Adverse reactions to monoclonal antibodies.*)

# Topoisomerase I inhibitors

*Topoisomerase I inhibitors* are derivatives of camptothecin and inhibit the enzyme topoisomerase I. These agents are derived from a naturally occurring alkaloid from the Chinese tree *Camptotheca acuminata*. Currently available topoisomerase I inhibitors include:
• irinotecan
• topotecan.

## Pharmacokinetics

Both irinotecan and topotecan are minimally absorbed and must be given I.V. Irinotecan undergoes metabolic changes to become the active metabolite SN-38. The half-life of SN-38 is about 10 hours; SN-38 is eliminated through biliary excretion. Topotecan is metabolized by the liver, although renal excretion is a significant path for elimination.

## Pharmacodynamics

Topoisomerase I inhibitors exert their cytotoxic effect by inhibiting topoisomerase I enzyme, an essential enzyme that mediates the relaxation of supercoiled DNA.

### It's all about that DNA

Topoisomerase inhibitors bind to the DNA topoisomerase I complex and prevent resealing, thereby causing DNA strand breaks. This results in impaired DNA synthesis.

## Pharmacotherapeutics

Topoisomerase I inhibitors act against both solid tumors and hematologic malignancies:
• Irinotecan is used to treat colorectal cancer and small-cell lung cancer.

*Warning!*

## Adverse reactions to monoclonal antibodies

All monoclonal antibodies are associated with infusion-related reactions that have occasionally been fatal. These include fever, chills, shortness of breath, low blood pressure, and anaphylaxis.

In addition, the following adverse reactions can occur:
• Alemtuzumab is associated with myelosuppression and an increased risk of opportunistic infections, such as pneumocystitis, pneumonia, and fungal and viral infections.
• Gemtuzumab ozogamicin is associated with significant myelosuppression and liver toxicity.
• Ibritumomab tiuxetan is associated with increased myelosuppression to rituximab.

• Topotecan is used to treat ovarian cancer, small-cell lung cancer, and acute myeloid leukemia.

## Drug interactions

Topoisomerase I inhibitors, particularly irinotecan, can interact with other drugs.
• Ketoconazole significantly increases SN-38 serum levels, thereby increasing the risk of irinotecan-associated toxicities.
• Irinotecan when taken with diuretics may exacerbate dehydration caused by irinotecan-induced diarrhea.
• Laxatives taken with irinotecan can induce diarrhea.
• Prochlorperazine administered with irinotecan can increase the incidence of extrapyramidal toxicities. (See *Adverse reactions to topoisomerase I inhibitors*.)

# Targeted therapies

A groundbreaking approach to anticancer therapies involves targeting proteins associated with the growth patterns of specific types of cancer. Drugs used for this new approach to cancer treatment include:
• bortezomib
• gefitinib
• imatinib.

## Pharmacokinetics

*Bortezomib* isn't absorbed orally and must be given I.V. It's extensively distributed into body tissues and metabolized by the liver.

*Gefitinib* is available in an oral form, and about half of the dose is absorbed. The drug is widely distributed in tissues. It undergoes hepatic metabolism with minimal urinary excretion.

*Imatinib* is also available in an oral form and is almost completely absorbed. It's 95% bound to plasma proteins and is extensively metabolized by the liver. The half-life of imatinib is about 15 hours.

## Pharmacodynamics

Bortezomib inhibits proteosomes, which are involved in integral cell-cycle function and promote tumor growth. Proteolysis by bortezomib results in disruption of the normal homeostatic mechanisms and leads to cell death.

*Warning!*

## Adverse reactions to topoisomerase I inhibitors

**Common reactions**
The more common adverse reactions to topoisomerase I inhibitors, particularly irinotecan, include:
• diarrhea (possibly severe)
• abdominal cramps
• hair loss or thinning
• increased sweating and production of saliva
• nausea, vomiting, and loss of appetite
• tiredness
• watery eyes.

**Additional reactions**
Occasionally, these reactions may occur:
• mouth sores and ulcers
• muscle cramps
• rashes, which may be itchy
• significant myelosuppression, especially with topotecan (rare)
• temporary effects on liver function test results.

## Too much of this...

Gefitinib inhibits the epidermal growth factor receptor-1 tyrosine kinase, which is overexpressed in such cancers as non–small-cell lung cancer. This inhibition blocks signaling pathways for growth, survival, and metastasis of cancer.

## ...too many of those

In patients with chronic myeloid leukemia, the BCR-ABL protein stimulates other tyrosine kinase proteins, causing an abnormally high production of WBCs. Imatinib binds to the adenosine triphosphate–binding domain of the BCR-ABL protein, effectively shutting down the abnormal WBC production.

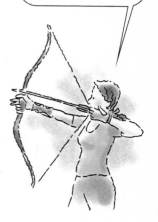

A new approach to treating cancer involves targeting the proteins that cause the growth of certain cancer types.

## Pharmacotherapeutics

Bortezomib is used to treat multiple myeloma that has relapsed after standard chemotherapy.

Gefitinib is used as a single agent for patients with non–small-cell lung cancer that hasn't responded to two standard chemotherapy regimens.

Imatinib is used to treat chronic myeloid leukemia, acute lymphoid leukemia, and GI stomal tumors.

## Drug interactions

Bortezomib, gefitinib, and imatinib have been associated with some drug interactions.

• Bortezomib when taken with drugs that inhibit cytochrome CYP3A4 (such as amiodarone, cimetidine, erythromycin, diltiazem, fluoxetine, verapamil, zafirlukast, and zileuton) or induce cytochrome CYP3A4 (such as amiodarone, carbamazepine, nevirapine, phenobarbital, phenytoin, and rifampin), could cause either toxicities or reduced efficacy of these drugs.

• Bortezomib when taken with oral hypoglycemics could cause hypoglycemia and hyperglycemia in patients with diabetes.

• Plasma levels of gefitinib and imatinib are reduced, sometimes substantially, when these drugs are given with carbamazepine, dexamethasone, phenobarbital, phenytoin, rifampin, or St. John's wort.

• High doses of ranitidine with sodium bicarbonate when taken with gefitinib reduce gefitinib levels.

• Administration of gefitinib or imatinib with warfarin causes elevations in the International Normalized Ratio, increasing the risk of bleeding.

• Clarithromycin, erythromycin, itraconazole, and ketoconazole, when taken with imatinibor may increase imatinib plasma levels.

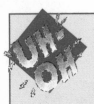

• Carbamazepine, dexamethasone, phenobarbital, phenytoin, or rifampin given with imatinib may increase metabolism of imatinib and decrease imatinib level.
• Imatinib given with simvastatin increases simvastatin levels about threefold.
• Imatinib increases plasma levels of other CYP3A4-metabolized drugs, such as triazolo-benzodiazepines, calcium channel blockers, and certain HMG-CoA reductase inhibitors. (See *Adverse reactions to targeted therapies.*)

# Unclassifiable antineoplastic drugs

Many other antineoplastic drugs can't be included in existing classifications. These drugs include:
• arsenic trioxide
• asparaginases
• procarbazine
• hydroxyurea
• interferon
• aldesleukin
• altretamine
• paclitaxel (taxane)
• docetaxel (taxane).

# Arsenic trioxide

*Arsenic trioxide* is a commercially available treatment for patients with acute promyelocytic leukemia (a rare form of acute myeloid leukemia). It's indicated when standard therapy has failed.

## Pharmacokinetics

Arsenic trioxide is administered I.V. because it's inadequately absorbed orally. The metabolism of arsenic trioxide involves reduction via arsenate reductase, with subsequent methylation to inactive metabolites in urine. Arsenic is distributed in the heart, liver, kidney, lung, hair, and nails. (See *Preventng the fatal effects of arsenic.*)

## Pharmacodynamics

Arsenic trioxide causes DNA fragmentation.

## Pharmacotherapeutics

Arsenic trioxide is used to treat acute promyelocytic leukemia that has relapsed after standard chemotherapy. It's also being investigated for treatment of multiple myeloma.

## Drug interactions

Giving arsenic trioxide with other drugs known to prolong the QT interval may increase the risk of cardiac arrhythmias. (See *Adverse reactions to arsenic trioxide.*)

*Warning!*

## Adverse reactions to arsenic trioxide

Arsenic trioxide can cause electrocardiogram abnormalities, which could progress to life-threatening cardiac arrhythmias. Other adverse reactions include:
• anxiety
• dizziness
• headache
• hypocalcemia
• insomnia
• liver damage
• muscle and bone aches
• nausea and vomiting
• rash
• tremor.

*Safe and sound*

## Preventing the fatal effects of arsenic

Arsenic trioxide has been linked to acute promyelocytic leukemia (APL) differentiation syndrome. To prevent its life-threatening effects, follow these guidelines:
• Monitor the patient for signs and symptoms of APL differentiation syndrome, including dyspnea, weight gain, pulmonary infiltrates, and pleural or pericardial effusion with or without leukocytosis.
• If you detect any of these signs or symptoms, notify the prescriber immediately.
• Expect to treat the syndrome with high doses of corticosteroids.

# Asparaginases

*Asparaginases* are cell cycle–specific and act during the G1 phase. They include:
- asparaginase
- pegaspargase.

## Pharmacokinetics

Asparaginase is administered parenterally. It's considered 100% bioavailable when administered I.V. and about 50% bioavailable when administered I.M.

### Distribution and metabolism

After administration, asparaginase remains inside the blood vessels, with minimal distribution elsewhere. The metabolism of asparaginase is unknown; only trace amounts appear in urine.

## Pharmacodynamics

Asparaginase and pegaspargase capitalize on the biochemical differences between normal cells and tumor cells.

*Tumor cells—eat your asparagine or else*

Most normal cells can synthesize asparagine, but some tumor cells depend on other sources of asparagine for survival. Asparaginase and pegaspargase help to degrade asparagine to aspartic acid and ammonia. Deprived of their supply of asparagine, the tumor cells die.

## Pharmacotherapeutics

Asparaginase is used primarily in combination with standard chemotherapy to induce remission in patients with acute lymphocytic leukemia.

*If allergic...*

Pegaspargase is used to treat acute lymphocytic leukemia in patients who are allergic to the native form of asparaginase.

## Drug interactions

Asparaginase drugs may interact with other drugs. Asparaginase and pegaspargase may reduce the effectiveness of methotrexate. Concurrent use of asparaginase with prednisone or vincristine increases the risk of toxicity. (See *Adverse reactions to asparaginase drugs.*)

**Warning!**

## Adverse reactions to asparaginase drugs

Many patients receiving asparaginase and pegaspargase develop nausea and vomiting. Fever, headache, abdominal pain, pancreatitis, coagulopathy, and liver toxicity may also occur.

**Rising risk**
Asparaginase and pegaspargase can cause anaphylaxis, which is more likely to occur with intermittent I.V. dosing than with daily I.V. dosing or I.M. injections. The risk of a reaction rises with each successive treatment.
   Hypersensitivity reactions may also occur.

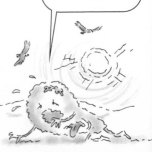

Without asparaginase, I'm finished!

# Procarbazine

*Procarbazine hydrochloride*, a methylhydrazine derivative with monoamine oxidase inhibitor (MAOI) properties, is used to treat Hodgkin's disease and primary and metastatic brain tumors.

## Pharmacokinetics

After oral administration, procarbazine is well absorbed. It readily crosses the blood-brain barrier and is well distributed into CSF.

### Metabolism and excretion

Procarbazine is metabolized rapidly in the liver and must be activated metabolically by microsomal enzymes. It's excreted in urine, primarily as metabolites. Respiratory excretion of the drug occurs as methane and carbon dioxide gas.

## Pharmacodynamics

An inert drug, procarbazine must be activated metabolically in the liver before it can produce various cell changes. It can cause chromosomal damage, suppress mitosis, and inhibit DNA, RNA, and protein synthesis. Cancer cells can quickly develop resistance to procarbazine.

## Pharmacotherapeutics

Procarbazine is used in the treatment of Hodgkin's disease, lymphoma, and brain cancer.

## Drug interactions

Interactions with procarbazine can be significant.
• It produces an additive effect when administered with CNS depressants.
• Taken with meperidine, it may result in severe hypotension and death.

### Mirroring MAO

Because of procarbazine's MAOI properties, hypertensive reactions may occur when it's administered concurrently with sympathomimetics, antidepressants, and tyramine-rich foods. (See *Adverse reactions to procarbazine*.)

**Warning!**

## Adverse reactions to procarbazine

Late-onset bone marrow suppression is the most common dose-limiting toxicity associated with procarbazine. Interstitial pneumonitis (lung inflammation) and pulmonary fibrosis (scarring) may also occur.

**A bad start**
Initial procarbazine therapy may induce flulike symptoms, including fever, chills, sweating, lethargy, and muscle pain.

**Gut reactions**
GI reactions include nausea, vomiting, stomatitis, and diarrhea.

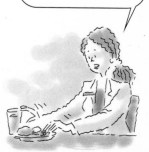

Procarbazine has MAOI properties. So watch out for tyramine-rich foods!

# Hydroxyurea

*Hydroxyurea* is used most commonly for patients with chronic myelogenous leukemia.

## When your neck is on the line

Hydroxyurea is also used for solid tumors and head and neck cancer.

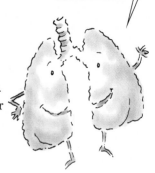

Fortunately, hydroxyurea can treat lung cancers!

## Pharmacokinetics

Hydroxyurea is readily absorbed and well distributed into CSF after oral administration. It reaches a peak serum level 2 hours after administration.

### Metabolism and excretion

About one-half of the dose is metabolized by the liver to carbon dioxide, which is excreted by the lungs, or to urea, which is excreted by the kidneys. The remaining one-half is excreted unchanged in urine.

## Pharmacodynamics

Hydroxyurea exerts its effect by inhibiting the enzyme ribonucleotide reductase, which is necessary for DNA synthesis.

## Divide and conquer

Hydroxyurea kills cells in the S phase of the cell cycle and holds other cells in the G1 phase, where they're most susceptible to irradiation.

## Pharmacotherapeutics

Hydroxyurea is used to treat selected myeloproliferative disorders. It may produce temporary remissions in some patients with metastatic malignant melanomas as well.

## Working with radiation

Hydroxyurea is also used in combination therapy with radiation to treat cancers of the head, neck, and lungs.

## Drug interactions

Cytotoxic drugs and radiation therapy enhance the toxicity of hydroxyurea. (See *Adverse reactions to hydroxyurea.*)

**Warning!**

## Adverse reactions to hydroxyurea

Treatment with hydroxyurea leads to few adverse reactions. Those that do occur include:
• bone marrow suppression
• drowsiness
• headache
• nausea and vomiting
• skin rash
• anorexia
• elevated uric acid levels, which require some patients to take allopurinol to prevent kidney damage.

# Interferons

A family of naturally occurring glycoproteins, *interferons* are so named because of their ability to interfere with viral replication. These drugs exhibit anticancer activity as well as activity against condylomata acuminata (soft, wartlike growths on the skin and mucous membrane of the genitalia caused by a virus). The three types of interferons are:

- *alfa interferons* derived from leukocytes

- *beta interferons* derived from fibroblasts (connective tissue cells)

- *gamma interferons* derived from fibroblasts and lymphocytes.

## Pharmacokinetics

After I.M. or subcutaneous administration, interferons are usually well absorbed. Information about their distribution is unavailable.

### Metabolism and excretion

Alfa interferons are filtered by the kidneys, where they're degraded. Liver metabolism and biliary excretion of interferons are negligible.

## Pharmacodynamics

Although their exact mechanism of action is unknown, interferons appear to bind to specific membrane receptors on the cell surface. When bound, they initiate a sequence of intracellular events that includes the induction of certain enzymes.

### Running interference

This process may account for the ability of interferons to:
- inhibit viral replication
- suppress cell proliferation
- enhance macrophage activity (engulfing and destroying microorganisms and other debris)
- increase cytotoxicity of lymphocytes for target cells.

## Pharmacotherapeutics

Alfa interferons have shown their most promising activity in treating blood malignancies, especially hairy cell leukemia. Their approved indications currently include:
- hairy cell leukemia

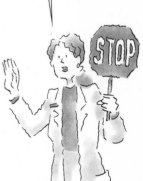

Interferons can put a stop to viral replication.

- AIDS-related Kaposi's sarcoma
- condylomata acuminata.

## Interfering in these areas as well...

Alfa interferons also demonstrate some activity against chronic myelogenous leukemia, malignant lymphoma, multiple myeloma, melanoma, and renal cell carcinoma.

### Drug interactions

Interferons interact with other drugs:
- They may enhance the CNS effects of CNS depressants and substantially increase the half-life of methylxanthines (including theophylline and aminophylline).
- Concurrent use with a live virus vaccine may potentiate replication of the virus, increasing the adverse effects of the vaccine and decreasing the patient's antibody response.
- Bone marrow suppression may be increased when an interferon is used with radiation therapy or a drug that causes blood abnormalities or bone marrow suppression.
- Alfa interferons increase the risk of kidney failure from interleukin-2. (See *Adverse reactions to interferons*.)

# Aldesleukin

*Aldesleukin* is a human recombinant interleukin-2 derivative that's used to treat metastatic renal cell carcinoma.

### Pharmacokinetics

After I.V. administration of aldesleukin, about 30% is absorbed into plasma and about 70% is absorbed rapidly by the liver, kidneys, and lungs. The drug is excreted primarily by the kidneys.

### Pharmacodynamics

The exact antitumor mechanism of action of aldesleukin is unknown. The drug may stimulate an immunologic reaction against the tumor.

### Pharmacotherapeutics

Aldesleukin is used to treat metastatic renal cell carcinoma. It may also be used in the treatment of Kaposi's sarcoma and metastatic melanoma.

**Warning!**

## Adverse reactions to interferons

Blood toxicity occurs in up to one-half of patients taking interferons and may produce leukopenia, neutropenia, thrombocytopenia, and anemia. Adverse GI reactions include anorexia, nausea, and diarrhea.

**Alfa concerns**
The most common adverse reaction to alfa interferons is the development of flulike symptoms, which may produce fever, fatigue, muscle pain, headache, chills, and joint pain.

**It catches your breath**
Coughing, difficulty breathing, hypotension, edema, chest pain, and heart failure have also been associated with interferon therapy.

## Drug interactions

Aldesleukin will interact with other drugs.

• Concomitant administration of aldesleukin and drugs with psychotropic properties (such as opioids, analgesics, antiemetics, sedatives, and tranquilizers) may produce additive CNS effects.

• Glucocorticoids may reduce aldesleukin's antitumor effects.

• Antihypertensive drugs may potentiate aldesleukin's hypotensive effects.

• Concurrent therapy with drugs that are toxic to the kidneys (such as aminoglycosides), bone marrow (such as cytotoxic chemotherapy drugs), heart (such as doxorubicin), or liver (such as methotrexate or asparaginase) may increase toxicity to these organs. (See *Adverse reactions to aldesleukin*.)

# Altretamine

*Altretamine* is a synthetic cytotoxic antineoplastic drug that's used as palliative treatment for patients with ovarian cancer.

## Pharmacokinetics

Altretamine is well absorbed after oral administration.

### Metabolism and excretion

Altretamine is metabolized extensively in the liver and excreted by the liver and kidneys. The parent compound is poorly bound to plasma proteins.

## Pharmacodynamics

The exact mechanism of action of altretamine is unknown. However, its metabolites are alkylating drugs.

## Pharmacotherapeutics

Altretamine is used as palliative treatment of persistent or recurring ovarian cancer after first-line therapy with cisplatin or an alkylating drug-based combination.

## Drug interactions

Altretamine has a few significant interactions with other drugs. Concomitant therapy with cimetidine may increase altretamine's half-life, increasing the risk of altretamine toxicity.

*Warning!*

## Adverse reactions to aldesleukin

During clinical trials, more than 15% of patients developed adverse reactions to aldesleukin. These include:

• pulmonary congestion and difficulty breathing

• anemia, thrombocytopenia, and leukopenia

• elevated bilirubin, transaminase, and alkaline phosphate levels

• hypomagnesemia and acidosis

• reduced or absent urinary output

• elevated serum creatinine level

• stomatitis

• nausea and vomiting.

## Don't mix with MAOI

Use with an MAOI may cause severe orthostatic hypotension (a drop in blood pressure upon rising). (See *Adverse reactions to altretamine*.)

# Paclitaxel and docetaxel

*Antineoplastic drugs* are used to treat metastatic ovarian and breast cancer after chemotherapy has failed. They include:
- paclitaxel
- docetaxel.

## Pharmacokinetics

After I.V. administration, paclitaxel is highly bound to plasma proteins. Docetaxel is administered I.V. with a rapid onset of action.

### Metabolism and excretion

Paclitaxel is metabolized primarily in the liver with a small amount excreted unchanged in urine. Docetaxel is excreted primarily in stool.

## Pharmacodynamics

Paclitaxel and docetaxel exert their chemotherapeutic effect by disrupting the microtubule network essential for mitosis and other vital cellular functions.

## Pharmacotherapeutics

Paclitaxel is used when first-line or subsequent chemotherapy has failed in treating metastatic ovarian cancer as well as metastatic breast cancer.

## Head, neck, and below

The taxanes may also be used for treating head and neck cancer, prostate cancer, and non–small-cell lung cancer. (See *Cultural considerations with docetaxel use*.)

## Drug interactions

Taxanes may interact with other drugs.
- Concomitant use of paclitaxel and cisplatin may cause additive myelosuppressive effects.
- Cyclosporine, ketoconazole, erythromycin, and troleandomycin may modify the metabolism of docetaxel.

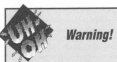

**Warning!**

## Adverse reactions to altretamine

More than 10% of patients using altretamine in clinical trials experienced adverse reactions, such as:
- nausea and vomiting
- neurotoxicity
- peripheral neuropathy
- anemia.

Bone marrow suppression is also common.

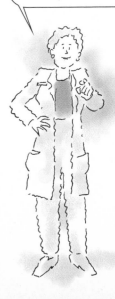

When other treatments fail, don't give up! Try paclitaxel to treat metastatic ovarian cancer and breast cancer.

## Yea or nay?

## Cultural considerations with docetaxel use

Clinical trials of docetaxel in Japanese and American patients with breast cancer revealed significant differences in the incidence of adverse effects between the two cultures.

**The results**

Japanese women were more likely to develop thrombocytopenia—14.4% versus 5.5%. However, the Japanese women in this study were less likely than the American patients (6% versus 29.1%) to develop many of the other adverse reactions such as hypersensitivity reactions.

Other results showed fewer incidences of fluid retention, neurosensory effects, muscle pain, infection, and development of anemia in the Japanese patients. The study also indicated that Japanese patients are more likely to develop fatigue and weakness than are American women.

**Putting it into a plan**

These results are important to consider when caring for patients receiving docetaxel and can provide clues for developing a care plan and for knowing what adverse reactions to expect.

## Warning!

## Adverse reactions to paclitaxel and docetaxel

During clinical trials, 25% or higher of patients experienced these adverse reactions to paclitaxel:
• bone marrow suppression
• hypersensitivity reactions
• abnormal EEG tracings
• peripheral neuropathy
• muscle pain and joint pain
• nausea, vomiting, and diarrhea
• mucous membrane inflammation
• hair loss.

**Docetaxel**

Adverse reactions to docetaxel include:
• hypersensitivity reactions
• fluid retention
• leukopenia, neutropenia, or thrombocytopenia
• hair loss
• stomatitis
• numbness and tingling
• pain
• weakness and fatigue.

• Phenytoin may decrease paclitaxel serum level, leading to a loss of efficacy.
• Quinupristin/dalfopristin may increase paclitaxel serum levels, increasing the risk of toxicity. (See *Adverse reactions to paclitaxel and docetaxel.*)

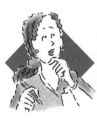

# *Quick quiz*

**1.** What's the major adverse reaction that's common to all alkylating drugs?
   A.   Photosensitivity
   B.   Nerve toxicity
   C.   Cardiac toxicity
   D.   Bone marrow suppression

*Answer:* D. Bone marrow suppression is a common adverse reaction to all alkylating drugs.

**2.** The drug likely to be administered with methotrexate to minimize its adverse effects is:

    A. fluorouracil.

    B. leucovorin.

    C. cladribine.

    D. trastuzumab.

*Answer:* B. Leucovorin is typically administered in conjunction with methotrexate to minimize adverse effects.

**3.** Before administering bleomycin to a patient, why should you administer an antihistamine and an antipyretic?

    A. To prevent fever and chills

    B. To prevent anaphylactic shock

    C. To prevent bone marrow suppression

    D. To prevent hypertension

*Answer:* A. An antihistamine and an antipyretic may be administered before bleomycin to prevent fever and chills.

## Scoring

☆☆☆ If you answered all three items correctly, extraordinary! You really mowed down the malignant neoplasms!

☆☆ If you answered two items correctly, congratulations! You're more than competent to combat cancer!

☆ If you answered fewer than two items correctly, give it another shot! Remember, this is your last crack at a quick quiz!

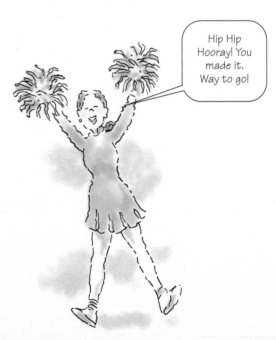

Hip Hip Hooray! You made it. Way to go!

# Appendices, references, and index

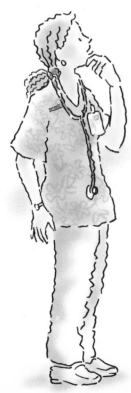

Other major drugs      414

Vaccines and treatment for
biological weapons exposure      421

Treatment and antidotes for
chemical weapons exposure      422

Herbal drugs      423

Selected references      426

Index      427

# Other major drugs

## OPHTHALMIC DRUGS

| Drug | Action | Treatment uses | Adverse reactions |
|------|--------|----------------|-------------------|
| **_Antiallergic agents_** | | | |
| Azelastine<br>Cromolyn<br>Emedastine<br>Ketotifen<br>Lodoxamide<br>Olopatadine | • Decrease irritation | • To treat allergic conjunctivitis<br>• To treat seasonal conjunctivitis<br>• To treat keratitis | • Tearing |
| **_Anesthetics_** | | | |
| Proparacaine<br>Tetracaine | • Prevent the initiation and transmission of nerve impulses | • To anesthetize the cornea, allowing application of instruments for measuring intraocular pressure (IOP) or removing foreign bodies<br>• To prepare for suture removal, conjunctival or corneal scraping, and tear duct manipulation | • Corneal inflammation<br>• Corneal opacities<br>• Delayed corneal healing<br>• Eye pain and redness<br>• Loss of visual acuity<br>• Scarring |
| **_Anti-infectives_** | | | |
| Ciprofloxacin<br>Erythromycin<br>Gentamicin<br>Levofloxacin<br>Natamycin<br>Norfloxacin<br>Ofloxacin<br>Sulfacetamide<br>Sulfisoxazole<br>Tobramycin<br>Trifluridine | • Kill bacteria or inhibit growth of bacteria or viruses | • To treat corneal ulcers or conjunctivitis caused by bacteria, fungus, or virus (each drug is specific to particular organisms) | • Secondary eye infections (with prolonged use)<br>• Severe hypersensitivity reactions |

## OPHTHALMIC DRUGS *(continued)*

| Drug | Action | Treatment uses | Adverse reactions |
|------|--------|----------------|-------------------|
| ***Anti-inflammatories*** | | | |
| *Steroidal anti-inflammatories*<br>Dexamethasone<br>Fluorometholone<br>Loteprednol<br>Prednisolone<br>Rimexolone | • Decrease leukocyte infiltration at inflammation sites, causing reduced oozing of fluids and reduced edema, redness, and scarring | • To treat inflammatory disorders and hypersensitivity-related conditions of the cornea, iris, conjunctiva, sclera, and anterior uvea | • Corneal ulceration<br>• Delayed corneal healing<br>• Increased susceptibility to viral or fungal corneal infection |
| *Nonsteroidal anti-inflammatories*<br>Diclofenac<br>Flurbiprofen<br>Ketorolac<br>Suprofen | • Decrease inflammation and itching | • To inhibit pupil constriction during surgery (flurbiprofen and suprofen)<br>• To reduce itching due to seasonal allergies (ketorolac)<br>• To treat inflammation after surgery | • Tearing, discomfort |
| ***Lubricants*** | | | |
| Methylcellulose<br>Polyvinyl alcohol | • Act as artificial tears<br>• Moisten cornea | • To protect cornea during diagnostic procedures<br>• To moisten contact lenses | • None |
| ***Miotics*** | | | |
| Carbachol<br>Pilocarpine | • Stimulate and contract the sphincter muscle of the iris, constricting the pupil<br>• Improve aqueous outflow | • To treat open-angle glaucoma, acute and chronic angle-closure glaucoma, and certain cases of secondary glaucoma resulting from increased IOP | • Blurred vision<br>• Bronchospasm<br>• Cataract formation<br>• Eye pain<br>• Photosensitivity<br>• Reversible iris cysts |
| ***Mydriatics*** | | | |
| Dipivefrin<br>Epinephrine<br>Hydroxyamphetamine<br>Phenylephrine | • Act on the iris to dilate the pupil<br>• Lower IOP | • To dilate the pupils for intraocular examinations<br>• To lower IOP in patients with glaucoma | • Blurred vision<br>• Confusion<br>• Dry skin<br>• Flushing<br>• Impaired ability to coordinate movement<br>• Irritation<br>• Rapid heart rate<br>• Transient burning sensations |

## OPHTHALMIC DRUGS *(continued)*

| Drug | Action | Treatment uses | Adverse reactions |
|---|---|---|---|
| ***Mydriatics and cycloplegics*** | | | |
| Atropine sulfate<br>Cyclopentolate hydrochloride<br>Homatropine hydrobromide<br>Tropicamide | • Act on the ciliary body of the eye to paralyze the fine-focusing muscles (thereby preventing accommodation for near vision) | • To perform refractive eye examinations in children before and after ophthalmic surgery<br>• To treat conditions involving the iris | • Same as for mydriatics |
| ***Other drugs to lower IOP*** | | | |
| *Adrenergic blockers (topical)*<br>Apraclonidine<br>Betaxolol<br>Brimonidine<br>Carteolol<br>Levobunolol<br>Metipranolol<br>Timolol maleate | • May reduce aqueous humor formation and slightly increase aqueous humor outflow | • To prevent and control elevated IOP, chronic open-angle glaucoma, and secondary glaucoma | • Bronchospasm<br>• Fatigue<br>• Headaches<br>• Slow heart rate |
| *Carbonic anhydrase inhibitors*<br>Acetazolamide<br>Brinzolamide<br>Dorzolamide | • Inhibit action of carbonic anhydrase, thus decreasing aqueous humor production | • To treat chronic open-angle glaucoma, acute angle-closure episodes, and secondary glaucoma | • Hemolytic or aplastic anemia<br>• Hypokalemia<br>• Leukopenia<br>• Nausea and vomiting |
| *Osmotic agents*<br>Glycerin<br>Isosorbide<br>Mannitol | • Reduce volume of vitreous humor<br>• Decrease IOP | • To prepare for intraocular surgery<br>• To treat acute glaucoma | • Hypokalemia<br>• Diuresis |
| *Prostaglandin analogues*<br>Bimatoprost<br>Latanoprost<br>Travoprost<br>Unoprostone | • Decrease IOP | • To treat glaucoma | • Irritation<br>• Tearing |

## OTIC DRUGS

| Drug | Action | Treatment uses | Adverse reactions |
|---|---|---|---|
| **_Anesthetics (local)_** | | | |
| Benzocaine | • Temporarily interrupt the conduction of nerve impulses | • To temporarily relieve ear pain | • Ear irritation or itching<br>• Edema<br>• Hives<br>• Masking of the symptoms of a fulminating middle ear infection |
| **_Anti-infectives_** | | | |
| Acetic acid<br>Boric acid<br>Chloramphenicol<br>Colistin sulfate<br>Neomycin sulfate<br>Polymyxin B sulfate | • Kill bacteria or inhibit bacterial growth<br>• Inhibit fungal growth (acetic acid and boric acid) | • To treat otitis externa<br>• To treat otitis media (colistin and polymyxin B sulfate) | • Burning<br>• Dermatitis<br>• Ear itching<br>• Hives |
| **_Anti-inflammatories_** | | | |
| Hydrocortisone<br>Dexamethasone-<br>   sodium phosphate | • Inhibit edema, capillary dilation, fibrin deposition, and phagocyte and leukocyte migration<br>• Reduce capillary and fibroblast proliferation, collagen deposition, and scar formation | • To treat inflammatory conditions of the external ear canal | • Masking or exacerbation of underlying otic infection<br>• Transient local stinging or burning sensations |
| **_Cerumenolytics_** | | | |
| Carbamide peroxide<br>Triethanolamine<br>   polypeptide | • Reduce hardened cerumen by emulsifying and mechanically loosening it | • To loosen and remove cerumen from the ear canal | • Mild, localized redness and itching |

## DERMATOLOGIC DRUGS

| Drug | Action | Treatment uses | Adverse reactions |
|---|---|---|---|
| *Anti-infectives* | | | |
| *Antibacterials*<br>Azelaic acid<br>Bacitracin<br>Clindamycin<br>Erythromycin<br>Gentamicin<br>Mafenide<br>Metronidazole<br>Mupirocin<br>Neomycin<br>Silver sulfadiazine<br>Sulfacetamide sodium<br>Tetracycline | • Kill or inhibit the growth of bacteria | • To treat infections caused by bacteria (each drug is specific to particular organisms; combination products may also be used) | • Contact dermatitis<br>• Rash<br>• Skin burning, itching, and redness<br>• Skin dryness<br>• Stinging |
| *Antifungals*<br>Amphotericin B<br>Butenafine<br>Ciclopirox<br>Clotrimazole<br>Econazole<br>Ketoconazole<br>Miconazole<br>Naftifine<br>Nystatin<br>Oxiconazole<br>Sulconazole<br>Terbinafine | • Kill or inhibit the growth of fungi | • To treat infections caused by fungi (each drug is specific to particular organisms) | • Same as for antibacterials |
| *Antivirals*<br>Acyclovir<br>Penciclovir | • Inhibit the growth of herpes virus | • To treat herpes genitalis or herpes labialis | • Same as for antibacterials |

## DERMATOLOGIC DRUGS *(continued)*

| Drug | Action | Treatment uses | Adverse reactions |
|---|---|---|---|
| ***Anti-inflammatories*** | | | |
| Alclometasone<br>Betamethasone<br>  dipropionate<br>Clobetasol<br>Clocortolone<br>Desonide<br>Desoximetasone<br>Dexamethasone<br>Diflorasone diacetate<br>Fluocinolone<br>Fluocinonide<br>Flurandrenolide<br>Fluticasone<br>Halcinonide<br>Halobetasol<br>Hydrocortisone<br>Mometasone<br>Triamcinolone<br>  acetonide | • Suppress inflammation by binding to intracellular corticosteroid receptors, initiating a cascade of anti-inflammatory mediators<br>• Cause vasoconstriction in inflamed tissue and prevent macrophages and leukocytes from moving into the area | • To relieve inflammation and itching in topical steroid-responsive disorders, such as eczema, psoriasis, angioedema, contact dermatitis, seborrheic dermatitis, atopic dermatitis, and hives | • Adrenal hormone suppression<br>• Stretch marks and epidermal atrophy (after 3 to 4 weeks of use) |
| ***Hair growth stimulants*** | | | |
| Minoxidil | • Stimulate hair growth by causing vasodilation, which increases blood flow to the skin (exact mechanism of action is unknown) | • To treat male and female pattern baldness | • Fluid retention<br>• Rapid heart rate<br>• Weight gain |
| ***Topical antiacne drugs*** | | | |
| *Keratolytics*<br>Acitretin<br>Adapalene<br>Isotretinoin<br>Tazarotene<br>Tretinoin | • Produce antibacterial effects<br>• Reduce inflammation | • To treat mild acne, oily skin, and acne vulgaris (oral antibiotic therapy used as needed for deep acne) | • Burning<br>• Hives<br>• Rash<br>• Scaling, blistering, and peeling<br>• Skin dryness<br>• Skin irritation<br>• Superinfection (with prolonged use) |

## DERMATOLOGIC DRUGS *(continued)*

| Drug | Action | Treatment uses | Adverse reactions |
|---|---|---|---|
| ***Topical antiacne drugs** (continued)* | | | |
| *Counterirritants*<br>Benzoyl peroxide | • Produce antibacterial effects<br>• Reduce inflammation | • To treat mild acne, oily skin, and acne vulgaris (oral antibiotic therapy used as needed for deep acne) | • Same as for keratolytics |
| *Antimicrobials*<br>Clindamycin<br>Doxycycline<br>Erythromycin<br>Minocycline<br>Tetracycline | • Produce antibacterial effects<br>• Reduce inflammation | • To treat mild acne, oily skin, and acne vulgaris (oral antibiotic therapy used as needed for deep acne) | • Same as for keratolytics<br>• Hypersensitivity reactions (oral)<br>• Candidal vaginitis (oral)<br>• Gram-negative pustular folliculitis (oral) |
| ***Scabicides and pediculicides*** | | | |
| Gamma benzene hexachloride<br>Lindane<br>Malathion<br>Permethrin | • Act on parasite nerve cell membranes to disrupt the sodium channel current, causing paralysis (some are also ovicidal) | • To treat scabies and lice | • Contact dermatitis<br>• Hypersensitivity reactions<br>• Respiratory allergy symptoms |

# Vaccines and treatment for biological weapons exposure

Listed here are potentially threatening biological (bacterial and viral) agents as well as treatments and vaccines currently available for conditions caused by biological agents.

Implement standard precautions for all cases of suspected exposure. For cases of smallpox, institute airborne precautions for the duration of the illness and until all scabs fall off. For pneumonic plague cases, institute droplet precautions for 72 hours after initiation of effective therapy.

| Biological agent (condition) | Treatment | Vaccine |
|---|---|---|
| *Bacillus anthracis* (anthrax) | • Ciprofloxacin, doxycycline, penicillin | • Limited supply of an inactivated cell-free product available; when used, shortens period of antimicrobial prophylaxis<br>• Not recommended in absence of exposure to anthrax |
| *Clostridium botulinum* (botulism)—Not contagious | • Supportive; may require endotracheal intubation and mechanical ventilation<br>• Passive immunization with equine antitoxin to lessen nerve damage | • Postexposure prophylaxis with equine botulinum antitoxin<br>• Botulinum toxoid available from the Centers for Disease Control and Prevention; recombinant vaccine under development |
| *Francisella tularensis* (tularemia)—Not contagious | • Gentamicin or streptomycin; alternatively, doxycycline, chloramphenicol, and ciprofloxacin | • Vaccination with live, attenuated vaccine currently under investigation and review by the Food and Drug Administration (FDA) |
| *Variola major* (smallpox)—Transmitted by inhalation of air droplets or aerosols; patient most infectious from onset of maculopapular rash through first 7 to 10 days | • No FDA-approved antiviral available; cidofovir may be therapeutic if administered 1 to 2 days after exposure | • Vaccine available as prophylaxis within 3 to 4 days of exposure |
| *Yersinia pestis* (plague)—Transmitted person to person via aerosol (pneumonic plague) | • Streptomycin or gentamicin; alternatively, doxycycline, ciprofloxacin, or chloramphenicol | • Vaccination no longer available; didn't protect against primary pneumonic plague |

# Treatment and antidotes for chemical weapons exposure

Listed here are potentially threatening chemical agents, treatments currently available, and antidotes.

In the event of chemical agent exposure, follow standard precautions and decontamination protocols, such as removing clothing and sealing it in plastic bags, irrigating the eyes, washing skin and hair using copious water, treating waste water as needed, and decontaminating the health care facility according to the specific agent involved.

| Chemical agent | Treatment | Antidote | Chemical agent | Treatment | Antidote |
|---|---|---|---|---|---|
| **Nerve agents**<br>Sarin<br>Soman<br>Tabun<br>VX | • Supportive care<br>• Diazepam or lorazepam to prevent seizures | • Atropine I.M. or I.V.<br>• Pralidoxime chloride I.M. or I.V. | **Pulmonary or choking agents**<br>Chlorine<br>Diphosgene<br>Phosgene<br>Sulfur dioxide | • Supportive care<br>• Oxygen therapy; possible ET intubation and mechanical ventilation with positive-end expiratory pressure | • None |
| **Cyanides**<br>Cyanogen chloride<br>Hydrogen cyanide | • Supportive care<br>• 100% oxygen by face mask; may need endotracheal (ET) intubation with 100% $FIO_2$<br>• Activated charcoal for conscious patient | • Amyl nitrite via inhalation<br>• Sodium nitrite I.V. and sodium thiosulfate I.V.; dosage based on patient's weight and hemoglobin level | **Ricin** (biotoxin isolated from castor bean oil extract) | • Supportive care<br>• For ingestion, activated charcoal | • None |
| **Vesicants or blister agents**<br>Lewisite<br>Mustard lewisite<br>Nitrogen mustard<br>Phosgene oxime<br>Sulfur mustard | • Thermal burn therapy<br>• Respiratory support and eye care | • No antidote available for mustards or phosgene oxime<br>• For lewisite and lewisite mustard mixtures: British Anti-Lewisite I.M. (rarely available) | **T-2 mycotoxins** (toxic compounds produced by fungi)<br>Fusarium<br>Myrotecium<br>Stachybotrys<br>Trichoderma<br>Verticimonosporium | • Supportive care<br>• For ingestion, activated charcoal<br>• Possible high-dose steroids | • None |

# Herbal drugs

The following table lists some common herbal drugs, their uses, and considerations to know when caring for patients taking these drugs.

| Herbal medicine | Common uses | Special considerations |
|---|---|---|
| Aloe | **Oral**<br>• Constipation<br>• Bowel evacuation<br>**Topical**<br>• Minor burns<br>• Skin irritation | • The laxative actions of aloe may take up to 10 hours after ingestion to be effective.<br>• Monitor the patient for signs of dehydration; geriatric patients are particularly at risk. |
| Chamomile | **Oral**<br>• Anxiety or restlessness<br>• Diarrhea<br>• Motion sickness<br>• Indigestion<br>**Topical**<br>• Inflammation<br>• Wound healing<br>• Cutaneous burns<br>**Teas**<br>• Sedation<br>• Relaxation | • People sensitive to ragweed and chrysanthemums or others in the Compositae family may be more susceptible to contact allergies and anaphylaxis.<br>• Patients with hay fever or bronchial asthma caused by pollens are more susceptible to anaphylactic reactions.<br>• Pregnant women shouldn't use chamomile.<br>• Chamomile may enhance anticoagulant's effect. |
| Cranberry | • Prophylaxis for urinary tract infection (UTI)<br>• Treatment of UTI<br>• Prevention of renal calculi | • Only the unsweetened form of cranberry prevents bacteria from adhering to the bladder wall and preventing or treating UTIs |
| Echinacea | • Supportive therapy to prevent and treat common cold and acute and chronic infections of the upper respiratory tract | • Echinacea is considered supportive therapy and shouldn't be used in place of antibiotic therapy. |
| Feverfew | • Prevention and treatment of migraines and headaches<br>• Hot flashes<br>• Rheumatoid arthritis<br>• Asthma<br>• Menstrual problems | • Avoid using in pregnant patients because feverfew is also an abortifacient.<br>• Feverfew may increase the risk of abnormal bleeding when combined with an anticoagulant or antiplatelet.<br>• Abruptly stopping feverfew may cause "postfeverfew syndrome" involving tension headaches, insomnia, joint stiffness and pain, and lethargy. |

| Herbal medicine | Common uses | Special considerations |
|---|---|---|
| Garlic | • Decrease cholesterol and triglyceride levels<br>• Prevent atherosclerosis<br>• Age-related vascular changes<br>• Prevent GI cancer<br>• Coughs, colds, fevers, and sore throats | • Odor of garlic may be apparent on breath and skin.<br>• Garlic may prolong bleeding time in patients receiving anticoagulants.<br>• Excess raw garlic intake may increase the risk of adverse reactions.<br>• Garlic shouldn't be used in patients with diabetes, insomnia, pemphigus, organ transplants, or rheumatoid arthritis or in those who have recently undergone surgery. |
| Ginger | • Nausea (antiemetic)<br>• Motion sickness<br>• Morning sickness<br>• GI upset (colic, flatulence, indigestion)<br>• Hypercholesteremia<br>• Liver toxicity<br>• Burns<br>• Ulcers<br>• Depression | • Ginger may increase the risk of bleeding, bruising, or nosebleeds.<br>• Pregnant women should obtain medical advice before using ginger medicinally.<br>• Ginger may interfere with the intended therapeutic effects of certain conventional drugs. |
| Ginkgo biloba | • "Memory" agent<br>• Alzheimer's disease<br>• Multi-infarct dementia<br>• Cerebral insufficiency<br>• Intermittent claudication<br>• Tinnitus<br>• Headache | • Adverse effects occur in less than 1% of patients; the most common is GI upset.<br>• Ginkgo biloba may potentiate anticoagulants and increase the risk of bleeding.<br>• Ginkgo extracts are considered standardized if they contain 24% flavonoid glycosides and 6% terpene lactones.<br>• Seizures have been reported in children after ingestion of more then 50 seeds.<br>• Treatment should continue for 6 to 8 weeks but for no more than 3 months. |
| Ginseng | • Fatigue<br>• Improve concentration<br>• Treat atherosclerosis<br>• Also believed to strengthen the body and increase resistance to disease after sickness or weakness | • Ginseng may cause severe adverse reactions when taken in large doses (more than 3 g per day for 2 years), such as increased motor and cognitive activity with significant diarrhea, nervousness, insomnia, hypertension, edema, and skin eruptions.<br>• Ginseng may potentiate anticoagulants and increase the risk of bleeding. |
| Green tea | • Prevent cancer<br>• Hyperlipidemia<br>• Atherosclerosis<br>• Dental caries<br>• Headaches<br>• Central nervous system (CNS) stimulant<br>• Mild diuretic | • Green tea contains caffeine.<br>• Avoid prolonged and high caffeine intake, which may cause restlessness, irritability, insomnia, palpitations, vertigo, headache, and adverse GI effects.<br>• Adding milk may decrease adverse GI effects of green tea.<br>• Green tea may potentiate anticoagulants and increase the risk of bleeding. |

| Herbal medicine | Common uses | Special considerations |
|---|---|---|
| Kava | • Antianxiety<br>• Stress<br>• Restlessness<br>• Sedation<br>• Promote wound healing<br>• Headache<br>• Seizure disorders<br>• Common cold<br>• Respiratory infections | • Kava is contraindicated in pregnancy and lactation.<br>• Kava shouldn't be used in combination with St. John's wort.<br>• Kava shouldn't be taken with other CNS depressants, monoamine oxidase inhibitors, levodopa, antiplatelets, alcohol, or anxiolytics.<br>• Kava can cause drowsiness and may impair motor reflexes and mental acuity; advise the patient to avoid hazardous activities.<br>• Effects should appear within 2 days of initiation of therapy. |
| St. John's wort | • Mild to moderate depression<br>• Anxiety<br>• Psychovegetative disorders<br>• Sciatica<br>• Viral infections | • Effects may take several weeks; however, if no improvement occurs after 4 to 6 weeks, consider alternative therapy.<br>• St. John's wort interacts with many different types of drugs.<br>• St. John's wort shouldn't be used in combination with prescription antidepressants or antianxiety medications. |
| Vitex | • Premenstrual syndrome | • Vitex should be taken in the morning with water.<br>• Vitex is a very slow acting substance; it may take several cycles to see an effect. |
| Yohimbine | • Impotence (works as an aphrodisiac) | • Yohimbine may cause CNS excitation, including tremor, sleeplessness, anxiety, increased blood pressure, and tachycardia.<br>• Don't use in patients with renal or hepatic insufficiency. |

# Selected references

*American Drug Index*, 50th ed. Philadelphia: Facts and Comparisons, 2006.

American Hospital Formulary Service. *AHFS Drug Information 2008*. Bethesda, Md.: American Society of Hospital Pharmacists, 2008.

Arana, G.W., et al. *Handbook of Psychiatric Drug Therapy*. Philadelphia: Lippincott Williams and Wilkins, 2006.

Bisno, A.L. "Practice Guidelines for the Diagnosis and Management of Skin and Soft-tissue Infections," *Clinical Infectious Disease* 41:1174-78, 2005.

Burke, M.B., and Wilkes, G.M. *2006 Oncology Nursing Drug Handbook*. Sudbury, Mass.: Jones & Bartlett Pubs., Inc., 2006.

Centers for Disease Control and Prevention. *www.cdc.gov*

Chong, O.T. "An Integrative Approach to Addressing Clinical Issues in Complementary and Alternative Medicine in an Outpatient Oncology Center," *Clinical Journal of Oncology Nursing* 10(1):83-88, February 2006.

Chu, E. *Physicians' Cancer Chemotherapy Drug Manual 2006*. Sudbury, Mass.: Jones & Bartlett Pubs., Inc., 2008.

Gensure, R., and Jüppner, H. "Parathyroid Hormone without Parathyroid Glands," *Endocrinology* 146(2):544-46, February 2005.

Golan, D., et al. *Principles of Pharmacology: The Pathophysiologic Basis of Drug Therapy*, 2nd ed. Philadelphia: Lippincott Williams & Wilkins, 2007.

Gutierrez, K. *Pharmacotherapeutics: Clinical Reasoning in Primary Care*, 2nd ed. Philadelphia: W.B. Saunders Co., 2008.

Houck, P.M., and Bratzler, D.W. "Administration of First Hospital Antibiotics for Community-Acquired Pneumonia: Does Timeliness Affect Outcomes?" *Current Opinion in Infectious Diseases* 18(2):151-56, April 2005.

Kanner, E.M., and Tsai, J.C. "Current and Emerging Medical Therapies for Glaucoma," *Expert Opinion on Emerging Drugs* 10(1):109-18 February 2005.

*Lippincott's Nursing Drug Guide 2008*. Philadelphia: Lippincott Williams & Wilkins, 2008.

Nolan, C.R. "Strategies for Improving Long-Term Survival in Patients with ESRD," *Journal of the American Society of Nephrology* 16(Suppl 2): S120-S127, November 2005.

*Nursing I.V. Drug Handbook*, 9th ed. Philadelphia: Lippincott Williams & Wilkins, 2006.

*Nursing2008 Drug Handbook*, 28th ed. Philadelphia: Lippincott Williams & Wilkins, 2008.

*Physician's Desk Reference*, 58th ed. Montvale, Md.: Thomson PDR, 2004.

*Professional Guide to Pathophysiology*, 2nd ed. Philadelphia: Lippincott Williams & Wilkins, 2007.

*Psychopharmacology*, 2nd ed. Arlington, Va.: American Psychiatric Publishing, Incorporated, 2006.

Roach, S., and Zorko, B.S. *Pharmacology for Health Professionals*. Philadelphia: Lippincott Williams & Wilkins, 2006.

Roach, S., and Ford, S.M. *Introductory Clinical Pharmacology*, 8th ed. Philadelphia: Lippincott Williams & Wilkins, 2007.

Salzman, C. *Clinical Geriatric Psychopharmacology*, 4th ed. Philadelphia: Lippincott Williams & Wilkins, 2005.

Sande, M.A., and Eliopoulos, G. *The Sanford Guide to HIV/AIDS Therapy*, 14th ed. Hyde Park, Vt.: Antimicrobial Therapy, Inc., 2005.

U.S. Food and Drug Administration: *www.fda.gov*

# Index

## A

Abacavir, 266-270
Abciximab, 165-169
Absorption, 7-9
    drug interactions and, 16
Acarbose, 342-345
Acebutolol, 43-47, 129-131
Acetaminophen, 96-98
    nonselective, safe use of, 99
    selective, risks of using, 98
Acetazolamide, 229, 368-369, 416t
Acetic acid, 417t
Acetohexamide, 342-345
Acetylcholine, 21, 22i, 23, 24, 26,
    27, 60, 61
Acetylcysteine, 190-191
Acidifying drugs, 368-369
Acitretin, 419t
Activated charcoal, 204-205, 422t
Active transport, 7
Acute therapy, 14
Acyclovir, 260-263, 418t
Adapalene, 419t
Additive effects, 16
Adenosine, 133-134
Adrenergic blocking drugs, 40-47
    topical, 416t
Adrenergic drugs, 32-39
    classifying, 32
    mechanism of action of, 33i
Adsorbent drugs, 204-205
Adverse drug reactions, 17-19
    dose-related, 17-18
    patient sensitivity–related, 18-19
Agonist, 12
Albuterol, 37-39, 176-177
Alclometasone, 419t
Aldesleukin, 408-409
Aldosterone, 301
Alemtuzumab, 398-399
Alfuzosin, 40-43
Alkalinizing drugs, 366-368
Alkylating drugs, 371-379
    mechanism of action of, 373i

Alkylating-like drugs, 378-379
Alkyl sulfonates, 374-375
Allopurinol, 307-309
Allylamine derivatives, synthetic,
    288-289
Almotriptan, 86-88
Aloe, 423t
Alosetron, 210
Alpha-adrenergic blockers, 40-43,
    141-142
    mechanism of action of, 41i
Alprazolam, 312-313, 314i, 315
Alprostadil, 231-232
Alteplase, 171-173, 172i
Altretamine, 409-410
Aluminum carbonate gel, 197-198
Aluminum-magnesium complex,
    197-198
Amantadine, 62-66, 264-266
Ambenonium, 24-27
Amikacin, 238-240
Amiloride, 227-228
Aminoglycosides, 238-240
1-(aminomethyl) cyclohexane–acetic
    acid, 78-79
Aminophylline, 183-185
Amiodarone, 131-132
Amitriptyline, 322-325
Amlodipine, 138-140
Ammonium chloride, 368-369
Amobarbital, 316-317
Amoxapine, 322-325
Amoxicillin, 196-197, 241-243
Amphetamine salts, mixed, 336-337
Amphotericin B, 280-283, 418t
Ampicillin, 241-243
Amprenavir, 272-275
Amylase, 206
Amyl nitrite, 135-136
Anakinra, 302-306
Anastrozole, 387-388
Androgens, 390-391
Anesthetic drugs, 108-115
    ophthalmic, 414t
    otic, 417t

Angiotensin-converting enzyme
    inhibitors, 144-145
Angiotensin II receptor blockers,
    146-147
Animals as drug sources, 3, 4
Antacids, 197-198
Antagonist, 12
    types of, 12-13
Antagonistic effect, 16
Anterior pituitary drugs, 349-350
Antiacne drugs, topical, 419-420t
Antiallergic agents as ophthalmic
    drugs, 414t
Antiandrogens, 391-392
Antianginal drugs, 134-140
    mechanism of action of, 134i
Antianxiety drugs, 318-319
Antiarrhythmic drugs, 123-134
Antibacterial drugs, 238-260
    dermatologic, 418t
Antibiotic antineoplastic drugs,
    385-386
Antibiotics, systemic, as gastrointesti-
    nal drugs, 196-197. See also An-
    tibacterial drugs.
Anticholinergic drugs, 27-32, 60-62,
    177-178
Anticholinesterase drugs, 24-27
    differentiating toxic response to,
        from myasthenic crisis, 24
    mechanism of action of, 22i
Anticoagulant drugs, 161-171
Anticonvulsant drugs, 68-85
Antidepressants, 320-329
    risks of, 322
Antidiabetic drugs, 339-345
Antidiarrheal drugs, 208-210
Antidiuretic hormone, 350-352
Antiemetics, 216-219
Antiestrogens, 388-390
Antiflatulent drugs, 205
Antifungal drugs, 280-289
    dermatologic, 418t
Antigout drugs, 306-309
Antihistamines, 216-219, 294-297

Antihypertensive drugs, 140-147
Anti-infective drugs, 237-290
   dermatologic, 418t
   ophthalmic, 414t
   otic, 417t
Anti-inflammatories
   dermatologic, 419t
   ophthalmic, 415t
   otic, 417t
Antilipemic drugs, 147-152
Antimetabolite drugs, 379-384
Antimicrobial drug, selecting, 237
Antimigraine drugs, 85-90
Antimycotic drugs, 280-289
Antineoplastic drugs, 371-411
   unclassifiable, 402-411
Antiparkinsonian drugs, 59-68
Antiplatelet drugs, 165-169
Antipsychotic drugs, 330-336
Antipyretics, 93-101
Antiretroviral drugs, 266-275
Antithymocyte globulin, 302-306
Antithyroid drugs, 355-356
Antitubercular drugs, 275-280
Antitussives, 188-189
Antiulcer drugs, 195-203
Antiviral drugs, 260-275
   dermatologic, 418t
Anxiolytics, 318-319
Apraclonidine, 416t
Argatroban, 169-170
Aripiprazole, 331-332
Aromatase inhibitors, 387-388
Arsenic trioxide, 403
Ascorbic acid, 368-369
Asparaginases, 404
Aspirin, 94-96, 166-169
Atazanavir, 272-275
Atenolol, 43-47, 137-138
Atorvastatin, 149-150
Atracurium, 56-58
Atropine, 27-32, 30i, 416t
Atypical antipsychotics, 331-332
Autonomic nervous system drugs,
   21-47
Azaspirodecanedione derivatives, 319
Azatadine, 294-295, 297
Azathioprine, 302-306

Azelaic acid, 418t
Azelastine, 414t
Azithromycin, 249-251
Aztreonam, 255-256

**B**
Bacitracin, 418t
Baclofen, 53-55
Barbiturates, 70-72, 110-112, 316-317
Basiliximab, 302-306
Beclomethasone, 178-180, 298-300
Belladonna, 27-32
Benazepril, 144-145
Bendroflumethiazide, 224-225
Benzocaine, 114-115, 417t
Benzodiazepines, 74-76, 110-112,
   312-313, 315
   mechanism of action of, 314i
Benzonatate, 188-189
Benzoyl peroxide, 420t
Benztropine, 27-32, 60-62
Benzyl alcohol, 114-115
Beta-adrenergic blockers, 43-47,
   129-131, 137-138
   cardioselective, 45
   mechanism of action of, 45i
   underuse of, in elderly patients, 46
Beta$_2$-adrenergic agonists, 176-177
Betamethasone, 298-300
Betaxolol, 43-47, 416t
Bethanechol, 21-24
Bicalutamide, 391-392
Bile-sequestering drugs, 147-148
Bimatoprost, 416t
Biological weapons exposure, vac-
   cines and treatment for, 421t
Biotransformation. *See* Metabolism.
Biperiden, 60-62
Bisacodyl, 214-215
Bisoprolol, 43-47
Bistriazole antimycotic drug, 285-287
Bitolterol, 37-39
Bivalirudin, 169-170
Bleomycin, 385-386
Boric acid, 417t
Bortezomib, 400-402
Brimonidine, 416t
Brinzolamide, 416t

Bromocriptine, 62-66
Brompheniramine, 294-295, 297
Buccal route of administration, 4
Buclizine, 216-219
Budesonide, 178-180
Bulk-forming laxatives, 212-213
Bumetanide, 225-227
Bupivacaine, 112-114
Buprenorphine, 105-107
Bupropion, 327-329
Buspirone, 319
Busulfan, 374-375
Butabarbital, 316-317
Butacaine, 114-115
Butenafine, 281, 418t
Butoconazole, 281
Butorphanol, 105-107

**C**
Calcium carbonate, 197-198
Calcium channel blockers, 138-140,
   142-143
   mechanism of action of, 139i
Calcium replacement, 361-363
Cancer, drugs and, 371
Candesartan cilexetil, 146-147
Capecitabine, 381-383
Captopril, 144-145
Carbachol, 21-24, 415t
Carbamazepine, 73-74
Carbamide peroxide, 417t
Carbapenems, 253-255
Carbenicillin, 241-243
Carbidopa-levodopa, 62-66
Carbonic anhydrase inhibitors,
   229, 416t
Carboplatin, 378-379
Carboxamides, 80-81
Carboxylic acid derivatives, 76-78
Cardiac glycosides, 120-122
Cardiovascular drugs, 119-152
Carisoprodol, 50-52
Carmustine, 375-376
Carteolol, 43-47, 416t
Carvedilol, 43-47, 141-142
Caspofungin, 287-288
Castor oil, 214-215
Catecholamines, 33-37

i refers to an illustration; t refers to a table.

Catechol-O-methyltransferase inhibitors, 66-68
Cefaclor, 243-246
Cefadroxil, 243-246
Cefazolin, 243-246
Cefdinir, 243-246
Cefepime, 243-246
Cefixime, 243-246
Cefotaxime, 243-246
Cefoxitin, 243-246
Cefpodoxime, 243-246
Cefprozil, 243-246
Ceftazidime, 243-246
Ceftibuten, 243-246
Ceftriaxone, 243-246
Cefuroxime, 243-246
Celecoxib, 98-100
Central-acting sympathetic nervous system inhibitors, 141-142
Centrally acting skeletal muscle relaxants, 50-52
Central nerve block, 113i
Cephalexin, 243-246
Cephalosporins, 243-246
   mechanism of action of, 245i
Cerumenolytics, 417t
Cetirizine, 294-295, 297
Cevimeline, 21-24
Chamomile, 423t
Chemical weapons exposure, treatment and antidotes for, 422t
Chloral hydrate, 317-318
Chlorambucil, 372-374
Chloramphenicol, 417t, 421t
Chlordiazepoxide, 312-313, 314i, 315
Chloroprocaine, 112-114
Chlorothiazide, 224-225
Chlorpheniramine, 294-295, 296i, 297
Chlorpromazine, 216-219, 333-336
Chlorpropamide, 342-345
Chlorthalidone, 224-225
Chlorzoxazone, 50-52
Cholesterol absorption inhibitors, 152
Cholestyramine, 147-148
Choline magnesium trisalicylate, 94-96
Cholinergic agonists, 21-24
   mechanism of action of, 22i
Cholinergic blocking drugs, 27-32, 60-62, 177-178

Cholinergic drugs, 21-27
   mechanism of action of, 22i
Choline salicylate, 94-96
Chorionic gonadotropin, 349-350
Ciclopirox, 281, 418t
Cidofovir, 421t
Cimetidine, 199, 200i, 201
Ciprofloxacin, 256-257, 277, 414t, 421t
Cisatracurium, 56-58
Cisplatin, 378-379
Citalopram, 320-322
Cladribine, 383-384
Clarithromycin, 196-197, 249-251
Class IA antiarrhythmics, 124-125
Class IB antiarrhythmics, 126-127
Class IC antiarrhythmics, 128-129
Class II antiarrhythmics, 129-131
Class III antiarrhythmics, 131-132
Class IV antiarrhythmics, 133-134. See also Calcium channel blockers.
Clemastine, 294-295, 297
Clindamycin, 248-249, 418t, 420t
Clioquinol, 281
Clobetasol, 419t
Clocortolone, 419t
Clomipramine, 322-325
Clonazepam, 74-76, 312-313, 314i, 315
Clonidine, 141-142
Clopidogrel, 165-169
Clorazepate, 74-76, 312-313, 314i, 315
Clotrimazole, 281, 418t
Clove oil, 114-115
Clozapine, 331-332
Cocaine, 112-115
Codeine, 102-105, 188-189
Colchicine, 307-309
Colesevelam, 147-148
Colestipol, 147-148
Colistin sulfate, 417t
Competitive drugs, 56-58
Competitive inhibition, 107
Corticosteroids, 178-180, 297-301
   special population concerns and, 179
Corticotropin, 349-350
Corticotropin repository, 349-350
Cortisone, 298-300
Cosyntropin, 349-350
Co-trimoxazole, 257-259

COX-2 inhibitors, 98-99, 100. See also Nonsteroidal anti-inflammatory drugs.
Cranberry, 423t
Cromolyn, 182, 414t
Cyanocobalamin, 158-159
Cyclizine, 216-219
Cyclobenzaprine, 50-52
Cyclopentolate, 416t
Cyclophosphamide, 302-306, 372-374
Cycloplegics, 416t
Cyclosporine, 302-306
Cyproheptadine, 294-295, 297
Cytarabine, 381-383

**D**
Dacarbazine, 376-377
Daclizumab, 302-306
Dactinomycin, 385-386
Dalteparin, 161-164
Dantrolene, 52-53
Darbepoetin alfa, 160-161
Darifenacin, 230-231
Darunavir, 272-275
Daunorubicin, 385-386
Decongestants, 191-193
Delavirdine, 270-271
Demecarium, 24-27
Demeclocycline, 247-248
Depolarizing blocking drugs, 58-59
Dermatologic drugs, 418-420t
Desflurane, 109-110
Desipramine, 322-325
Desloratadine, 294-295, 297
Desmopressin, 350-352
Desonide, 419t
Desoximetasone, 419t
Dexamethasone, 298-300, 415t, 417t, 419t
Dexchlorpheniramine, 294-295, 297
Dextroamphetamine, 336-337
Dextromethorphan, 188-189
Diazepam, 53-55, 74-76, 312-313, 314i, 315, 422t
Diazoxide, 142-143
Dibucaine, 114-115
Diclofenac, 98-100, 415t
Dicloxacillin, 241-243
Dicyclomine, 27-32

i refers to an illustration; t refers to a table.

Didanosine, 266-270
Dietary fiber, 212-213
Diflorasone, 419t
Diflunisal, 94-96
Digestive drugs, 206
Digoxin, 120-122
Digoxin toxicity, signs and symptoms of, 122
Dihydroergotamine, 89-90
Diltiazem, 133-134, 138-140
Dimenhydrinate, 216-219, 294-295, 297
Diphenhydramine, 60-62, 216-219, 294-295, 297
Diphenidol, 218
Diphenoxylate with atropine, 208-209
Dipivefrin, 415t
Dipyridamole, 165-169
Direct-acting skeletal muscle relaxants, 52-53
Directly observable therapy, 276
Direct thrombin inhibitors, 169-170
Direct vasodilators, 142-143
Disopyramide, 124-125
Distribution, 9-10
    drug interactions and, 16
Diuretics, 224-229
Divalproex, 76-78
Dobutamine, 33-37
Docetaxel, 410-411
Docusate salts, 213-214
Dofetilide, 131-132
Dolasetron, 216-219
Donepezil, 24-27
Dopamine, 33-37
Dopaminergic drugs, 62-66
Dorzolamide, 416t
Dose-response curve, 13, 14i
Doxazosin, 40-43, 141-142
Doxepin, 322-325
Doxorubicin, 385-386
Doxycycline, 247-248, 420t, 421t
Dronabinol, 218
Drotrecogin alfa, 289-290
Drug administration routes, 4-5
    effect of, on absorption, 7-8
Drug allergy, 18-19
Drug dependence, 15

Drug effect, 12
Drug interactions, 15-17
Drug nomenclature, 2
Drug potency, 13
Drug sources, 2-4
Drug tolerance, 15
Duloxetine, 320-322
Duration of action, 12
Dyclonine, 114-115

**E**
Echinacea, 423t
Echinocandins, 287-288
Echothiophate, 24-27
Econazole, 281, 418t
Edrophonium, 24-27
    toxic drug response versus myasthenic crisis and, 24
Efavirenz, 270-271
Electrolyte replacement drugs, 359-366
Eletriptan, 86-88
Emedastine, 414t
Emetics, 219-220
Emollient laxatives, 213-214
Empiric therapy, 14
Emtricitabine, 266-270
Enalapril, 144-145
Enalaprilat, 144-145
Endocrine drugs, 339-356
Enflurane, 109-110
Enoxaparin, 161-164
Entacapone, 66-68
Ephedrine, 37-39, 191-193
Epidural infusion, 5
Epinephrine, 33-37, 415t
Epoetin alfa, 160-161
Eprosartan, 146-147
Eptifibatide, 165-169
Erectile dysfunction therapy drugs, 231-232
Ergoloid mesylates, 40-43
Ergotamine, 40-43
Ergotamine preparations, 89-90
Ertapenem, 253-255
Erythromycin, 249-251, 414t, 418t, 420t
Erythropoietin agents, 160-161
Escitalopram, 320-322
Esmolol, 43-47, 129-131
Esomeprazole, 201-202

Estazolam, 312-313, 314i, 315
Estradiol, 347-348
Estramustine, 372-374
Estrogenic substances, conjugated, 347-348
Estrogens, 347-348
    esterified, 347-348
Estropipate, 347-348
Eszopiclone, 317-318
Ethacrynic acid, 225-227
Ethambutol, 276-280
Ethinyl estradiol, 233-234, 347-348
Ethosuximide, 82-83
Ethotoin, 69-70
Ethyl chloride, 114-115
Ethylenimines, 377-378
Ethynodiol diacetate, 233-234
Etodolac, 98-100
Etomidate, 110-112
Etoposide, 396-397
Excretion, 11
    drug interactions and, 16
Exemestane, 387-388
Expected therapeutic response, 17
Expectorants, 187
Ezetimibe, 152

**F**
Factor Xa inhibitor drugs, 170-171
Famciclovir, 260-263
Famotidine, 199, 200i, 201
Fenofibrate, 148-149
Fenoprofen, 98-100
Fentanyl, 102-105, 110-112
Ferrous fumarate, 156-157
Ferrous gluconate, 156-157
Ferrous sulfate, 156-157
Feverfew, 423t
Fexofenadine, 294-295, 297
Fibric acid derivatives, 148-149
First-pass effect, 8
Flavoxate, 230-231
Flecainide, 128-129
Floxuridine, 381-383
Fluconazole, 285-287
Flucytosine, 283-284
Fludarabine, 383-384

Fludrocortisone, 301
Flunisolide, 178-180
Fluocinolone, 419t
Fluocinonide, 419t
Fluorometholone, 415t
Fluoroquinolones, 256-257, 277
Fluorouracil, 381-383
Fluoxetine, 320-322
Fluoxymesterone, 390-391
Fluphenazine, 333-336
Flurandrenolide, 419t
Flurazepam, 312-313, 314i, 315
Flurbiprofen, 98-100, 415t
Flutamide, 391-392
Fluticasone, 178-180
Fluvastatin, 149-150
Fluvoxamine, 320-322
Folic acid, 159-160
Folic acid analogues, 380-381
Fondaparinux, 170-171
Food, drug interactions and, 17
Food and Drug Administration, new
    drug development and, 5-6
Formoterol, 37-39, 176-177
Fosamprenavir, 272-275
Foscarnet, 264
Fosinopril, 144-145
Fosphenytoin, 69-70
Frovatriptan, 86-88
Fulvestrant, 388-390
Furosemide, 225-227

**G**
Gabapentin, 78-79
Galantamine, 24-27
Gamma benzene hydrochloride, 420t
Ganciclovir, 260-263
Garlic, 423t
Gastric route of administration, 4
Gastrointestinal drugs, 195-220
Gefitinib, 400-402
Gemcitabine, 381-383
Gemfibrozil, 148-149
Gemtuzumab ozogamicin, 398-399
Genitourinary drugs, 223-234
Gentamicin, 238-240, 414t, 418t, 421t
Ginger, 423-424t
Ginkgo biloba, 424t

Ginseng, 424t
Gliclazide, 342-345
Glimepiride, 342-345
Glipizide, 342-345
Glucagon, 345, 346i
Glucan synthesis inhibitors, 287-288
Glucocorticoids, 298-300
Glyburide, 342-345
Glycerin, 211-212, 416t
Glycopyrrolate, 27-32
Gonadotropin-releasing hormone
    analogues, 393-395
Goserelin, 393-395
Granisetron, 216-219
Green tea, 424t
Griseofulvin, 281
Guaifenesin, 187
Guanadrel, 141-142
Guanethidine, 141-142
Guanidine, 24-27

**H**
Hair growth stimulants, 419t
Halcinonide, 419t
Half-life, 11
Halobetasol, 419t
Haloperidol, 333-336
Haloprogin, 281
Halothane, 109-110
Hematinic drugs, 155-161
Hematologic drugs, 155-173
Heparin, 161-164
    partial thromboplastin time monitor-
        ing and, 163
Herbal drugs, 423-424t
Histamine-1 receptor antagonists,
    294--297
Histamine-2 receptor antagonists,
    199, 201
    mechanism of action of, 200i
HMG-CoA reductase inhibitors,
    149-150
Homatropine, 27-32, 416t
Homeostasis, drugs and, 359
Hormonal antineoplastic drugs,
    386-395
Hormonal contraceptives, 233-234
Hormone modulators, 386-395

Hormone replacement therapy, heart
    disease and, 348
5-HT$_1$-receptor agonists, 86-88
    contraindications to, 88
5-HT$_3$ receptor antagonists, 210
Hydantoins, 69-70
Hydralazine, 142-143
Hydrochlorothiazide, 224-225
Hydrocodone, 102-105, 188-189
Hydrocortisone, 178-180, 298-300,
    417t, 419t
Hydroflumethiazide, 224-225
Hydromorphone, 102-105
Hydroxocobalamin, 158-159
Hydroxyamphetamine, 415t
5-Hydroxy-3-methylglutaryl coenzyme
    A reductase inhibitors, 149-150
Hydroxyprogesterone, 392-393
Hydroxyurea, 406
Hydroxyzine, 216-219, 294-295, 297
Hyoscyamine sulfate, 27-32
Hyperglycemic drug, 345, 346i
Hyperosmolar laxatives, 211-212
Hypersusceptibility, 18
Hypoglycemic drugs, 339-345

**IJ**
Iatrogenic effects, 18
Ibritumomab tiuxetan, 398-399
Ibuprofen, 98-100
Ibutilide, 131-132
Idarubicin, 385-386
Idiosyncratic response, 19
Ifosfamide, 372-374
Imatinib, 400-402
Imidazole, 284-285
Iminostilbenes, 73-74
Imipenem-cilastatin, 253-255
Imipramine, 322-325
Immune system drugs, 293-309
Immunosuppressants, 302-306
Inamrinone, 122-123
Indapamide, 224-225
Indinavir, 272-275
Indomethacin, 98-100
Influenza A drugs, 264-266
Inhalation anesthetics, 109-110
Inotropics, 119-123

Insulin, 340-342, 341i
Interferons, 407-408
Intra-articular infusion, 5
Intradermal route of administration, 4
Intramuscular route of administration, 4, 8
Intraocular pressure, drugs to lower, 416t
Intraosseous infusion, 5
Intraperitoneal infusion, 5
Intrapleural infusion, 5
Intrathecal infusion, 5
Intravenous anesthetics, 110-112
Intravenous route of administration, 5, 7
Intrinsic activity, 12
Investigational new drug, approval process for, 5-6
Ipecac syrup, 219-220
Ipratropium, 176-177
Irbesartan, 146-147
Irinotecan, 399-400
Iron, 156-157
    parenteral, testing for sensitivity to, 157
Iron dextran, 156-157
Irritant cathartics, 214-215
Isoetharine, 37-39
Isoflurane, 109-110
Isoniazid, 276-280
Isoproterenol, 33-39
Isosorbide, 135-136, 416t
Isotretinoin, 419t
Itraconazole, 285-287

**K**

Kanamycin, 238-240
Kaolin and pectin, 209-210
Kava, 424t
Ketamine, 110-112
Ketoconazole, 284-285, 418t
Ketoprofen, 98-100
Ketorolac, 98-100, 415t
Ketotifen, 414t

**L**

Labetalol, 43-47, 141-142
Lactulose, 211-212

Lamivudine, 266-270
Lamotrigine, 79-80
Lansoprazole, 201-202
Latanoprost, 416t
Laxatives, 211-216
Lepirudin, 169-170
Letrozole, 387-388
Leucovorin, 160
Leukotriene modifiers, 180-182
Leuprolide, 393-395
Levalbuterol, 37-39, 176-177
Levarterenol, 33-37
Levetiracetam, 84-85
Levobunolol, 43-47, 416t
Levobupivacaine, 112-114
Levodopa, 62-66
    pros and cons of, 64
Levofloxacin, 256-257, 414t
Levorphanol, 102-105
Levothyroxine, 352-354
Lidocaine, 112-115, 126-127
    mechanism of action of, 127i
Lincomycin derivatives, 248-249
Lindane, 420t
Liothyronine, 352-354
Liotrix, 352-354
Lipase, 206
Lisdexamfetamine, 336-337
Lisinopril, 144-145
Lithium, 329-330
Local anesthetics, 112-114
Lodoxamide, 414t
Lomustine, 375-376
Loop diuretics, 225-227
Loperamide, 208-209
Lopinavir, 272-275
Loratadine, 294-295, 297
Lorazepam, 74-76, 312-313, 314i, 315, 422t
Losartan, 146-147
Loteprednol, 415t
Lovastatin, 149-150
Loxapine, 333-336
Lubricant laxatives, 215-216
Lubricants, ophthalmic, 415t
Lymphocyte immune globulin, 302-306

**M**

Macrolides, 249-251
Mafenide, 418t
Magaldrate, 197-198
Magnesium hydroxide and aluminum hydroxide, 197-198
Magnesium replacement, 363-365
Magnesium salts, 211-212
Maintenance therapy, 14
Malathion, 420t
Mannitol, 228, 416t
Maprotiline, 327-329
Margin of safety, 13
Mast cell stabilizers, 182
Mechlorethamine, 372-374
Meclizine, 216-219, 294-295, 297
Medroxyprogesterone, 392-393
Megestrol, 392-393
Meloxicam, 98-100
Melphalan, 372-374
Menotropins, 349-350
Menthol, 114-115
Meperidine, 102-105
Mephobarbital, 70-72, 316-317
Mepivacaine, 112-114
Mercaptopurine, 383-384
Meropenem, 253-255
Mesoridazine, 333-336
Mestranol, 233-234
Metabolism, 10-11
    drug interactions and, 16, 17
Metaproterenol, 37-39, 176-177
Metaxalone, 50-52
Metformin, 342-345
Methadone, 102-105
Methazolamide, 229
Methimazole, 355-356
Methocarbamol, 50-52
Methohexital, 110-112
Methotrexate, 380-381
Methscopolamine, 27-32
Methsuximide, 82-83
Methyclothiazide, 224-225
Methylcellulose, 212-213, 415t
Methyldopa, 141-142
Methylphenidate, 336-337
Methylprednisolone, 178-180, 298-300, 299i

Methylxanthines, 183-185
Metipranolol, 43-47, 416t
Metoclopramide, 218
Metolazone, 224-225
Metoprolol, 43-47, 137-138
Metronidazole, 196-197, 418t
Mexiletine, 126-127
Miconazole, 281, 418t
Midazolam, 110-112
Miglitol, 342-345
Milrinone, 122-123
Mineralocorticoids, 301
Mineral oil, 215-216
Minerals as drug sources, 3
Minocycline, 247-248, 420t
Minoxidil, 142-143, 419t
Miotics, 415t
Mirtazapine, 327-329
Misoprostol, 202-203
    dangers of using, during preg-
        nancy, 203
Mitomycin 385-386
Mitoxantrone, 385-386
Mixed alpha- and beta-adrenergic
        blockers, 141-142
Mixed opioid agonist-antagonists,
        101, 105-107
Modafinil, 336-337
Moexipril, 144-145
Molindone, 333-336
Mometasone, 419t
Monoamine oxidase inhibitors,
        325-327
Monobactams, 255-256
Monoclonal antibodies, 186-187,
        398-399
Montelukast, 180-182
Mood stabilizer drugs, 329-330
Moricizine, 128-129
Morphine sulfate, 102-105
Motor end plate, neuromuscular
        blocking drugs and, 56i
Moxifloxacin, 256-257
Mucolytics, 189-191
Mupirocin, 418t
Muromonab-CD3, 302-306
Mycophenolate mofetil, 302-306
Mydriatics, 415-416t

**N**
Nabumetone, 98-100
Nadolol, 43-47, 137-138
Nafcillin, 241-243
Naftifine, 281, 418t
Nalbuphine, 105-107
Naloxone, 107-108
Naltrexone, 107-108
    for drug addiction, 108
Naproxen, 98-100
Naratriptan, 86-88
Narcotic agonists. *See* Opioid
        agonists.
Natamycin, 414t
Nateglinide, 342-345
Natural antineoplastic drugs, 395-397
Nedocromil, 182
Nefazodone, 327-329
Negative chronotropic effect, 120
Negative dromotropic effect, 120
Nelfinavir, 272-275
Neomycin, 238-240, 417t, 418t
Neostigmine, 24-27
Neuromuscular blocking drugs, 55-59
    motor end plate and, 56i
    safe use of, 57
Nevirapine, 270-271
New drug development, 5-6
Niacin, 150-151
Nicardipine, 138-140
Nicotinic acid, 150-151
Nifedipine, 138-140
Nilutamide, 391-392
Nitrates, 135-136
Nitrofurantoin, 259-260
Nitrogen mustards, 372-374
Nitroglycerin, 135-136
Nitroprusside, 142-143
Nitrosoureas, 375-376
Nitrous oxide, 109-110
Nizatidine, 199, 200i, 201
Nonbenzodiazepines-nonbarbiturates,
        317-318
Noncatecholamines, 37-39
Nondepolarizing blocking drugs, 56-58
Non-nucleoside reverse transcriptase
        inhibitors, 270-271
Nonopioid analgesics, 93-101

Nonselective drug, 13
Nonsteroidal anti-inflammatory drugs,
        98-100
    risks of using, 98
Norepinephrine, 33-37
Norepinephrine depletors, 141-142
Norfloxacin, 256-257, 414t
Nortriptyline, 322-325
Nucleoside analogue reverse tran-
        scriptase inhibitors, 266-270
Nucleosides, synthetic, 260-263
Nucleotide analogue reverse tran-
        scriptase inhibitors, 271-272
Nystatin, 280-282, 418t

**O**
Obesity drugs, 207-208
Ofloxacin, 256-257, 277, 414t
Olanzapine, 331-332
Olmesartan, 146-147
Olopatadine, 414t
Omalizumab, 186-187
Omeprazole, 201-202
Ondansetron, 216-219
Onset of action, 11
Ophthalmic drugs, 414-416t
Opioid agonists, 101, 102-105
    pain control and, 104i
    safe use of, 102
Opioid antagonists, 101, 107-108
Opioid-related drugs as antidiarrheals,
        208-209
Oral anticoagulants, 164-166
Oral antidiabetic drugs, 342-345
Oral route of administration, 5, 8
Orlistat, 207-208
Orphenadrine, 50-52
Osmotic agents, 416t
Osmotic diuretics, 228
Otic drugs, 417t
Overdose, 18
Oxacillin, 241-243
Oxaliplatin, 378-379
Oxaprozin, 98-100
Oxazepam, 312-313, 314i, 315
Oxcarbazepine, 80-81
Oxiconazole, 281, 418t
Oxybutynin, 27-32, 230-231

i refers to an illustration; t refers to a table.

Oxycodone, 102-105
Oxymorphone, 102-105
Oxytocin, 350-352

**P**
Paclitaxel, 410-411
Pain medications, 93-115
Paliperidone, 331-332
Palliative therapy, 15
Pancreatic enzymes, 206
Pancreatin, 206
Pancrelipase, 206
Pancuronium, 56-58
Pantoprazole, 201-202
Parasympatholytic drugs, 60-62
Parasympathomimetic drugs. *See*
     Cholinergic drugs.
Paromomycin, 238-240
Paroxetine, 320-322
Partial agonists, 44
Passive transport, 7
Pathogen resistance, preventing,
     237-238
Patient sensitivity–related reactions,
     18-19
Patient's response to drug, factors that
     affect, 15
Peak concentration, 11-12
Pediculicides, 420t
Pegaspargase, 404
Penbutolol, 43-47
Penciclovir, 418t
Penicillin-binding proteins, 241-242
Penicillins, 241-243, 421t
Pentazocine, 105-107
Pentobarbital, 316-317
Pentostatin, 383-384
Peptic ulcer drugs, 195-203
Peripheral vascular resistance, 136
Permethrin, 420t
Perphenazine, 216-219, 333-336
Pharmacodynamics, 12-13, 14i
Pharmacokinetics, 7-12
Pharmacologic class, 2
Pharmacotherapeutics, 14-15
Phenazopyridine hydrochloride,
     100-101

Phenelzine, 325-327
Phenobarbital, 70-72, 316-317
Phenothiazines, 216-219
Phenoxybenzamine, 40-43
Phentermine, 207-208
Phentolamine, 40-43, 141-142
Phenylephrine, 37-39, 191-193, 415t
Phenyltriazines, 79-80
Phenytoin, 69-70
Phosphodiesterase inhibitors, 122-123
Physostigmine, 24-27
Pilocarpine, 21-24, 415t
Pimozide, 333-336
Pindolol, 43-47
Pinocytosis, 7
Pioglitazone, 342-345
Pirbuterol, 37-39, 176-177
Piroxicam, 98-100
Pituitary drugs, 348-352
Plants as drug sources, 3
Podophyllotoxins, 396-397
Polycarbophil, 212-213
Polyenes, 280-283
Polyethylene glycol, 211-212
Polymyxin B sulfate, 417t
Polythiazide, 224-225
Polyvinyl alcohol, 415t
Positive inotropic effect, 119-120
Posterior pituitary drugs, 350-352
Potassium replacement, 360-361
Potassium-sparing diuretics, 227-228
Potentiation, 16
Pramipexole, 62-66
Pramoxine, 114-115
Pravastatin, 149-150
Prazosin, 40-43, 141-142
Prednisolone, 178-180, 298-300, 415t
Prednisone, 178-180, 298-300
Prilocaine, 112-114
Primidone, 70-72
Probenecid, 306-307
Procainamide, 124-125
Procaine, 112-114
Procarbazine, 405
Prochlorperazine, 216-219
Procyclidine, 60-62
Prodrug, 10
Progestins, 392-393

Promethazine, 216-219, 294-295, 297
Propafenone, 128-129
Propantheline, 27-32
Proparacaine, 414t
Propofol, 110-112
Propoxyphene, 102-105
Propranolol, 43-47, 129-131, 137-138
Propylthiouracil, 355-356
Prostaglandin analogues, 416t
Protease, 206
Protease inhibitors, 272-275
Protirelin, 349-350
Proton pump inhibitors, 201-202
Protriptyline, 322-325
Pseudoephedrine, 191-193
Psychotropic drugs, 311-337
Psyllium hydrophilic mucilloid, 212-213
Purine analogues, 383-384
Pyrazinamide, 276-280
Pyridostigmine, 24-27
Pyrimidine analogues, 381-383
     mechanism of action of, 382
Pyrophosphate analogues, 264
Pyrrolidines, 84-85

**Q**
Quazepam, 312-313, 314i, 315
Quetiapine, 331-332
Quinapril, 144-145
Quinidine, 124-125

**R**
Rabeprazole, 201-202
Radioactive iodine, 355-356
Ramelton, 317-318
Ramipril, 144-145
Ranitidine, 199, 200i, 201
Rasagiline, 62-66
Recombinant human activated protein
     C, 289-290
Rectal route of administration, 5
Remifentanil, 102-105
Repaglinide, 342-345
Replacement therapy, 15
Reserpine, 141-142
Respiratory drugs, 175-193
Respiratory route of administration, 5

i refers to an illustration; t refers to a table.

Reteplase, 171-173
Ribavirin, 264-266
Rifampin, 276-280
Rimantadine, 264-266
Rimexolone, 415t
Risperidone, 331-332
Ritonavir, 272-275
Rituximab, 398-399
Rivastigmine, 24-27
Rizatriptan, 86-88
Rocuronium, 56-58
Ropinirole, 62-66
Ropivacaine, 112-114
Rosiglitazone, 342-345
Rosuvastatin, 149-150

**S**
Salicylates, 94-96
    safe use of, 96
Saline compounds, 211-212
Salmeterol, 37-39, 176-177
Salsalate, 94-96
Saquinavir, 272-275
Scabicides, 420t
Scopolamine, 27-32, 218
Secobarbital, 316-317
Secondary effects, 18
Sedative-hypnotic drugs, 311-318
Selective serotonin reuptake in-
        hibitors, 320-322
    discontinuation syndrome and, 321
Selegiline, 62-66
Senna, 214-215
Serotonin 5-HT$_3$ receptor antagonists,
        216-219
Sertraline, 320-322
Sevoflurane, 109-110
Sibutramine, 207-208
Side effects, 17-19
Sildenafil, 231-232
Silver sulfadiazine, 418t
Simethicone, 197-198, 205
Simvastatin, 149-150
Sirolimus, 302-306
Skeletal muscle relaxants, 49-55
Sleep agents, warning about, 318
Sodium bicarbonate, 366-368
Sodium biphosphate, 211-212

Sodium citrate, 366-368
Sodium ferric gluconate complex,
        156-157
Sodium lactate, 366-368
Sodium phosphate, 211-212
Sodium replacement, 365-366
Sodium salicylate, 94-96
Solifenacin, 230-231
Somatrem, 349-350
Somatropin, 349-350
Sotalol, 43-47, 131-132
Spironolactone, 227-228
St. John's wort, 424t
Stabilizing drugs, 56-58
Stable iodine, 355-356
Statins, 149-150
Stavudine, 266-270
Stimulant laxatives, 214-215
Stimulants, 336-337
Stool softeners, 213-214
Streptokinase, 171-173
Streptomycin, 238-240, 276-280, 421t
Streptozocin, 375-376
Subcutaneous route of administration,
        5, 8
Sublingual route of administration, 4, 7
Succinimides, 82-83
Succinylcholine, 58-59
Sucralfate, 202-203
Sufentanil, 102-105, 110-112
Sulconazole, 281, 418t
Sulfacetamide, 414t, 418t
Sulfadiazine, 257-259
Sulfamate-substituted monosaccha-
        rides, 82
Sulfamethoxazole and trimethoprim,
        257-259
Sulfinpyrazone, 165-169, 306-307
Sulfisoxazole, 414t
Sulfonamides, 83-84, 257-259
Sulindac, 98-100
Sumatriptan, 86-88
Supplemental therapy, 15
Supportive therapy, 15
Suprofen, 415t
Sympatholytic drugs, 40-47, 141-142
Sympathomimetic drugs. *See* Adren-
        ergic drugs.

Syncytial virus drugs, 264-266
Synthetic drug sources, 2, 3-4

**T**
Tacrine, 24-27
Tacrolimus, 302-306
Tadalafil, 231-232
Tamoxifen, 388-390
    risks versus benefits of, 389
Tamsulosin, 40-43
Targeted therapies, 400-402
Target organs, 23
Tazarotene, 419t
Telmisartan, 146-147
Temazepam, 312-313, 314i, 315
Tenecteplase, 171-173
Teniposide, 396-397
Tenofovir, 271-272
Terazosin, 40-43, 141-142
Terbinafine, 281, 288-289, 418t
Terbutaline, 37-39, 176-177
Terconazole, 281
Testolactone, 390-391
Testosterone, 390-391
Tetracaine, 112-115, 414t
Tetracycline, 196-197, 418t, 420t
Tetracyclines, 247-248
Theophylline, 183-185
Therapeutic class, 2
Therapeutic index, 13
Thiazide and thiazide-like diuretics,
        224-225
Thiethylperazine, 216-219
Thioguanine, 383-384
Thiopental, 110-112
Thioridazine, 333-336
Thiotepa, 377-378
Thiothixene, 333-336
Thrombolytic drugs, 171-173
Thymoglobulin, 302-306
Thyroglobulin, 352-354
Thyroid antagonists, 355-356
Thyroid drugs, 352-354
Thyroid-stimulating hormone, 349-350
Thyroid USP (desiccated), 352-354
Thyrotropin, 349-350
Ticarcillin, 241-243
Ticlopidine, 165-169

i refers to an illustration; t refers to a table.

Timolol, 43-47, 416t
Tinzaparin, 161-164
Tioconazole, 281
Tipranavir, 272-275
Tirofiban, 165-169
Tizanidine, 50-52
Tobramycin, 238-240, 414t
Tolazamide, 342-345
Tolbutamide, 342-345
Tolcapone, 66-68
Tolnaftate, 281
Tolterodine, 27-32, 230-231
Topical anesthetics, 114-115
Topical route of administration, 5
Topiramate, 82
Topoisomerase I inhibitors, 399-400
Topotecan, 399-400
Toremifene, 388-390
Trandolapril, 144-145
Translingual route of administration, 4
Tranylcypromine, 325-327
Trastuzumab, 398-399
Travoprost, 416t
Trazodone, 327-329
Tretinoin, 419t
Triacetin, 281
Triamcinolone, 178-180, 298-300, 419t
Triamterene, 227-228
Triazenes, 376-377
Triazolam, 312-313, 314i, 315
Triazoles, synthetic, 285-287
Tricyclic antidepressants, 322-325
Triethanolamine polypeptide, 417t
Trifluoperazine, 333-336
Trifluridine, 414t
Trihexyphenidyl, 27-32, 60-62
Trimethobenzamide, 216-219
Trimipramine, 322-325
Triptans. *See* 5-HT$_1$-receptor agonists.
Triptorelin, 393-395
Tromethamine, 366-368
Tropicamide, 416t
Trospium, 230-231
Tuberculosis
    directly observable therapy for, 276
    drug regimens for treating, 276-280
Typical antipsychotics, 333-336

**U**
Undecylenic acid, 281
Unfractionated heparin, 161-164
Unoprostone, 416t
Urea, 228
Uricosurics, 306-307
Urinary tract antispasmodics, 230-231
Urokinase, 171-173

**V**
Vaginal route of administration, 5
Valacyclovir, 260-263
Valganciclovir, 260-263
Valproate, 76-78
Valproic acid, 76-78
Valsartan, 146-147
Vancomycin, 251-253
Vardenafil, 231-232
Vasodilating drugs, 142-143
Vasopressin, 350-352
Vecuronium, 56-58
Venlafaxine, 320-322, 327-329
Verapamil, 133-134, 138-140
Vinblastine, 395-396
Vinca alkaloids, 395-396
Vincristine, 395-396
Vinorelbine, 395-396
Vitamin B$_{12}$, 158-159
Vitex, 424t
Voriconazole, 285-287

**W**
Warfarin, 164-166
    monitoring levels of, 165

**X**
Xanthines, 183-185

**Y**
Yohimbine, 424t

**Z**
Zafirlukast, 180-182
Zaleplon, 317-318
Zidovudine, 266-270, 268i
Zileuton, 180-182
Ziprasidone, 331-332
Zolmitriptan, 86-88

Zolpidem, 317-318
Zonisamide, 83-84

i refers to an illustration; t refers to a table.

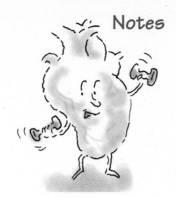

Notes

Notes

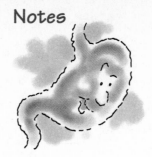